T0252384

Clinical Trials with Missing Data

STATISTICS IN PRACTICE

Statistics in Practice is an important international series of texts which provide detailed coverage of statistical concepts, methods and worked case studies in specific fields of investigation and study.

With sound motivation and many worked practical examples, the books show in down-to-earth terms how to select and use an appropriate range of statistical techniques in a particular practical field within each title's special topic area.

The books provide statistical support for professionals and research workers across a range of employment fields and research environments. Subject areas covered include medicine and pharmaceutics; industry, finance and commerce; public services; the earth and environmental sciences, and so on.

The books also provide support to students studying statistical courses applied to the above areas. The demand for graduates to be equipped for the work environment has led to such courses becoming increasingly prevalent at universities and colleges. It is our aim to present judiciously chosen and well-written workbooks to meet everyday practical needs. Feedback of views from readers will be most valuable to monitor the success of this aim.

A complete list of titles in this series appears at the end of the volume.

Clinical Trials with Missing Data

A Guide for Practitioners

Michael O'Kelly

Senior Strategic Biostatistics Director
Quintiles Ireland Ltd, Ireland

Bohdana Ratitch

Statistical Scientist, Quintiles, Montreal, Canada

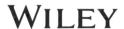

This edition first published 2014
© 2014 John Wiley & Sons, Ltd

Registered office
John Wiley & Sons Ltd, The Atrium, Southern Gate, Chichester, West Sussex, PO19 8SQ, United Kingdom

For details of our global editorial offices, for customer services and for information about how to apply for permission to reuse the copyright material in this book please see our website at www.wiley.com.

Library of Congress Cataloging-in-Publication Data

O'Kelly, Michael, author.
   Clinical trials with missing data : a guide for practitioners / Michael O'Kelly, Bohdana Ratitch.
      p. ; cm. – (Statistics in practice)
   Includes bibliographical references and index.
   ISBN 978-1-118-46070-2 (hardback)
   I. Ratitch, Bohdana, author.   II. Title.   III. Series: Statistics in practice.
   [DNLM: 1. Clinical Trials as Topic.   2. Bias (Epidemiology)   3. Models, Statistical.   4. Research Design. QV 771.4]
   R853.C55
   610.72′4–dc23

                                        2013041088

A catalogue record for this book is available from the British Library.

ISBN: 978-1-118-46070-2

Set in 10/12pt Times by Aptara Inc., New Delhi, India

1   2014

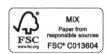

To Raymond Kearns, teacher and Linda O'Nolan, partner.
—Michael O'Kelly

To my family, with love and gratitude for inspiration and support.
—Bohdana Ratitch

Contents

6   Multiple imputation

Bohdana Ratitch

8   Doubly robust estimation   369
Belinda Hernández, Ilya Lipkovich and Michael O'Kelly

Preface

The aim of this book is to explain the difficulties that arise with the credibility and interpretability of clinical study results when there is missing data; and to provide practical strategies to deal with these difficulties. We try to do this in straightforward language, using realistic clinical trial examples.

This book is written to serve the needs of a broad audience of pharmaceutical industry professionals and regulators, including statisticians and non-statisticians, as well as academics with an interest in or need to understand the practical side of handling missing data. This book could also be used for a practical course in methods for handling missing data. For statisticians, this book provides mathematical background for a wide spectrum of statistical methodologies that are currently recommended to deal with missing data, avoiding unnecessary complexity. We also present a variety of examples and discussions on how these methods can be implemented using mainstream statistical software. The book includes a framework in which the entire clinical study team can contribute to a sound design of a strategy to deal with missing data, from prevention, to formulating clinically plausible assumptions about unobserved data, to statistical analysis and interpretation.

In the past, missing data was sometimes viewed as a problem that can be taken care of within statistical methodology without burdening others with the technicalities of it. While it is true that sophisticated statistical methods can and should be used to conduct sound analyses in the presence of missing data, all these methods make assumptions about missing data that clinical experts should help to formulate – assumptions that should be clinically interpretable and plausible. Moreover, it is important to understand that some assumptions about missing data are *always* being made, be it explicitly or implicitly. Even a strategy using only observed data for analysis carries within it certain implicit assumptions about subjects with missing data, and these assumptions are being implicitly made part of study conclusions. Clinicians fully participate in the effort to select carefully the type of data (clinical endpoints) that could best serve as evidence for efficacy and safety of a treatment. Their clinical expertise is invaluable for the choice of data that is collected in a clinical trial and subsequently used as observed data. Similarly, it is only natural to expect that the same level of clinical expertise would be provided to make choices for "hidden data" – the assumptions that would be used in place of missing data as an integral part of the overall body of evidence. Parts of this book (Chapters 1–4) contain non-technical material that can be easily understood by non-statisticians, and we hope that it will help clinicians and statisticians to build a common ground and a common language in order to tackle appropriately the problem of missing data together. Chapter 2 is dedicated entirely to prevention of missing data, which is the best way to deal with the problem, albeit not sufficient by itself in reality. Everyone involved in the planning and conduct of clinical trials would benefit from the ideas presented in this chapter.

Chapters 5 through 8 are aimed primarily at statisticians and cover well-understood methods that are presently regarded as statistically sound ways of conducting analyses in the presence of missing data and which can provide clinically meaningful estimands of treatment effect. In particular, this book covers direct likelihood methodology for longitudinal data with repeated correlated measurements; multiple imputation; pattern-mixture models; and inverse weighting and doubly robust methods. We discuss in detail how these methodologies can be applied under a variety of clinical assumptions about unobserved data, both in the context of primary and sensitivity analyses. Aspects that are covered more briefly include selection models and non-parametric approaches. Examples cover both continuous outcomes and binary responses (e.g., treatment success/failure). Missing data problems in other contexts, such as time-to-event analyses, are not covered in this book.

Along with algebraic basics and plain language explanations of statistical methodology, this book contains numerous examples of practical implementations using SAS®. Throughout the book, as well as in supplemental material, we provide fragments of SAS code that would be sufficient for readers to use as templates or at least good starting points to implement all analyses mentioned in this book. We also provide pointers and explanations for a number of SAS macros publicly available at www.missingdata.org.uk, developed by members of the Drug Information Association Scientific Working Group on Missing Data. Both authors of this book are members of this Working Group. We note that alternative software solutions exist in other programming environments, including free packages such as R. Other authors, for example, Carpenter and Kenward (2013) and van Buuren (2012), have provided tools that the readers would be able to use in order to implement general analysis principles discussed in this book.

Examples of realistic clinical trial data featured in this book provide illustrations of how reasonable missing data strategies can be designed in several different clinical indications, each with some specific challenges and characteristics. All examples have two treatment arms – experimental and control – but the methodology discussed in this book can be applied in more general settings with more than two arms in a straightforward manner.

We have also endeavored to make the book suitable for casual use, allowing the professional statistician with a particular need to use a particular section without having to be familiar with the whole book. Therefore, each chapter begins with a list of key points covered; abbreviations are expanded on first appearance in each chapter; references are listed at the end of each chapter; explanations of particular points may be repeated if it helps to make a passage readable (although there are many cross-references between chapters too); where a book is referenced, we try to give page numbers if we think this might be helpful; and for some references to journal papers we also give web links to enable fast reference to abstracts and to enable downloading for those who may have electronic subscriptions.

Finally, we would like to stress that the problem of missing data unfortunately does not have a one-fits-all solution. A clinical research team must evaluate their strategy for missing data in the context of a specific clinical indication, subject population, expected mechanism of action of the experimental treatment, control treatment used in the study, and standards of care that would be available to subjects once they leave the trial. This book aims at providing the reader with a good general understanding of the issues involved and a tool box of methods from which to select the ones that would be the most appropriate for a study at hand.

References

Carpenter JR, Kenward MG (2013) *Multiple Imputation and its Application.* John Wiley & Sons Ltd, West Sussex.

Van Buuren S (2012) *Flexible Imputation of Missing Data.* Chapman & Hall/CRC Press, Boca Raton, FL.

SAS and all other SAS Institute Inc. product or service names are registered trademarks or trademarks of SAS Institute Inc. in the United States and other countries.® indicates USA registration.

Acknowledgments

We thank the contributors to this book, Sonia Davis, Sara Hughes, Belinda Hernndez and Ilya Lipkovich, for their clear contributions and constant helpfulness.

We have found the scholars and experts on missing data to be friendly, approachable and willing to share ideas and expertise. As many who learn from him will tell you, James Roger epitomizes this spirit of willingness to spark ideas off others and to share the fruits of applied mathematics and elegant programming. It is likely that much of our work on sensitivity analyses in this book would not have been done without Roger's inspiration and example. It seems typical of those who work on missing data that much material from one of our favorite books on the subject was made freely available on the internet by authors James Carpenter and Mike Kenward. We thank these two scholars. Gary Koch first pointed us to Roger's ideas on sensitivity analyses; Gary also suggested the usefulness of sequential multiple imputation; over many years he has answered our questions on the direction of our work. Craig Mallinckrodt has genially chaired the Scientific Working Group for Missing Data and we thank him for fostering co-operation between pharmaceutical companies and academia, all with the aim of improving our handling of missing data. Geert Molenberghs gave thought-provoking answers to our queries; he also reviewed this book and we thank him for his helpful comments. Thank you to John Preisser, Willem Koetse, Forrest DeMarcus, and David Couper for reviews and contributions to Chapter 5. We thank Quintiles' Judith Beach for her legal review and general advice; we thank Quintiles' Kevin Nash for his review also. The errors that remain are ours. From our employers, Quintiles, we thank especially Olga Marchenko, who championed the research; Tom Pike and King Jolly for their encouragement; and Andy Garrett and Yves Lalonde who supported Bohdana Ratitch in making time for the book. We also pay tribute to Quintiles for its remarkable support for the development of its employees – Michael O'Kelly owes his entire post-graduate education to the support of Quintiles, and in particular to the support of Imelda Parker when she was head of the Quintiles Dublin statistics department. Thanks to Ilaria Meliconi from Wiley who first encouraged us to think of writing the book; and to Wiley's Debbie Jupe who guided us as the book progressed, with help from Richard Davies and Heather Kay. Finally, we thank our spouses and family for their support.

Notation

Throughout this book, algebraic notation will be as described below. Occasionally, the same symbol may be used for different purposes in different chapters following well-established conventions in respective domains. We will define specific meanings of such symbols in each relevant chapter; we note some variants in use here.

Notation conventions

Index letter	Index range	Description
i	$1, \ldots, N$	Subject
t	$1, \ldots, T$	Treatment allocated to the individual subject
j	$1, \ldots, J$	Time point or visit number
c	$1, \ldots, T$	Reference or control treatment, used when necessary to identify control vs. experimental treatment arm
l	$0, \ldots, L$	Withdrawal visit: the visit at which the last observation is made for the individual subject (0 for those with no observed post-baseline data and $L = J$ for those with complete data)
p	$1, \ldots, P$	Pattern: group of subjects; can be defined in many ways, depending on analysis
s	$0, \ldots, S$	Time-invariant (baseline) covariate; may be extended to include auxiliary covariables in multiple imputation, depending on context
v	$1, \ldots, V$	Post-baseline covariate V is also used for variance–covariance matrix in Chapter 5
m	$1, \ldots, M$	Imputation number for multiple imputation
k	Context dependent	Indexes model parameters; range may be $0, \ldots, S$, $0, \ldots, V$ or $0, \ldots, S + V$, depending on the context

Notation conventions

Variable letter	Highest index number(s)	Description
Y	N and J	A set of outcome variables, e.g., Y_j represents outcome at time point j; in the context of the imputation model for multiple imputation, may refer to both primary outcome and post-baseline auxiliary variables
X	S	A set of covariates; usually baseline covariates, but may also include observed post-baseline covariates, depending on the context
W	Context dependent	Effects included in a statistical model; may include X, Y and their interactions
β	Context dependent	Regression model coefficients
θ	Context dependent	Parameters of a statistical model, usually in a joint probability distribution
R	N and J	A set of missingness indicators, e.g., $R_j = 0$ represents observation missing at time point j, $R_j = 1$ represents observation available at time point j R is also used for residuals covariance matrix in Chapter 5
F	None	A set of missingness model covariates
ψ	None	Missingness model regression coefficients

Additional conventions:

- Letter in upper case with an index refers to a variable at an individual visit (not its value), for example, in a context of a model, $Y_1, \ldots, Y_J$.

- Letter in upper case without indices refers to a set of variables (not their values), for example, $Y = (Y_1, \ldots, Y_J)$.

- Letter in lower case with indices refers to a value of an individual variable for an individual subject, for example, y_{ij} – value of a variable Y_j for subject i.

- Letter in lower case, with an index, and bolded refers either to

    o values of an individual variable for a set of subjects, for example, $\boldsymbol{y}_j = (y_{1j}, \ldots, y_{Nj})$ – values of a variable Y_j for subjects $i = 1, \ldots, N$ or

    o values of a set of variables for a subject, for example, $\boldsymbol{y}_i = (y_{i1}, \ldots, y_{iJ})$ – values at all time points $j = 1, \ldots, J$ for subject i.
    Specific meaning is described in each context where this notation is used.

- Letter in either upper or lower case, without indices, and bolded refers to values of a set of variables for a set of subjects, for example, Y or $y = (y_1, \ldots, y_J)$ – data matrix, values of all variables Y for all subjects.

- Y_{obs} and Y_{mis} refer to the set of observed values and the set of missing values of a data matrix Y, respectively.

Table of SAS code fragments

Contributors

Chapter 5 by:

Sonia M. Davis, Collaborative Studies Coordinating Center, Professor of the Practice, Department of Biostatistics, University of North Carolina, USA.

Chapter 8 by:

Belinda Hernández, School of Mathematical Sciences (Discipline of Statistics) and the School of Medicine and Medical Science, University College Dublin, Ireland.

Chapter 2 by:

Sara Hughes, Head of Clinical Statistics, GlaxoSmithKline, UK.

Contributions to and review of Chapter 8 by:

Ilya Lipkovich, Center for Statistics in Drug Development, Quintiles Innovation, Morrisville, North Carolina, USA.

Michael O'Kelly: authored chapters 1, 3, 4 and 7, contributed research for Chapter 8, and reviewed all chapters.

Bohdana Ratitch: authored Chapter 6, contributed to chapters 1, 4 and 7, contributed research for chapters 4 and 7, and reviewed all chapters.

1

What's the problem with missing data?

Michael O'Kelly and Bohdana Ratitch

"For when they reach the scene of crime – Macavity's not there!"
Macavity the Mystery Cat, TS Eliot*

Key points

- Missing data for the purposes of this book are data that were planned to be recorded during a clinical trial but are not available. Non-monotone or intermediate missing data occur when a subject misses a visit but contributes data at later visits. Monotone missing data, where all data for a subject is missing after a certain time-point due to early withdrawal from the study, is the more serious problem in interpreting the results of a trial.

- The most important thing about missing data is that it is missing: we can never be sure whether the assumptions made about it are true.

- An example illustrates the potential bias of using only observed data in an analysis (a favorable subset of subjects); and of using a subject's last available

---

Clinical Trials with Missing Data: A Guide for Practitioners, First Edition. Michael O'Kelly and Bohdana Ratitch.
© 2014 John Wiley & Sons, Ltd. Published 2014 by John Wiley & Sons, Ltd.

observation or baseline observation in place of missing values (bias varies and may be difficult to predict).

- Assuming that data are missing at random (i.e., that given the data and the model, missingness is independent of the unobserved values) allows one to use study data to infer likely values for missing data, but is likely biased in that it assumes that subjects who withdrew from the study have results like similar subjects who remained in the study.

- Given that we can never be sure whether the assumptions made about missingness in the primary analysis are true, sensitivity analyses are needed to stress-test the trial results for robustness to assumptions about missing data: sensitivity analyses will help the reader of the clinical study report to assess the credibility of a trial with missing data.

1.1   What do we mean by missing data?

This book is about missing data in clinical trials. In a clinical trial, missing data are data that were planned to be recorded but are not present in the database. No matter how well designed and conducted a trial is, some missing data can almost always be expected. Missingness may be absolutely unrelated to the subject's medical condition and study treatment. For example, data could be missing due to a human error in recording data; due to a scheduling conflict that prevented the subject from attending the study visit; or due to a subject's moving to a region outside of the study's remit. On the other hand, data may be missing for reasons that are related to subject's health and the experimental treatment he/she is undergoing. For example, subjects may decide to discontinue from study prematurely if their condition worsens or fails to improve, or if they experience adverse reactions or adverse events (AEs). A contrary situation is also possible, although probably less common, where a subject is cured and observations are missing because the subject is not willing to bother with the rest of the study assessments. Apart from missingness due to missed visits, missing data can arise simply due to the nature of the measurement or the nature of the disease. An example of data that would be missing because not meaningful is a quality-of-life score for a subject who has died. Those cases where missingness is related to the subject's underlying condition and study treatment have the greatest potential to undermine the credibility of a trial. Sometimes, a subject's data collected prior to discontinuation reflects the reason for withdrawal (e.g., worsening, improvement or toxicity), but subjects can also discontinue without providing that crucial information that would have enabled us to assess the reason for missingness and thus incorporate it in our analysis. Such cases potentially hide some important information about treatment efficacy and/or safety, without which study conclusions may be biased.

When a subject has provided data over the course of the study, but some assessments, either in the middle of the trial or at the primary time point, are missing for any reason, their data can be referred to as partial subject data. In this book, we explore the implications of this partial data and ways to minimize the potential bias.

In many clinical trials, collected data are longitudinal in nature, that is, data about the same clinical parameter is collected on multiple occasions (e.g., during study visits or through subject diaries). In such studies, a primary endpoint (clinical parameter used to evaluate the primary objective of the trial at a specific time point) is typically required to be measured at the end of the treatment period or a period at the end of which the clinical benefit is expected to be attained or maintained, with assessments performed at that point as well as on several prior occasions, thus capturing subject's progress after the start of the treatment. This is in contrast with another type of trial, where the primary endpoint is event-driven, for example, based on such events as death or disease progression. In this book, we focus primarily on the former type of the trials, and we look at various ways in which partial subject data can be used for analysis.

Most of this book is about ways to handle missing data once it occurs, but it is also important to prevent missing data insofar as this is possible. Chapter 2 discusses this in detail, and describes some ways in which the statistician can contribute to prevention strategies. We now put some of the discussion above somewhat more formally.

1.1.1   Monotone and non-monotone missing data

A subject who completes a clinical trial may have data missing for a measurement because he/she failed to turn up for some visits in the middle of the trial. Such a measurement is said to have "non-monotone missing," "intermediate missing" or "intermittent missing" data, because the status of the measurement for a subject can switch from missing to non-missing and back as the patient progresses through the trial. In many clinical trials, this kind of missingness is more likely to be unrelated to the study condition or treatment. However, in some trials, it may indicate a temporary but important worsening of the subject's health (e.g., pulmonary exacerbations in lung diseases).

In contrast, monotone missingness occurs when data for a measurement is not available for a subject after some given time point; in the case of monotone missingness, once a measurement starts being missing, it will be missing for the subsequent visits in the trial, even though it had been planned to be collected. Subjects that discontinue early from the study are the usual source of monotone missing data. In most trials, the amount of monotone missing data is much greater than the amount of non-monotone missing data. In trials where the primary endpoint is based on a measurement at a specific time point, prior intermittent missing data will have a smaller impact on the primary analysis, compared to monotone missing data. Nevertheless, even in these cases, non-monotone missing data can affect study conclusions. This can happen if the intermediate data are utilized in a statistical model for analysis – the absence of such intermediate data may bias the estimates of the statistical model parameters. In this book, however, we will focus mostly on the problem of monotone missing data, because monotone missing data tend to pose more serious problems than non-monotone when estimating and interpreting trial results. For a more detailed discussion of handling non-monotone missing data, see Section 6.2.1. In this chapter, to introduce some of the concepts and problems in handling missing data, we will look at some common methods of handling monotone missing data in clinical trials, and examine the implications of each method.

In Section 4.2.1, we will also briefly discuss situations where subject discontinues study treatment prematurely, but may stay on study and provide data at the time points as planned originally, despite being off study treatment. These cases need special consideration when including data after treatment discontinuation in the analysis, so that the interpretation of results takes into account possible confounding factors incurred after discontinuation (e.g., alternative treatments).

1.1.2 Modeling missingness, modeling the missing value and ignorability

In the missing data methodology, we often use two terms: *missing value* and *missingness* (or *missingness mechanism*). It will be helpful to clarify what these terms refer to as they both play important and distinct roles in the statistical analysis. Missing value refers to a datum that was planned to be collected but is not available. A datum may be missing because, for example, the measurement was not made or was not collected. Missing and non-missing data may also be referred to as unobserved and observed, respectively. Missingness refers to a binary outcome (Yes/No), that of the datum being missing or not missing at a given time point. Missingness mechanism refers to the underlying random process that determines when data may be missing. In other words, missingness mechanism refers to the probability distribution of the binary missingness event(s). The missingness mechanism may depend on a number of variables, which themselves may be observed or not observed. In the analysis, we can use one model (often referred to as a substantive model) for the values of the clinical parameter of interest (some values of which in reality will be missing), and another model for the distribution of a binary missingness indicator variable (datum missing or not). The missingness model may not be of interest in itself, but in some situations it may influence estimation of the substantive model and would need to be taken into account in order to avoid bias. Some analyses make use of both of these models.

1.1.3 Types of missingness (MCAR, MAR and MNAR)

The classifications of missing data mechanisms introduced by Rubin (1976; 1987) and Little and Rubin (2002) provide a formal framework that describes how missingness mechanism may affect inferences about the clinical outcome. A value of a clinical outcome variable is said to be missing completely at random (MCAR) when its missingness is independent of observed and unobserved data, that is, when observed outcomes are a simple random sample from complete data; missing at random (MAR) when, given the observed outcomes and the statistical model, missingness is independent of the unobserved outcomes; and missing not at random (MNAR) when missingness is not independent of unobserved data, even after accounting for the observed data. When data are missing for administrative reasons, the missingness mechanism could be MCAR, because the reason for missingness had nothing to do with the outcome model and its covariates. Dropout due to previous lack of efficacy could be MAR, because in some sense predictable from the observed data in the model. It is important to note that MAR is not an intrinsic characteristic of the data or missingness mechanism itself, but is closely related to the analysis model: if we include all the factors on which missingness depends in our model, we will be operating under MAR; otherwise, our analysis would not conform to MAR assumptions. Dropout after a sudden *unrecorded* drop in efficacy could be MNAR, since missingness would be dependent on unobserved data and would not be predictable from the observed data alone. Of these assumptions, MCAR is strongest and least realistic; while MNAR is the least restrictive. However, the very variety of assumptions possible under MNAR may be regarded as a problem: it has been argued that it would be difficult to pre-specify a single definitive MNAR analysis (Mallinckrodt *et al.*, 2008).

We can test for dependence of missingness on observed outcomes, and so test for MAR versus MCAR. However, we cannot test whether the mechanism is MAR versus MNAR, because that would require testing for a relationship between missingness and unobserved data. Unobserved data, we think it is no harm to repeat, is not there, and so the relationship with missingness cannot be tested.

See Appendix 1.A at the end of this chapter for formal definitions of MCAR, MAR and MNAR.

Under some assumptions, missingness can be shown to be *ignorable*. Missingness is classified as ignorable if a valid estimate of the outcome can be calculated without taking the missingness mechanism into account. In his first paper addressing the problem of missing data, Rubin (1976) showed that, when using Bayesian or direct likelihood methods to estimate any parameter θ related to the clinical outcome, missing data are ignorable when the missingness mechanism is MAR and θ "is 'distinct' from" the parameter of the missing data process (missingness mechanism). Rubin put the word "distinct" in quotation marks because the distinctness condition is a very particular one. The missingness parameter is distinct from θ "if there are no *a priori* ties, via parameter space restrictions or prior distributions, between (the missingness parameter) and θ." Thus while we might often expect the same observed data to contribute to the modeling of both missingness and the outcome, θ and the missingness parameter will still probably be distinct in such cases, and the missingness ignorable.

1.1.4   Missing data and study objectives

Clinical trial researchers and regulatory authorities are concerned about the effect of missing data on two aspects of the clinical data analysis: the estimates of the difference between experimental and control treatments, and the variance of this estimate. With respect to the difference between treatments, missing data can affect (and can bias) the magnitude of that estimate and make the experimental treatment look more or less clinically efficacious than it is (in the extreme cases even reverse a true comparison) or obscure an important interplay between treatment efficacy and tolerability. With regard to the variance of this estimate, missing data can either compromise the power of the study or, on the contrary, lead to underestimation of the variance, depending on the method chosen for analysis. Regulatory authorities require reasonable assurances that the chosen method of analysis in the presence of missing data is not likely to introduce an important bias in favor of the experimental treatment and will not underestimate the variance.

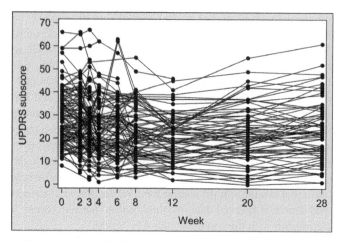

Figure 1.1   Available data in Parkinson's disease dataset.

1.2   An illustration

To start our exploration of missing data, consider the following illustrative dataset that is patterned after typical Parkinson's disease clinical data as available, for example, in Emre *et al.* (2004) and Parkinson Study Group (2004a, 2004b). We suppose our trial had two treatment arms, an experimental arm and a placebo control arm, and that the trial had nine visits, with baseline at Visit 0, and the primary efficacy endpoint at Week 28. Fifty-seven subjects were enrolled in each treatment group. The primary measure of efficacy was a sub-score of the Unified Parkinson's Disease Rating Scale (UPDRS). For a general description of this illustrative dataset, see Section 1.10.1. A "spaghetti plot" of the complete dataset (Figure 1.1), although showing no strong distinct patterns, allows us to see the mass of data that can be available in a typical longitudinal trial.

A high score here indicates poor subject outcome. Parkinson's disease is progressive, and for most treatments of the disease, one would expect to see a return to worsening after three to six months treatment seen in Emre *et al.* (2004) and Parkinson Study Group (2004a, 2004b) just cited. In other words, some transient improvement may be achieved and progression may be delayed for some time by treatment, but progression is not expected to stop completely. The reader may be able to see from Figure 1.1 that indeed, while many subjects in the illustrative dataset improved slightly (lower scores), subjects tended to revert to disease progression towards the end of the trial (higher scores).

In our example dataset, nearly 38% of subjects discontinued early, 18 (32%) and 25 (44%) subjects in the control and experimental arms, respectively, giving rise to substantial amounts of monotone missing data. Figure 1.2 highlights those subjects.

The large proportion of missing data for the primary endpoint in this example (38% of subjects discontinued) is troubling with regard to its impact on the power

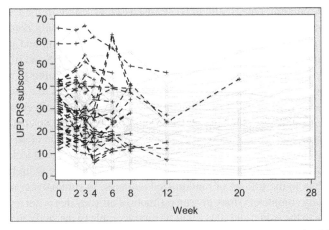

Figure 1.2   Parkinson's disease dataset: early discontinuations highlighted.

of the study. Also, the difference between treatment arms in the proportion of withdrawals (12% more in the experimental arm compared to placebo) is large enough to suggest that the reason for discontinuation depends on treatment. Both of these observations should motivate a careful consideration of the impact missing data may have on study conclusions. The statistician will want to consider ways to make inference from available study data while minimizing a possibility of bias that would unfairly favor the experimental treatment.

What options are available to proceed with analysis in the presence of missing data? The most obvious and easiest choice is to use only subjects with data available for the primary endpoint – study completers for whom assessments were performed at the final study visit. A second approach to consider would be to use all available longitudinal data (from all visits), including partial data from study dropouts, with the hope that this partial data could contribute in a meaningful way to the overall statistical analysis. Finally, we can impute missing data of discontinued subjects in some principled way, taking into account the information we have about these subjects prior to their dropout. We will discuss these three basic options in more detail below.

1.3   Why can't I use only the available primary endpoint data?

Sometimes, only the subjects with available data for the primary endpoint (study completers) are used in the primary study analysis and test. Could we discard the data from subjects who discontinued early, use only available data at Week 28, and still have an unbiased estimate of treatment effect? If we are interested in estimating the treatment effect *in the kind of subject who would complete the nine trial visits*, then the data available at the ninth visit (Visit 8, Week 28) can be the basis of an unbiased estimate. What is to be estimated – the estimand – is important in assessing how to handle missing data. Estimands are discussed at length in the U.S. National Research Council report, *The prevention and treatment of missing data in clinical trials,* commissioned by the U.S. Food and Drug Administration and published in 2010. A variety of estimands are discussed in Section 4.1.1, and US and EU regulatory guidance are discussed in Chapter 3. Usually, however, it is desired to estimate not just the treatment effect among the "elite" selection of subjects that completed the trial, but something more widely applicable such as the treatment effect in all subjects of the type randomized to the clinical trial (including both completers and subjects who discontinued early). The reasons recorded for discontinuation often suggest that many subjects discontinue either because of side effects or because of lack of efficacy. Thus, there is often good reason to believe that the efficacy score would be better in completers than in the full set of randomized subjects. In summary, complete cases (data from study completers) may give an estimate of efficacy that is not representative of all subjects in the study, and likely will be too favorable to the study treatments. An approach that is applicable to all subjects randomized will generally be more useful and more acceptable to the regulator. This approach where results are applicable to all subjects randomized is known as the "intent-to-treat" (ITT) approach. According to the ITT principle, all subjects that were included (randomized) in the trial should be included in the analysis, regardless of their compliance with treatment.

The use of data from completers only has an additional drawback that partial data from subjects that discontinued early, but still provided some information prior to withdrawal, is completely wasted.

In our dataset, Figure 1.3 illustrates the somewhat poorer efficacy scores that can pertain to subjects who discontinue early, taking as an example subjects whose last observation was at Week 6 or 8, (10 discontinuations each in the control and experimental treatment groups). Early withdrawals in the control group had higher (worse) mean efficacy scores from the start, compared to completers in their own

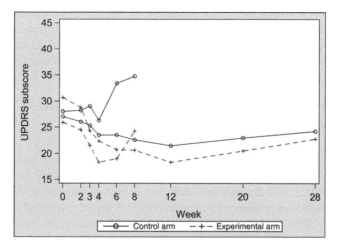

Figure 1.3   Parkinson's disease dataset: mean efficacy score at each time point for completers and for subjects whose last observation was at Visit 4 or 5 (Week 6 or 8).

treatment group. Early withdrawals in the experimental treatment group had a lower (better) mean score at baseline; by Visit 4 (Week 6) the gap between the completers and withdrawals had narrowed, and at Visit 5 (Week 8) the withdrawals now had a higher (worse) score than completers. In Section 1.10.1, Figure 1.9 shows that, taking all subjects, for this illustrative dataset, withdrawals tended to have worse UPDRS scores than completers, but not at all visits. However, very often in our experience, completers tend to have more favorable trajectories than subjects who discontinue early, and thus tend not to be representative of efficacy for all subjects who were randomized to the trial.

Perhaps there may be cases where the scores of completers are better than the scores of dropouts to a similar extent in both arms, and the estimated difference between treatment groups may be unaffected? We can never be sure that this will be true, and in many trials the proportion of early discontinuations, and the reasons for discontinuation, vary substantially between treatment groups. If reasons for discontinuation do vary by treatment group, then efficacy in completers will likely vary between treatment groups also, biasing the "available cases" estimate of the difference between treatment groups. In our example study, a higher proportion of subjects discontinued early due to adverse events (AEs) in the experimental arm compared to the control arm (Table 1.2). Excluding dropouts from analysis would likely favor the experimental arm to a greater extent than the control arm, if AEs are associated with poorer efficacy scores. With this kind of difference in discontinuation between treatment groups, it would be very difficult to interpret an estimate based only on completers. Such an estimate could not with credibility be applied to the general Parkinson's population. As noted above, another disadvantage of analyzing completers only is that we are not making use of information from subjects who were partially observed. Thus, a statistical test based on completers would tend, all other things being equal, to have less power than a test which makes use in a principled way of data from withdrawals.

1.4   What's the problem with using last observation carried forward?

Until recently, the most common method of handling missing data was to estimate the treatment effect using the last available measurement for a subject. This method has been known as "last observation carried forward," or LOCF. The argument can be made for LOCF, that the observation just before a subject discontinues is likely to give evidence unfavorable to the study treatment – because the subject is likely to have left the study when his/her health was at a low point (unless he/she left for reasons unrelated to the condition under study). Last observation carried forward could thus be regarded as leading to a conservative estimate of efficacy for a treatment. To examine the LOCF method further, we plot some typical trajectories from our example study (Figure 1.4).

Figure 1.4 shows two typical trajectories of the efficacy score for completers and two typical trajectories for subjects who discontinued early. As is common in studies of Parkinson's disease, the completer on the control arm shows a small

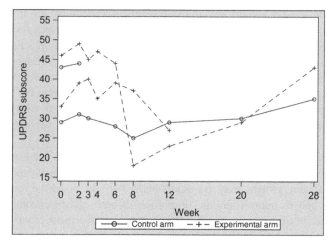

Figure 1.4   Parkinson's disease dataset: four selected trajectories.

improvement and finishes the study close to his/her baseline value. The completer in the experimental arm also improves, and then reverts to a UPDRS value close to baseline. The two trajectories of early discontinuations are selected to show some implications of the method of handling missing data. Here, the control arm data are of a subject who discontinued very early, and experimental arm data are of a subject who discontinued after the midpoint of the study.

The efficacy score for the subject in the control group had changed little from baseline when he/she discontinued, and so LOCF imputes for Visit 8 (Week 28) a value almost unchanged since baseline (Figure 1.5). The subject in the experimental arm had a somewhat improved (lower) UPDRS score by Visit 6 (Week 12) when he/she discontinued. The values imputed by LOCF here do not seem very unreasonable,

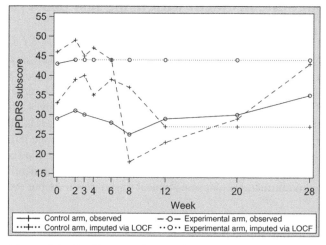

Figure 1.5   Parkinson's disease dataset: LOCF imputation.

except that the tendency of subjects to worsen late in the study is not reflected in the imputation.

For LOCF to provide valid estimates of efficacy at the primary time point (e.g., the last scheduled visit), a very particular MNAR assumption would need to hold, namely that with a probability of one, no matter what the general trend of outcomes in the study, a future outcome is equal to a subject's last available outcome. Molenberghs and Kenward (2007, pp. 45–47) point out how strong and unrealistic the LOCF assumption is. Verbeke and Molenberghs (1997, Chapter 5) show how much at variance LOCF is with the linear mixed model, with breaches of the usual assumptions about group differences and evolution over time. In summary, the LOCF assumption is not often clinically plausible; LOCF is unlikely in general to give a sensible estimate of a subject's efficacy at the study endpoint.

It is striking that LOCF makes no use of the information about the likely trajectory of discontinuations that is available from other subjects in this study. For example, Figure 1.3 tells us that, among completers, there is a slight worsening (increasing) in the mean efficacy score from Visit 5 (Week 8) onwards, in both treatment groups, perhaps reflecting the progressive nature of Parkinson's disease. No such worsening (increase) is included in LOCF imputations. Since LOCF fails to take account of the general worsening observed in subjects with Parkinson's disease, LOCF is likely to favor treatment arms that have more discontinuations, especially for subjects who discontinue mid-study when mean efficacy score is lowest (best). We see this to some extent in the case of the subject from the experimental arm that discontinued at Week 12. Should efficacy at Week 28 not be somewhat worse than efficacy at Week 12, given the progressive nature of Parkinson's disease as seen in the study trend? We note that our example here is not one that will often be found in a real clinical trial, as LOCF is generally considered not appropriate for progressive diseases, precisely because LOCF does not take progression into account. But even for other indications where the outcomes tend to improve with time or for chronic diseases, there are other problems with this method that we will discuss later in the book.

Our uncertainty about missing values in the previous paragraph brings us to another widely expressed objection to LOCF and similar methods such as baseline observation carried forward (BOCF). LOCF and BOCF are known as single imputation methods. They posit a single imputed value for the missing value, and thereafter treat the imputed value as though it were "real" data. The objection to single imputation methods is that they fail to reflect uncertainty about missing data. Regulators have voiced particular concern with regard to this unrealistic lack of variability in single imputation methods, and this concern is described further in Chapter 3, which summarizes the regulatory documents; Chapter 6 discusses this issue further in the context of multiple imputation.

1.5   Can we just assume that data are missing at random?

Would an MAR assumption give more credible results than LOCF for an estimate of efficacy at Visit 8 (Week 28)? If we accept the MAR assumption, we take it that observed data can in some sense account for missing values. Thus, if we assume MAR, missingness of the outcomes Y is independent of unobserved data conditional on the observed outcomes Y_{obs} and other covariables in the statistical model used. The MAR assumption states, as was defined earlier, that probability of missingness does not depend on unobserved data, given observed outcomes. It is helpful to understand that this assumption has an implication for the distribution of unobserved "potential" outcomes, given observed outcomes (or in the repeated measures context, as distribution of future outcomes given earlier outcomes). Informally, MAR can be shown (Verbeke and Molenberghs, 2000, Section 20.2.1, Theorem 20.1, p. 334) to be equivalent to the assumption that the conditional distribution of potential (missing) outcomes for dropouts given their observed outcomes, is the same as the conditional distribution of observed outcomes for patients who continued. As a result, the estimate of treatment effect that we get from the likelihood-based (ignorable) inference under MAR is essentially the estimate of what would have happened, had all the patients who discontinued remained on their respective treatments. See Section 4.2.2.3 for further discussion on what is estimated by MAR, and Section 4.1.1 on what it may be desired to estimate.

Thus under MAR we use all relevant study data, including partial data from discontinued subjects, to infer plausible values for missing data. Chapter 5 shows in detail how to do this in SAS® (SAS Institute Inc., 2011) using a direct likelihood method known as mixed models for repeated measures (MMRM). Direct likelihood approaches can include models of repeated measures for binary and other non-normal outcomes, as well as continuous, normally distributed outcomes. Chapter 6 gives details about how to implement the same MAR assumptions using multiple imputation (MI) When their statistical models are the same, the two methods – MI and MMRM – in theory should give similar results, and in our experience, they usually do. However, we note that with MI, the model used to impute missing values may be distinct from the primary analysis model used to estimate treatment effect. The model used to impute the missing values must have the same explanatory variables as the model of the primary analysis, but can have extra variables in addition to those. MI can even include post-baseline variables to help model the outcome. In contrast, direct likelihood methods such as MMRM, make inferences about missing values and in the same step estimate the treatment effect; inclusion of post-baseline covariables in this single step would almost certainly lead to confounding of the estimate of treatment effect, and so in practice direct likelihood approaches cannot make use of post-baseline variables other than the outcome being modeled. Thus, MI can use more information than direct likelihood approaches in handling missing data, which may in some circumstances give it an advantage over direct likelihood approaches.

Both methods – direct likelihood modeling and MI – use partially observed study data to make inferences with missing data under MAR and have an advantage over single-imputation LOCF in that they take account of the uncertainty pertaining to missing data. Generally speaking, the confidence intervals provided by MI and by direct likelihood methods such as MMRM depend on the amount of missing information with respect to the estimated parameters, whereas for the single-imputation LOCF estimates this is not the case. Thus, our uncertainty about the missing data is

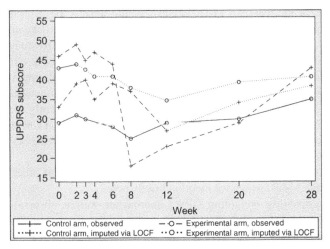

Figure 1.6   Parkinson's disease dataset: MAR imputation for selected trajectories.

reflected in the summary statistics from MMRM and MI, but we cannot depend upon this being so when we use single imputation methods, such as LOCF or BOCF.

Chapter 6 describes how, in place of the missing data, MI uses a number of draws from the posterior distribution of the missing observation, given the observed data. The variability between the MI draws, calculated and incorporated using Rubin's rules (Rubin, 1987) reflects the uncertainty about the missing data. Figure 1.6 shows values imputed under the MAR assumption for the trajectories of the two selected subjects that discontinued early, using MI. MI uses all the data in Figure 1.1 to estimate the posterior distribution of the missing data. Imputed values shown on Figure 1.6 represent the mean of 100 draws from the posterior distribution. (For convenience, the variability of the draws is not indicated in the plot, but it would of course be taken into account in subsequent analysis with imputed data). We can see that the slight worsening (increase) in efficacy scores found in the study from Visit 6 (Week 12) onwards is reflected in the MAR estimates for the two subjects who discontinued early. We also see that the study pattern of modest improvement in efficacy scores followed by return to disease progression is reflected in the imputation of the subject from the control group who discontinued shortly after the start of the study. Thus, MAR includes the likely trajectory of symptoms in its inference about missing values.

There is a wide variety of opinion about applicability of the MAR assumption. Many argue that it is "often reasonable" to assume that clinical trial data are MAR, see, for example, Mallinckrodt *et al.* (2008). Because it assumes that discontinuations follow the pattern of completers, some argue that MAR gives a kind of per-protocol estimate of treatment effect, albeit capable of being applied to the ITT population. In Chapter 3, we will see that the US and EU regulatory guidances point to this limitation of methods that assume MAR. Kenward (2011) similarly talks (broadly speaking) of MAR giving a *de jure* estimate of treatment effect. Section 4.2.3.3 describes a case where, at the least, an MAR analysis would need to be carefully justified. However, while one acknowledges that MAR uses study data to make inferences for missing data, such use of study data is not always as favorable to study treatments as it sounds. We often find that subjects who discontinue early have efficacy scores that are worse than the study average. Since MAR models missing values using study data, MAR models the missing values of early discontinuations on similar poorly performing subjects who completed the study. Consequently MAR's use of observed study outcomes to model later missing outcomes may result in acceptably unfavorable estimates of efficacy for subjects who discontinue. See Section 4.2.2.4 for further discussion of these points.

In addition to direct likelihood and MI, there are a number of other approaches that can assume MAR, which we mention briefly here.

Inverse probability weighting (IPW) approaches weight observations by the inverse of the probability of their being observed, and thus "even up" the estimate to give adequate emphasis to the kind of subject associated with missing data. Logistic regression can be used to estimate the probability of an observation being observed, using baseline data or trial data prior to dropout. Since this approach uses study data to take account of missing data, it can give valid estimates assuming MAR. The approach using generalized estimating equations (GEEs) takes account of explanatory variables such as treatment and baseline score, but does not take modeled account of pre-discontinuation outcomes and thus assumes MCAR; but GEEs can use IPW weighting, and thus weighted GEEs can also be valid under the MAR assumption. These weighted GEEs can be further augmented with functions of the observed data and configured so as to be doubly robust in that inference will be valid if at least one model – either the model for missingness or the model for the missing values - is correct, but not necessarily both. Carpenter and Kenward (2006) discuss the theory and practice of this method. Vansteelandt *et al.* (2010) usefully describe a number of ways of implementing doubly robust estimation. Chapter 8 discusses weighted and doubly robust estimation and shows how to implement Vansteelandt *et al.*'s version of doubly robust estimation via SAS code and using a SAS macro.

1.6   What can be done if data may be missing not at random?

However, sometimes we may feel we cannot justify the assumption of MAR clinically. In other instances, the regulator may judge that MAR is too favorable an assumption with regard to the experimental arm, and an outcome worse than that assumed by MAR should be imputed.

Selection models take into account the probability of observations being missing by modeling this probability along with the outcome, using a joint likelihood. The missingness of MNAR data is by definition dependent on unobserved outcomes. Selection models can model MNAR assumptions by modeling this dependence. For example, assumptions about the degree of dependence can be modeled by forcing the coefficient for the relationship between the unobserved data and missingness to have a specified value. Shared parameter models posit a latent variable, given which the missingness is often assumed to be independent of the unobserved values. The model's estimate of the magnitude and/or statistical significance of the latent variable is thought by some to give evidence about the strength of a putative MNAR link between missingness and unobserved values of the outcome. We do not give a full treatment of selection models and shared parameter models, but note them among the tools available to the statistician in Chapter 4 and discuss them briefly; while a further description of the two methods, with SAS code and an example, is provided in Appendices 7.I and 7.J.

Both MI and MMRM can also be used to implement analyses based on MNAR assumptions, using pattern-mixture models (PMMs). We have used PMMs with such MNAR assumptions for a primary analysis. An example where this may be appropriate is a trial where the indication is chronic pain. Here, it may be reasonable to assume for purposes of estimating treatment effect that discontinuations do worse than similar subjects who remain in the study, and thus that MAR would not be suitable.

Most sensitivity analyses assume some form of MNAR. We will describe how to use MI for this purpose in detail in the chapter on sensitivity analyses, Chapter 7; use of MMRM-type estimates for PMMs is also noted in Chapter 7. Our next section discusses in more detail how PMMs can be used to facilitate sensitivity analyses.

1.7   Stress-testing study results for robustness to missing data

One of the things we know for certain about missing data is that it's not there – we cannot be sure of what the missing data might have been. Ultimately, we do not know the level of bias that may result from a particular assumption about missing data. Could a few subjects have discontinued due to sudden worsening of disease that was not recorded, and thus have data MNAR? Even if a small proportion of data is MNAR, the assumptions of a standard MAR analysis such as MMRM will be incorrect. We would argue that the unknown bias due to missing values is not just a nuisance parameter or a crack in the evidence that may be papered over. The fact that a subject discontinues early from a study is in itself an important piece of evidence about the study treatment. The US and EU guidance (see Chapter 3) strongly advises that results from MAR analyses should be "stress tested" for robustness to the MAR assumption.

Chapter 7 describes approaches for testing study conclusions for robustness to missing data. We think such tests of robustness are an essential part of handling missing data, whether MCAR, MAR or indeed MNAR is assumed.

1.8   How the pattern of dropouts can bias the outcome

For the subject in Figure 1.5 who discontinued at Week 12 in the experimental arm, LOCF assumed no worsening – even though on average efficacy scores did worsen after Week 12 in the study. For progressive disease, LOCF thus tends inappropriately to favor early discontinuations. Does this mean that LOCF is "anti-conservative?" Not necessarily. If for a trial in progressive disease we expect more or earlier discontinuations in the control arm than in the experimental arm, LOCF could be regarded as "conservative" in estimating the difference between treatment groups in that LOCF will be expected to favor the control group. However, LOCF-based estimates would still paint an overly optimistic picture of disease progression within each arm. We may begin to see that, for a given estimand, bias due to missing data will depend upon the interplay between

- the assumptions we make (LOCF, MAR, etc.)

- the expected trajectory of outcome over time

- relative timing and proportion of missing data in experimental arm and control arm

- reasons for discontinuation in experimental arm and control arm

- objective of the study (superiority, non-inferiority)

Among these factors that contribute to our assessment of bias, the MAR assumption can often, by its nature, take account of the second factor – the expected trajectory of outcome over time. In Figure 1.6, we see how the disease trajectory can usually be modeled well from the observed study data. Thus if, for example, subjects with a particular indication tend to worsen over time (whatever their treatment), MAR will model this in its imputation of their missing values. In general, then, MAR methods allow for disease trajectory in their inference about missing data. Because of this, disease trajectory is often less important in determining the bias of MAR methods. This does not take away from the weakness of the MAR assumption noted in Section 1.5, that it infers that subjects who stop treatment will have symptoms like similar subjects who remain in the study and on treatment. Thus, while MAR will often correctly model the "natural" disease trajectory, it may well model a continuing effect of treatment after the subject has stopped taking the treatment in a way that is not clinically realistic. As noted, this could be a particular problem, for example, in studies of chronic diseases, where symptoms are known to return to baseline when treatment stops. In such cases, MAR may erroneously infer that the symptoms of subjects who stop treatment will maintain a smooth trajectory similar to subjects who remain on treatment.

1.9   How do we formulate a strategy for missing data?

It is not possible to predict bias accurately, and no approach for handling missing data will be perfect. This fact is recognized in the wording of the EU guidance: the primary analysis should be chosen that "would … provide a point estimate that is unlikely to be biased in favor of experimental treatment to an important degree (under reasonable assumptions)" (European Medicines Agency, 2010). Because we cannot be sure that the assumptions of the primary analysis are true, a comprehensive report of study results must include sensitivity analyses that stress-test the primary study result, to assess its robustness when those assumptions do not hold. Sensitivity analyses usually implement pre-specified MNAR assumptions that can be demonstrated to be likely to be more unfavorable to the experimental treatment than those of the primary analysis. We have noted that statistical frameworks for implementing sensitivity analyses include selection models, shared parameter models and PPMs. Our Chapter 7 concentrates on the use of PMMs to implement a variety of sensitivity analyses.

The strategy for missing data must be chosen and justified individually for each trial. Chapter 2 shows how steps can be taken when both designing and implementing a trial to prevent missing data in the first place. Chapter 4 maps the process of how to identify justifiable approaches to missing data. The choice of both main analysis and sensitivity analyses can take into account the likely patterns of outcome and of missingness in the trial data, using historic data about the efficacy and safety trajectory of the indication, and the likely effects of treatment. Those historic data, if they exist, will be needed to support a scientific justification of the chosen strategy in the study protocol. Historic data can also suggest sensitivity analyses that stress-test the study result by including assumptions that are likely to be unfavorable to the experimental arm, with regard to missing data, while remaining clinically plausible.

There is no one strategy that is best for missing data. Nevertheless, we propose the following pointers:

- a plan should be devised to prevent or minimize missing data in the design and implementation of a trial;

- the MAR assumption can in many, but not all, cases offer an estimate that is "unlikely to be biased to an important degree";

- but the MAR approach is likely to have some bias;

- the likely extent of bias due to missing values would need to be assessed on a study by study basis;

- an MNAR approach may be warranted for the primary analysis in some cases;

- sensitivity analyses to assess robustness to the assumptions of the primary analysis are always warranted;

- the study design and analyses should make assumptions about missing data that are clinically meaningful, transparent and easily understood;

- in a growing number of cases, regulators have in their advice and their approvals been following the latest regulatory documents issued in the United States or the EU; on occasion, however, particular regulatory views, sometimes linked to a strong tradition for a therapeutic area, can dictate primary and even sensitivity analyses that do not follow the current guidances or the reasoning we have presented in this chapter; in this case, of course, agreement must be reached on the best strategy taking regulatory views into account.

A detailed guide to planning a strategy for handling missing data will be presented in Chapter 4.

The examples in this book are drawn from phase II and phase III trials, but we note that it will be helpful to pay attention to missing data in early-phase trials not only for the sake of those trials, but also because this will make for a more informed strategy for missing data in later confirmatory trials. Exploration of missing data patterns should be included in the clinical study report of early-phase trials.

Finally, missing data is not only the statistician's problem – the whole team needs to take part in discussions pertaining to assumptions and prevention.

1.10   Description of example datasets

This section describes three example datasets that are used throughout the book to illustrate various approaches for dealing with missing data.

1.10.1   Example dataset in Parkinson's disease treatment

The illustrative example described in this section has been patterned after typical Parkinson's disease data, for example, in Emre *et al.* (2004) and Parkinson Study Group (2004a, 2004b). The dataset represents a randomized, double-blind trial designed to compare two treatment arms – experimental and placebo, with 57 subjects per arm. The primary efficacy endpoint is a sub-score of the UPDRS with lower values representing less severe symptoms. Time points included in our example dataset represent study visits scheduled to occur at baseline (Visit 0), and then at post-baseline Weeks 2, 3, 4, 6, 8, 12, 20 and 28 (a total of eight post-baseline visits).

In our example, 68% of subjects in the placebo arm completed the study versus 56% of subjects in the experimental arm. Table 1.1 summarizes (cumulative) percentages of subjects discontinued from the trial by visit. For example, this table shows that 19% of subjects in the placebo arm discontinued at or before Visit 4

Table 1.1   Parkinson's disease dataset, subjects completing and discontinuing from the trial by visit of discontinuation.

Visit (Time Point)	Placebo arm	Experimental arm
	Discontinued Subjects (Cumulative)	
1 (Week 2)	4%	7%
2 (Week 3)	9%	16%
3 (Week 4)	9%	21%
4 (Week 6)	19%	32%
5 (Week 8)	26%	39%
6 (Week 12)	30%	44%
7 (Week 20)	32%	44%
	Study Completers	
	68%	56%

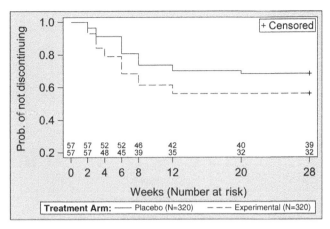

Figure 1.7   Parkinson's disease dataset, Kaplan-Meier plot of time to discontinua-tion from the study in each treatment arm. The two rows of numbers within the plot at the bottom are counts of those "at risk" of discontinuation at each time point.

(Week 6). Overall, there were considerably more subjects who discontinued from the experimental arm compared to the placebo arm.

Figure 1.7 presents a Kaplan-Meier plot of probability of continuing in the study in both treatment arms. It further highlights in a visual manner the difference in the proportion of discontinuations between the arms, which started to become quite apparent from around Week 4 and was sustained until the end of the study. Larger proportions of subjects withdrew up to Week 6 from the experimental arm; after Week 6 the probability curves remained mostly parallel throughout the rest of the study. This suggests that there may have been a group of subjects who were not able to tolerate the experimental treatment relatively early in the study and discontinued for this reason, while the withdrawals at the later stages were similar in both arms.

Figure 1.8 summarizes mean change from baseline (CFB) in UPDRS sub-score values by time point for study completers and a number of dropout cohorts (corre-sponding to the time point of discontinuation) for each treatment arm. Most discon-tinuation cohorts contain a relatively small number of subjects, so one can expect the means to have more diverse trajectories, compared to the trajectory for study com-pleters. In the placebo arm, we can see that subjects who discontinued at Week 6 and 12 showed on average some improvement prior to discontinuation, while, for exam-ple, those who discontinued at Week 8 and 20 experienced both improvement and worsening. In the experimental arm, the slope of the trajectory of most discontinued subjects was initially close to the slope of completers in their arm, although those that discontinued at Weeks 6 and 8 had worsening of symptoms prior to discontinuation after some initial improvement.

Figure 1.9 summarizes the CFB by grouping all subjects who discontinued at any point versus completers in each treatment arm. It appears that, on average, withdrawals from the experimental arm are very similar to placebo completers prior

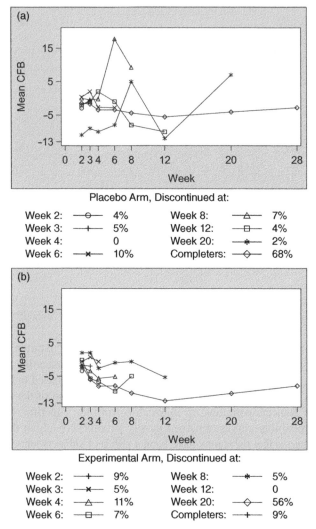

Figure 1.8   Parkinson's disease dataset, summary of mean change from baseline (CFB) in UPDRS sub-score by time point across dropout cohorts (grouped by time of discontinuation) and study completers.

to discontinuation, while placebo dropouts were on all but one visit doing worse compared to placebo completers.

Table 1.2 also clearly suggests that withdrawals differed between treatment arms: 38% of subjects discontinued from the experimental treatment due to an adverse event (AE) versus 9% in the placebo arm, indicating that the experimental treatment toxicity was an important factor in subjects' inability to continue on treatment. In the placebo arm, 16% of subjects discontinued due to lack of efficacy, while no subjects discontinued due to this reason from the experimental treatment. The proportion

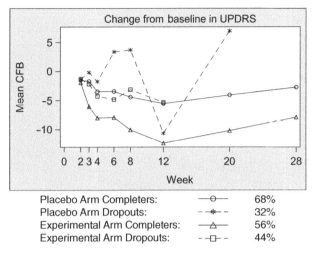

Placebo Arm Completers: —○—   68%
Placebo Arm Dropouts: – –＊– –   32%
Experimental Arm Completers: —△—   56%
Experimental Arm Dropouts: – –□– –   44%

Figure 1.9   Parkinson's disease dataset, summary of mean change from baseline (CFB) in UPDRS sub-score by time point for study dropouts and completers in each treatment arm.

of subjects discontinuing due to other reasons (such as loss to follow-up, protocol violation, withdrawal of consent) is similar in the two arms.

Figure 1.10 summarizes mean CFB across time by discontinuation status/reason in each treatment arm. In the experimental arm, subjects who withdrew for reasons other than AE did so quite early in the study. Those who discontinued due to AEs stayed on study longer and showed some modest improvement (comparable to that of placebo subjects) before adverse reactions led to the decision to discontinue treatment. In the placebo arm, these data show a tendency towards worsening among subjects who discontinued due to AEs and other reasons. Interestingly, in the group of placebo subjects who had a primary reason for discontinuation recorded as lack of efficacy, CFB during the interval just prior to discontinuation at Week 12 appeared as favorable. A situation like this may indicate that there is another (e.g., secondary) efficacy parameter that played an important role in the decision to discontinue, while the primary efficacy endpoint does not directly correlate with the recorded primary reason.

In SAS code examples provided throughout this book, we will refer to variables as contained in this dataset and used for analysis. Depending on the analysis performed,

Table 1.2   Parkinson's disease dataset, reasons for discontinuing from the trial.

Reason for Discontinuation	Placebo arm	Experimental arm
	Discontinued Subjects	
Adverse Event	9%	39%
Lack of Efficacy	16%	0%
Other Reasons	7%	5%

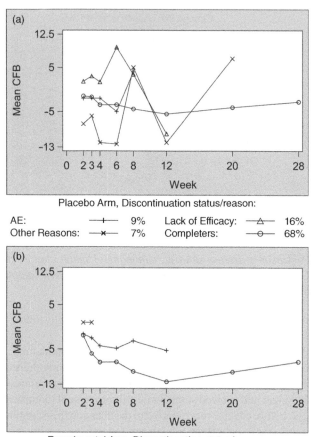

Placebo Arm, Discontinuation status/reason:

AE: ———+———   9%   Lack of Efficacy: ——△——   16%
Other Reasons: ——✕——   7%   Completers: ——○——   68%

Experimental Arm, Discontinuation status/reason:

AE: ———+———   38%   Lack of Efficacy: ——△——   0
Other Reasons: ——✕——   6%   Completers: ——○——   56%

Figure 1.10   Parkinson's disease dataset, summary of mean CFB in UPDRS sub-score by time point for study completers and dropouts by reason for discontinuation.

we may utilize either a vertically structured or a horizontally structured dataset. Variables that are common in both of these structures are as follows:

- *subjid* – subject number;

- *region* – geographic region;

- *trt* – treatment arm (with 1 representing placebo arm, and 2 – the experimental arm);

- *lastvis* – last study visit subject attended (taking the value of 0 for baseline, and values 1 through 8 for post-baseline Weeks 2, 3, 4, 6, 8, 12, 20 and 28, respectively);

- *reasond* – primary reason for discontinuation (taking values Adverse Event; Lack of Efficacy; and Other Reasons).

A dataset with a vertical structure contains one record per subject and visit, and has the following additional variables:

- *visit* – study visit (taking the value of 0 for baseline, and values 1 through 8 for post-baseline Weeks 2, 3, 4, 6, 8, 12, 20 and 28);

- *upd* – subjects' UPDRS sub-score for a given visit;

- *base_upd* - subjects' UPDRS sub-score at baseline;

- *inv* – investigator site.

A dataset with a horizontal structure contains one record per subject with the following variables representing analysis values at different visits:

- *upd_0, upd_1, ..., upd_8* – subjects' UPDRS sub-scores for baseline and Visit 1 through 8 (or Weeks 2, 3, 4, 6, 8, 12, 20, and 28) respectively.

1.10.2   Example dataset in insomnia treatment

Data introduced in this section have been patterned after typical clinical trials in an adult population with an insomnia indication, for example, in Krystal *et al.* (2008); Roth *et al.* (2005); Purdue Pharma LP (2007); Eli Lilly and Company (2008). Our dataset represents a randomized, double-blind trial with 320 subjects in each of the two arms – experimental and placebo. The primary efficacy endpoint is the mean total sleep time (TST) per night measured in minutes. We also consider another efficacy parameter, morning sleepiness, commonly measured in insomnia trials. This parameter, which we refer to as the morning sleepiness score (MSS), is evaluated on a 0 to 10 scale, with lower values representing less sleepiness and thus a more favorable outcome. Additionally, this dataset contains another sleep-related parameter – sleep quality score (SQS), which we will make use of in some analyses. Typically, TST, MSS and SQS are recorded by subjects daily, while the analysis endpoints represent averages of these daily values over the period of time between clinic visits. Time points included in our example dataset represent study visits scheduled to occur prior to the commencement of the study treatment (referred to as baseline or Week 0), and then at post-baseline Weeks 1, 2, 4, 6, and 8. In other words, an analysis value for the TST endpoint at Visit k for a given subject in our dataset is the average of daily TST values recorded between Visits $k - 1$ and k. For a baseline time point ($k = 0$), it is assumed that subjects recorded their daily values between a screening visit and a Week 0 visit and the average over the days between these visits is used as baseline. Analysis values for the morning sleepiness score represent similar between-visit averages of daily scores for each subject.

In our example, 82% of subjects in the placebo arm completed the study versus 80% of subjects in the experimental arm. Table 1.3 summarizes (cumulative) percentages of subjects discontinued from the trial by visit. For example, this table shows that 15% of subjects in each arm discontinued at or before Visit 3 (Week 4). Percentages of dropouts are fairly similar across the two treatment arms for all time points.

Table 1.4 provides a summary of reasons for discontinuation. In this example dataset, there is not much difference between the treatment arms in this respect.

Table 1.3   Insomnia dataset, subjects completing and discontinuing from the trial by visit.

Visit (Time Point)	Placebo arm	Experimental arm
	Discontinued Subjects (Cumulative)	
1 (Week 1)	6%	6%
2 (Week 2)	9%	10%
3 (Week 4)	15%	15%
4 (Week 6)	18%	20%
	Study Completers	
	82%	80%

Figure 1.11 contains a Kaplan-Meier plot of probability of remaining in the study by treatment arm. The probability curves are very similar in both treatment arms and show only a very small difference towards the end of the study. The rate of discontinuation was very similar at different stages of the trial, with approximately 5% of subjects dropping out after each visit.

Figure 1.12 and 1.13 summarize mean CFB in TST and MSS values by time point for study completers and different dropout cohorts (corresponding to the time point of discontinuation) for each treatment arm. Upon examining these figures, we can see that while subjects that discontinued from the experimental arm look similar to completers in their TST and MSS, subjects that discontinued from the placebo arm are noticeably different from placebo completers, in terms of the CFB in TST and MSS. Placebo subjects discontinued after Weeks 2 and 6 had little improvement or worsening in TST. Those who discontinued after Week 4, seem to have improved in terms of TST, but less so in terms of MSS. If we examine baseline values (see Table 1.5), we can see that mean baseline TST seemed substantially worse in this group of dropouts compared to other subjects (220 min vs. 337 min for completers).

Table 1.4   Insomnia dataset, reasons for discontinuing from the trial.

Reason for Discontinuation	Placebo arm	Experimental arm
	Discontinued Subjects	
Adverse Event	4%	5%
Consent Withdrawn	3%	4%
Lack of Efficacy	1%	0%
Lost to Follow-up	5%	6%
Protocol Violated	4%	2%
Other Reasons	1%	3%

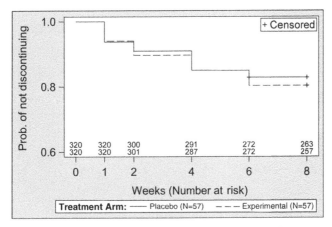

Figure 1.11 Insomnia dataset, Kaplan-Meier plot of time to discontinuation from the study in each treatment arm. The two rows of numbers within the plot at the bottom are counts of those "at risk" of discontinuation at each time point.

Similarly, the mean baseline morning sleepiness score in this group of subjects was the highest (equal to 5.9), while, for example, completers had a baseline mean of 5.1. This seems to indicate that even though these subjects showed improvement in terms of TST and, to some extent, MSS, it might not have been a satisfactory one given their more severe symptoms at baseline. Overall, the trajectory of TST and MSS values prior to withdrawal as well as baseline values seem to be correlated with dropout in the placebo arm, and may suggest that an MAR assumption would be plausible, at least for the placebo arm.

However, as already noted, compared to the placebo arm, discontinuations from the experimental arm appear to be somewhat more similar to completers in their arm, in terms of their trajectory prior to dropout. Nevertheless, experimental arm subjects last observed at Weeks 1, 2, or 6 showed little improvement from baseline in term of TST. Subjects last observed at Weeks 1 and 6 had changes in MSS that showed trends similar to those in TST. For experimental arm subjects who were last observed at Week 4, the picture is less clear. They seem to have improved both in terms of TST and especially MSS. Their baseline TST and MSS values are, on average, somewhat worse than those of other subjects but to a less important degree than in the case of placebo subjects.

Primary reasons for discontinuation do not seem to shed any more light: reasons are distributed similarly for the two treatment groups. Discontinuation after an apparent improvement in the primary and key secondary efficacy parameter may either indicate that subjects were reasonably satisfied with their achieved sleep pattern and did not consider that further treatment was necessary, or it may be suggestive of an MNAR mechanism.

In SAS code examples provided throughout this book, we will refer to variables as contained in the datasets we used for analysis. Depending on the analysis performed,

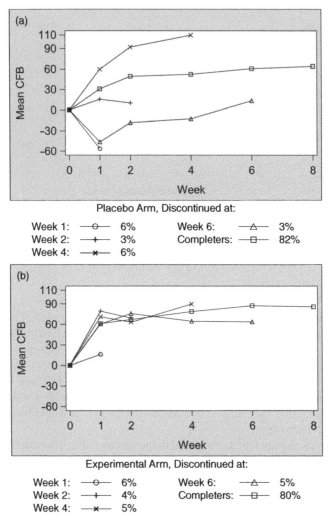

Figure 1.12   Insomnia dataset, summary of mean CFB in total sleep time (minutes) by time point across dropout cohorts (grouped by time of discontinuation) and study completers.

we utilize either a vertically structured or a horizontally structured dataset. Variables that are common in both of these structures are as follows:

- *subjid* – subject number;

- *agegrp* – subject's age group at study entry(taking value of 1 through 5 for age groups of <30 years, 30–34 years, 35–44 years, 45–54 years and ≥55 years);

- *sex* – subject's sex;

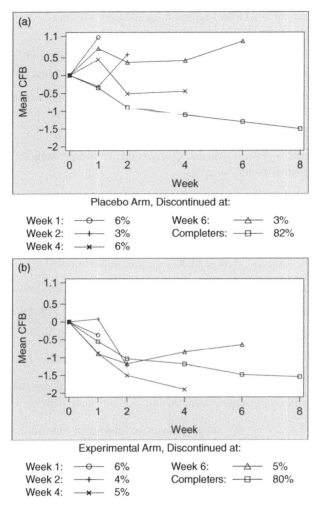

Figure 1.13 Insomnia dataset, summary of mean change from baseline (CFB) in morning sleepiness score (0 to 10) by time point across dropout cohorts (grouped by time of discontinuation) and study completers.

Table 1.5 Insomnia dataset, summary of baseline values of efficacy endpoints.

Subjects discontinued at visit (Time point)	Baseline TST Mean (±STD)		Baseline MSS Mean (±STD)	
	Placebo	Experimental	Placebo	Experimental
1 (Week 1)	345 (±113)	336 (±38)	4.6 (±1.8)	4.8 (±1.2)
2 (Week 2)	345 (±115)	363 (±77)	5.2 (±0.6)	4.5 (±1.2)
3 (Week 4)	220 (±142)	298 (±96)	5.9 (±1.3)	5.4 (±1.0)
4 (Week 6)	383 (±68)	295 (±145)	3.7 (±1.8)	4.6 (±1.8)
Completers	337 (±79)	322 (±80)	5.1 (±1.5)	4.9 (±1.5)

- *trt* – treatment arm (with 1 representing placebo arm, and 2 – the experimental arm);

- *lastvis* – last study visit subject attended (taking the value of 0 for baseline, and values 1 through 5 for post-baseline Weeks 1, 2, 4, 6 and 8 respectively);

- *reasond* – primary reason for discontinuation (taking values Adverse Event; Consent Withdrawn; Lack of Efficacy; Lost to Follow-up; Protocol Violated; and Other Reasons).

A dataset with a vertical structure contains one record per subject and visit, and has the following additional variables:

- *visit* – study visit (taking the value of 0 for baseline, and values 1 through 5 for post-baseline Weeks 1, 2, 4, 6 and 8);

- *tst* – subjects' average total sleep time value for a given visit;

- *base_tst* - subjects' average total sleep time value at baseline;

- *mss* – subjects' average morning sleepiness score for a given visit;

- *base_mss* – subjects' average morning sleepiness score at baseline;

- *sqs* – subject's average sleep quality score for a given visit;

- *base_sqs* – subject's average sleep quality score at baseline.

A dataset with a horizontal structure contains one record per subject with the following variables representing analysis values at different visits:

- *tst_0, tst_1, ..., tst_5* – subjects' average total sleep time values for baseline and Visit 1 through 5 (or Weeks 0, 1, 2, 4, 6, and 8) respectively;

- *mss_0, mss_1, ..., mss_5* – subjects' average morning sleepiness scores for baseline and Visit 1 through 5 (or Weeks 0, 1, 2, 4, 6, and 8) respectively;

- *sqs_0, sqs_1, ..., sqs_5* – subjects' average sleep quality scores for baseline and Visit 1 through 5 (or Weeks 0, 1, 2, 4, 6, and 8) respectively.

1.10.3 Example dataset in mania treatment

The example dataset described in this section has been patterned after typical trials in mania treatment, for example, Bowden *et al.* (2010); Lipkovich *et al.* (2008); Post *et al.* (2005). Our dataset represents a randomized, double-blind, two-arm trial comparing an experimental treatment to placebo, with 550 subjects randomized to each arm. The primary efficacy endpoint is a total score from the Young Mania Rating Scale (YMRS) based on the subject's evaluation of his/her clinical condition over the past 48 hours using 11 items evaluating severity of a variety of symptoms. The YMRS score can take values between 0 and 88, with higher scores representing more severe symptoms. Time points included in our example dataset represent study visits

Table 1.6   Mania dataset, subjects completing and discontinuing from the trial by visit of discontinuation.

Visit (Time Point)	Placebo arm	Experimental arm
	Discontinued Subjects (Cumulative)	
0 (Baseline)	1%	1%
1 (Day 4)	5%	4%
2 (Day 7)	8%	10%
3 (Day 14)	21%	18%
4 (Day 21)	30%	25%
	Study Completers	
5 (Day 28)	70%	75%

scheduled to occur at baseline (Visit 0), and then at post-baseline Days 4, 7, 14, 21, and 28 (a total of five post-baseline visits).

In this example dataset, 70% of subjects in the placebo arm completed the study versus 75% of subjects in the experimental arm. Table 1.6 summarizes (cumulative) percentages of subjects discontinued from the trial by visit. For example, this table shows that 21% of subjects in the placebo arm discontinued at or before Visit 3 (Day 14). The overall proportion of subjects who discontinued from the placebo arm was somewhat larger (by 5%), and the difference in the proportion of discontinuations between the two arms increased towards the end of the trial.

Figure 1.14 shows a Kaplan-Meier plot of probability of not withdrawing from the study for each treatment arm. The probability curves of the two arms are very

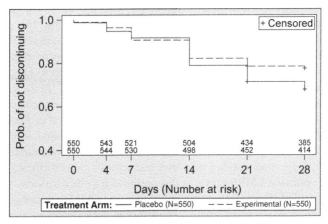

Figure 1.14   Mania dataset, Kaplan-Meier plot of time to discontinuation from the study in each treatment arm. The two rows of numbers within the plot at the bottom are counts of those "at risk" of discontinuation at each time point.

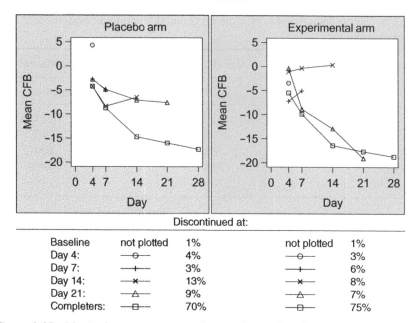

Figure 1.15 Mania dataset, summary of mean change from baseline (CFB) in YMRS score by time point across dropout cohorts (grouped by time of discontinuation) and study completers.

close until a midpoint of the study (Day 14), with the probability of discontinuation increasing more rapidly in the placebo arm from that point on.

Figure 1.15 summarizes mean CFB in YMRS score by time point for study completers and a number of dropout cohorts (corresponding to the time point of discontinuation for each treatment arm). In this dataset, 1% of subjects in each arm discontinued before providing any post-baseline assessments; this group is not depicted on the plots of mean CFB. In the placebo arm, we can see that subjects who discontinued tended to experience worsening or small improvement compared to placebo completers. Mean improvement in YMRS score up to Day 28 is quite pronounced among placebo completers (strong placebo effect). In the experimental arm, subjects who discontinued at or before Day 14 also experienced either a very small improvement or worsening. Subjects that discontinued after Day 21 (7% of subjects), on the contrary, showed an important improvement, similar to completers in their arm. Only a small number of subjects in this cohort discontinued due to an adverse event, suggesting that they may have had deterioration on efficacy parameters other than the primary YMRS score, or discontinued for other reasons.

The left panel of Figure 1.16 summarizes observed CFB by grouping all subjects who discontinued at any point versus completers in each treatment arm. From this plot, for example, it is apparent that using an approach such as last observation carried forward could favor the experimental arm because of the cohort of experimental arm withdrawals that had a significant improvement prior to discontinuing after Day 21.

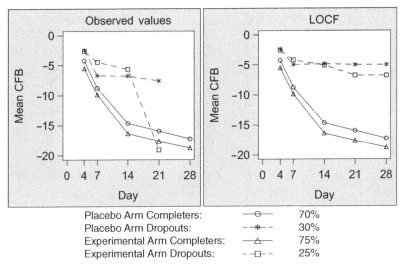

Figure 1.16   Mania dataset, summary of mean CFB in YMRS score by time point for study dropouts and completers in each treatment arm, based on observed values (left panel) and LOCF-imputed values (right panel).

This is illustrated on the right panel of Figure 1.15 which depicts mean CFB using LOCF-imputed values. In this case, LOCF imputation makes placebo withdrawals look bad and some experimental withdrawals look good. Thus, LOCF may be viewed as anti-conservative, especially if a rapid deterioration of mania symptoms after premature treatment discontinuation is clinically plausible between Day 21 and 28. Nevertheless, we shall see in Section 4.2.3.2 that it is possible to implement the assumption that LOCF applies only to the experimental arm while assuming MAR for the control arm, and that this could be a sufficiently conservative approach with this illustrative dataset (based on the fact that there are more withdrawals in the placebo group, so more of them will be favored by MAR, and not all experimental improved before discontinuation, so LOCF will not favor all in the experimental arm).

Table 1.7 summarizes discontinuations by reason for discontinuation. In this dataset, percentage of subjects discontinuing due to an AE is very small in both treatment arms (1% in placebo and 3% in experimental), indicating that the experimental

Table 1.7   Mania dataset, reasons for discontinuing from the trial.

Reason for Discontinuation	Placebo arm	Experimental arm
	Discontinued Subjects	
Adverse Event	1%	3%
Consent Withdrawn or Decision of Investigator	18%	16%
Other Reasons	11%	6%

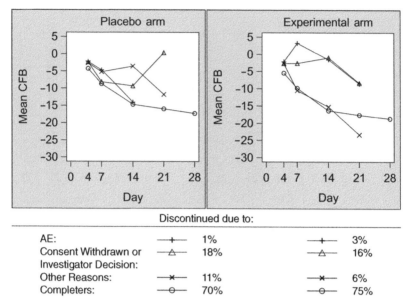

Figure 1.17   Mania dataset, summary of mean change from baseline (CFB) in YMRS score by time point for study completers and dropouts by reason for discontinuation.

treatment was, in general, well tolerated. The majority of subjects discontinued due to an investigator decision or withdrawal of consent, in proportions that are similar in both arms (18% in placebo and 16% in experimental). Approximately 5% more of subjects withdrew from the placebo arm due to other reasons compared to the experimental arm.

Figure 1.17 summarizes mean CFB across time in each treatment arm by reason for discontinuation. In both arms, subjects who withdrew consent or discontinued due to an investigator decision did not show adequate improvement in the YMRS score. Subjects who withdrew due to other reasons did improve, especially those in the experimental arm.

In SAS code examples provided throughout this book, we will refer to variables as contained in this dataset and used for analysis. Depending on the analysis performed, we may utilize either a vertically structured or a horizontally structured dataset. Variables that are common in both of these structures are as follows:

- *subjid* – subject number;

- *trt* – treatment arm (with 1 representing placebo arm, and 2 - the experimental arm);

- *lastvis* – last study visit subject attended (taking the value of 0 for baseline, and values 1 through 5 for post-baseline Days 4, 7, 14, 21, and 28 respectively);

- *reasond* – primary reason for discontinuation (taking values Adverse Event; Consent Withdrawn or Investigator Decision; and Other Reasons).

A dataset with a vertical structure contains one record per subject and visit, and has the following additional variables:

- *visit* – study visit (taking the value of 0 for baseline, and values 1 through 5 for post-baseline Days 4, 7, 14, 21, and 28);
- *ymrs* – subjects' YMRS score for a given visit;
- *base_ymrs* – subjects' YMRS score at baseline;
- *inv* – investigator site.

A dataset with a horizontal structure contains one record per subject with the following variables representing analysis values at different visits:

- *ymrs_0, ymrs_1, …, ymrs_5* – subjects' YMRS scores for baseline and Visit 1 through 5 (or Days 4, 7, 14, 21, and 28) respectively.

Appendix 1.A: Formal definitions of MCAR, MAR and MNAR

Missing data mechanisms are often classified as missing completely at random (MCAR), missing at random (MAR) or missing not at random (MNAR) as per the terminology introduced by Rubin (1976) and Little and Rubin (2002). These types of missingness can be formally defined as follows, using notation similar to that of Molenberghs and Kenward (2007). Consider the full data density of the study outcome (including both missing and observed outcomes):

$$f(y, r | W, F, \theta, \psi) = f(y | W, \theta) f(r | y, F, \psi) \tag{1.1}$$

where y is a matrix of outcomes, r is the matrix of missingness indicators, W and F are the design matrices for y and r, respectively, and the corresponding parameter vectors are θ and ψ. Under MCAR, missingness is independent of outcomes, and we can transform (1.1) as follows:

$$\begin{gathered} f(y, r | W, F, 0, \psi) = f(y | W, \theta) f(r | F, \psi) \\ \text{and consequently} \\ f(y_{obs}, r | W, F, \theta, \psi) = f(y_{obs} | W, \theta) f(r | F, \psi) \end{gathered} \tag{1.2}$$

where y_{obs} is the observed subset of outcomes y. In this case, we can treat y as independent of the missingness r.

Under MAR, y is independent of missingness r, given the observed subset of outcomes y_{obs}:

$$\begin{gathered} f(y, r | W, F, \theta, \psi) = f(y | W, \theta) f(r | y_{obs}, F, \psi) \\ \text{and consequently} \\ f(y_{obs}, r | W, F, \theta, \psi) = f(y_{obs} | W, \theta) f(r | y_{obs}, F, \psi) \end{gathered} \tag{1.3}$$

Under MNAR, missingness depends on unobserved outcomes, and we cannot transform (1.1) using independent factors for observed outcomes and missingness as we can under the MCAR and MAR assumptions. In this case, the joint distribution has to be treated as follows:

$$f(y_{obs}, r \,|\, W, F, \theta, \psi) = \int f(y \,|\, W, \theta) f(r \,|\, y, F, \psi) \, dy_{mis} \qquad (1.4)$$

These definitions of the types of missingness are conditional on the statistical model used. Some authors (including Little and Rubin as cited) do not make the definitions conditional on the statistical model, but since the correctness of the model is important in practice, we follow Verbeke and Molenberghs (2000) and Molenberghs and Kenward (2007) in including it in the definition.

References

Bowden C, Mosolov S, Hranov L, Chen E, Habil H, Kongsakon R, Manfredi R, Lin H-N (2010) Efficacy of valproate versus lithium in mania or mixed mania: a randomized, open 12-week trial. *International Clinical Psychopharmacology* **25**: 60–67.

Carpenter JR, Kenward MG (2006) A comparison of multiple imputation and doubly robust estimation for analyses with missing data. *Journal of the Royal Statistical Society Series A* **169**: 571–584.

Eli Lilly and Company (2008) *An Efficacy Study of Compound LY2624803 in the Treatment of Patients With Chronic Insomnia (SLUMBER)*, in ClinicalTrials.gov [Internet]. National Library of Medicine, Bethesda (MD). http://clinicaltrials.gov/show/NCT00784875, accessed 18 June 2013.

Emre M, Aarsland D, Albanese A, Byrne J, Deuschl G, De Deyn P, Durif F, Kulisevsky J, van Laar T, Lees A, Poewe W, Robillard A, Rosa M, Wolters E, Quarg P, Tekin P, Lane R (2004) Rivastagmine for dementia associated with Parkinson's disease. *New England Journal of Medicine* **351**: 2509–2518.

European Medicines Agency (2010) *Guideline on Missing Data in Confirmatory Clinical Trials. EMA/CPMP/EWP/1776/99 Rev.1.* http://www.ema.europa.eu/docs/en_GB/document_library/Scientific_guideline/2010/09/WC500096793.pdf, accessed 23 June 2013.

Kenward MG (2011) Handling dropout and withdrawal in longitudinal clinical trials, presented at *Biostatistics Network Symposium: "Contemporary statistical methods in medical research"*, 15th September 2011. http://www.ucl.ac.uk/statistics/biostatistics-network/talks/TalkKenward.pdf, accessed 17 July 2013.

Krystal A, Erman M, Zammit G, Soubrane C, Roth T; on behalf of the ZOLONG Study Group (2008) Long-term efficacy and safety of zolpidem extended-release 12.5 mg, administered 3 to 7 nights per week for 24 weeks, in patients with chronic primary insomnia: a 6-month, randomized, double-blind, placebo-controlled, parallel-group, multicenter study. *Sleep* **31**: 79–90.

Lipkovich I, Houston J, Ahl J (2008) Identifying patterns in treatment response profiles in acute bipolar mania: a cluster analysis approach. *BMC Psychiatry* **8**: 65, available at http://www.ncbi.nlm.nih.gov/pmc/articles/PMC2515837, accessed 18 June 2013.

Little RJA, Rubin DB (2002) *Statistical Analysis with Missing Data*, 2nd edn. John Wiley & Sons, Ltd., New York.

Mallinckrodt CH, Lane PW, Schnell D, Peng Y, Mancuso J (2008) Recommendation for the primary analysis of continuous endpoints in longitudinal clinical trials. *Drug Information Journal* **42**: 303–319.

Molenberghs G, Kenward MG (2007) *Missing Data in Clinical Studies*. John Wiley & Sons Ltd., West Sussex.

National Research Council. Panel on Handling Missing Data in Clinical Trials. Committee on National Statistics, Division of Behavioral and Social Sciences and Education (2010) *The Prevention and Treatment of Missing Data in Clinical Trials*. The National Academies Press, Washington, DC, available at http://www.nap.edu/catalog.php?record_id=12955, accessed 16 July 2013.

Parkinson Study Group (2004a) A controlled, randomized delayed-start study of rasagiline in Early Parkinson Disease. *Arch Neurol.* **61**: 561–566.

Parkinson Study Group (2004b) Levodopa and the progression of Parkinson's disease. *New England Journal of Medicine* **351**: 2498–24508.

Post R, Altshuler L, Frye M, Suppes T, McElroy S, Keck P, Leverich G, Kupka R, Nolen W, Luckenbaugh D, Walden J, Grunze H (2005) Preliminary observations on the effectiveness of levetirecetam in the open adjunctive treatment of refractory bipolar disorder. *Journal of Clinical Psychiatry* **66**: 370–374.

Purdue Pharma LP (2007) *A Study of Zolpidem Tartrate Sublingual Tablet in Adult Patients With Insomnia*, in ClinicalTrials.gov [Internet]. National Library of Medicine, Bethesda (MD), available from http://clinicaltrials.gov/ct2/results?term=NCT00466193&Search= Search, accessed 18 June 2013.

Roth T, Walsh J, Krystal A, Wessel T, Roehrs T (2005) An evaluation of the efficacy and safety of eszopiclone over 12 months in patients with chronic primary insomnia. *Sleep Medicine* **6**: 487–495.

Rubin DB (1976) Inference and missing data. *Biometrika* **63**: 581–592.

Rubin DB (1987) *Multiple Imputation for Nonresponse in Surveys*. John Wiley & Sons, Ltd., New York.

SAS Institute Inc. (2011) *SAS/STAT® 9.3 User's Guide*. SAS Institute Inc., Cary, NC.

Tohen M, Greil W, Calabrese J, Sachs G, Yatham L, Oerlinghauser B, Koukopoulos A, Cassano G, Grunze H, Licht R, Dell'Osso L, Evans A, Risser R, Baker R, Crane H, Dossenbach M, Bowden C (2005) Olanzapine versus lithium in the maintenance treatment of bipolar disorder: a 12-month, randomized, double-blind, controlled clinical trial. *American Journal of Psychiatry* **162**: 1281–1290.

Vansteelandt S, Carpenter J, Kenward MG (2010) Analysis of incomplete data using inverse probability weighting and doubly robust estimators. *Methodology: European Journal of Research Methods for the Behavioral and Social Sciences* **6**(1): 37–48.

Verbeke G, Molenberghs G (1997) *Linear Mixed Models in Practice: A SAS-Oriented Approach. Lecture Notes in Statistics 126*. Springer-Verlag, New York.

Verbeke G, Molenberghs G (2000) *Linear Mixed Models for Longitudinal Data*. Springer-Verlag, New York.

2

The prevention of missing data

Sara Hughes

Key points

- The impact of missing data can be wide-ranging; for example, it could lead to a perceived or real reduction in trial quality and validity, reductions in statistical power or increases in study size.

- All the members of the team involved in the design and execution of a clinical trial – including the statistician – have a role to play in increasing retention and reducing missing data. An increased focus on missing data prevention at the study design stage is a worthwhile investment.

- An example illustrates four activities the statistician should lead at the study design stage with respect to missing data prevention: (i) quantifying the amount of missing data in previous trials of a disease, and its resultant impact; (ii) identifying subgroups of subjects who require an increased level of trial retention support (when appropriate); (iii) translating statistical analysis of previous trial data into information to inform future subject care; (iv) education of the clinical trial team and participation in the creation of missing data prevention plans.

2.1 Introduction

Advancing the statistical methodology for the handling of missing data has been a significant research area for the statistical community during recent years, and indeed forms the major part of this book. In contrast, there has been much less focus on

---

Clinical Trials with Missing Data: A Guide for Practitioners, First Edition. Michael O'Kelly and Bohdana Ratitch.
© 2014 John Wiley & Sons, Ltd. Published 2014 by John Wiley & Sons, Ltd.

proactive intervention prior to clinical trial initiation, and during trial conduct, aimed at reducing the level of missing data for analysis although some examples exist (e.g., Senturia *et al.*, 1998; Cassidy *et al.*, 2001; Walter and Hart, 2001; Moreno-Black *et al.*, 2004; Robinson *et al.*, 2007; Villacorta *et al.*, 2007; Magruder *et al.*, 2009; Secd *et al.*, 2009; Zook *et al.*, 2010). There is considerable potential to improve the clarity and quality of study results and also increase statistical power and efficiency, if clinical trial teams assess at the trial initiation stage the typical impact of missing data for the disease under study, and investigate ways in which to reduce dropouts. Proactive approaches to missing data prevention are also being sought by the regulatory agencies. For example, the National Research Council (NRC) report on missing data commissioned by the U.S. Food and Drug Administration (FDA) devotes 26 of its 145 pages to the topic of missing data prevention (National Research Council, 2010). While the European Medicines Agency's (EMA's) Guideline on Missing Data is more concise, it also conveys the same message: *". . . by careful planning it is possible to reduce the amount of data that are missing. This is important because missing data are a potential source of bias when analyzing data from clinical trials. Interpretation of the results of a trial is always problematic when the proportion of missing values is substantial. When this occurs, the uncertainty of the likely treatment effect can become such that it is not possible to conclude that evidence of efficacy has been established."* (European Medicines Agency, 2010).

The focus of this chapter is to examine ways in which missing data can be reduced by improving subject retention in clinical trials. Clearly missing data also occurs for other reasons (e.g., intermittent missed visits). The discussion that follows will be equally relevant for reducing missing data due to these other reasons. It is also important to clarify that while this chapter focuses on methods for improving subject retention, we need to distinguish between trial discontinuations that are related to treatment and are thus unavoidable versus those which are not related to treatment and are thus potentially preventable (e.g., due to a subject being lost to follow-up). It is clearly inappropriate to try to influence the decision of a subject or investigator to discontinue treatment when that treatment is in some way unacceptable for the subject and the focus of efforts to reduce missing data should be with respect to potentially preventable discontinuations. As discussed throughout this book, the amount of missing data is not the only concern, as any amount of informative missingness can lead to biased conclusions. Nevertheless, reducing the level of missing data is a very important element and should be the first item in the overall strategy, with the statistical mitigation approaches planned for what is truly unpreventable.

2.2   The impact of "too much" missing data

There are various possible implications of a substantial level of missing data within a trial. The impact can be statistical, financial, or be either a perceived or real reduction in trial quality and validity. Three examples follow in order to illustrate some of the various possible impacts.

2.2.1   Example from human immunodeficiency virus

In the study of antiretroviral drugs for the treatment of Human Immunodeficiency Virus (HIV), the primary efficacy endpoint in large-scale trials is typically the proportion of subjects whose HIV virus (as measured in plasma) is suppressed at a specified time point. All the commonly used algorithms for deriving this binary endpoint, including the algorithm mandated by the FDA for their assessment, classify all subjects who have discontinued from the trial prior to that time point (and therefore have missing data at that time point) as failures. This failure classification is regardless of the reason for discontinuation, and regardless of whether a subject's HIV virus was suppressed or not at the point of discontinuation. For any binary endpoint, one of the key drivers of sample size and statistical power is the response rate anticipated in both the test and control arms – and thus for this HIV endpoint the number of dropouts directly influences these items. A high dropout rate reduces the response rate, which in turn leads to the requirement of larger trials with more patients exposed to experimental drugs.

Further, a high discontinuation rate will affect the quality of the data from these trials as it is not known whether lost patients are "true" failures: individuals for whom the drug is ineffective or intolerable. For non-inferiority trials, as are typically required currently for HIV drug registration, a low "lost to follow-up" rate is essential to meet regulatory requirements. The EMA's Guideline on HIV drug development explicitly states that "*If a non-inferiority margin can be scientifically justified and non-inferiority is a reasonable clinical objective, such studies are acceptable.... a low 'lost to follow-up' rate is essential and sensitivity analyses are expected*" (European Medicines Agency, 2008). This also underlines the importance of maximizing retention and minimizing missing data.

Additional problems arise if different research groups have differing abilities to retain subjects in their trials. In this instance, researchers performing naïve comparisons of various drugs' efficacy across trials by comparing response rates may draw incorrect conclusions even when the drugs are equally efficacious in each study. For example, consider Sponsor A who performs a clinical trial comparing two HIV drugs, drug 1 versus drug 2, and the average lost to follow-up rate in Sponsor A's clinical trials is 5%. Now consider another trial by Sponsor B, who performs a clinical trial comparing two other HIV drugs, drug 3 versus drug 4, but the average lost to follow-up rate in Sponsor B's clinical trials is 15%. Regardless of the efficacy of any of the four drugs being examined, response rates for drug 3 and drug 4 can be no higher than 85%, given that all the lost to follow-up subjects will be classed as failures, whereas response rates for drug 1 and drug 2 could be as high as 95%. Thus, a cursory cross-trial assessment of the efficacy of drug 1 versus drug 3 may conclude that the efficacy of drug 3 is inferior to drug 1 when in fact the only difference may be the lost to follow-up rate.

2.2.2   Example from acute coronary syndrome

The above example illustrated the impact that a high lost to follow-up rate (and therefore a high level of missing data) can have on clinical trial size, clinical trial cost and the validity of cross-trial comparisons. It also illustrated the theoretical risk of trial data being deemed as uninterpretable and unacceptable to regulatory agencies. However, on occasion, this latter risk becomes a reality. In May 2012, an FDA Advisory Committee voted against supporting a new indication for Xarelto (rivaroxaban). Xarelto was proposed to reduce the risk of thrombotic cardiovascular events in patients with Acute Coronary Syndrome. The vote followed a review of a single Phase 3 trial, ATLAS, which achieved both its primary endpoint and several secondary endpoints. The key rationale for the negative vote was the extent of missing data which was considered too much to overcome (Cardiovascular & Renal Drugs Advisory Committee Bulletin, 2012). A total of 9% of ATLAS subjects had unknown vital status at the end of the study and members of the Advisory Committee told the sponsor company that the level of missing data was unacceptable. One panelist who voted against approval commented that the level of missing data was "troubling and concerning" (Medpage Today Bulletin, 2012).

2.2.3 Example from studies in pain

There have been several instances on public record over the past few years of New Drug Application reviews performed by the Division of Anesthesia, Analgesia and Addiction Products (DAAAP) at the FDA for diseases such as neuropathy and fibromyalgia in which the analysis they favored was Baseline Observation Carried Forward (BOCF). The motivation behind this approach was an attempt to avoid treatment-related dropouts being assigned what they viewed as inappropriately favorable outcomes. However, as in the HIV example above, the resultant impact is that all subjects who drop out from a clinical trial prematurely – regardless of reason – are assigned an extremely poor outcome (i.e., their baseline value). For example, the medical review and evaluation for Pfizer's diabetic peripheral neuropathy drug, Lyrica (pregabalin), in 2004 stated that *"The shortcomings of the LOCF approach in pain studies have been discussed extensively within the Division and the Agency. It is noted that patients achieving adequate symptom control but experiencing intolerable side effects often terminate the study with 'good' pain scores, which are carried forward in the LOCF analysis. However, these subjects are true treatment failures because they were unable to tolerate the dose necessary to achieve symptom control. Therefore the LOCF analysis overestimates the benefit of the drug. Consequently, the Agency prospectively expressed a primary interest in an analysis . . . using a BOCF imputation strategy for missing data . . . "* (U.S. Food and Drug Administration, 2004).

Other, more recent reviews by DAAAP have continued to take the same approach. While this continues to be the case, the conservative impact on the results in the presence of a substantial amount of non-treatment related dropout is clear.

2.3 The role of the statistician in the prevention of missing data

At first glance it may not be self-evident that statisticians have a role to play in the prevention of missing data. Clinical trial site staff are the individuals who directly interact with trial subjects, and as such their role in the retention of those subjects is immediately clear. However, all the members of the team involved in the design and execution of a clinical trial – including the statistician – have a role to play in increasing retention and reducing missing data.

Statisticians have a key role to play in four areas of missing data prevention as follows:

1. **Quantifying the amount of missing data in previous trials of a disease and its resultant impact**

   Statisticians are able to explore data from previous clinical trials in a disease area to gain an understanding of the likely extent of both treatment-related and treatment-unrelated discontinuations in future trials of that disease. Statisticians also have a clear understanding of the potential impact of missing data for the trial being designed and can communicate that to other study team members. In Chapter 4, we shall see how the statistician will need to use historic data to also plan the statistical analysis.

2. **Identifying subgroups of subjects who require an increased level of trial retention support**

   For some diseases and trial endpoints, identifying groups of subjects at higher retention risk, and prioritizing retention efforts in those specific groups will not be appropriate. For example, in clinical trials of illnesses such as depression with subjective efficacy endpoints, retention interventions such as increased patient support may in themselves impact a subject's depression rating. In situations such as this, the drive to decrease missing data should be applied to all trial subjects rather than to particular subgroups of subjects. However, in those diseases where targeted retention efforts will not influence the outcome measure of interest statisticians can explore data from previous trials in a disease area in order to identify whether there are particular subgroups of subjects who are at increased risk of missing data (e.g., of being lost to follow-up) in order to prioritize increased efforts to retain those subjects within new trials. It is important to note, however, that one unintentional consequence of this type of investigation could be that future trial recruitment of these patient subgroups would decrease (either due to planners of future studies amending entry criteria, or site staff not considering these subject groups for trial participation), which is contrary to the need for demographic diversity in order to ensure generalizability of trial results. Thus one important aspect when sharing results of this type of analysis is to reinforce the importance of recruiting a trial population which reflects the disease burden as a whole, and that analysis results should only be used in order to allow retention efforts to be prioritized to specific subject groups.

3. **Translating statistical analysis of previous trial data into information to inform future subject care**

   Traditional summary statistics and statistical analysis is the critical first step in understanding the quantity of, and nature of, missing data in previous clinical trials. However, in order to be most useful for clinical trial person-nel of new studies, this needs to be translated into information regarding what is expected to happen with a future individual subject, in order that site staff can assess how best to care for each new clinical trial subject they are presented with.

4. **Education of the clinical trial team and participation in the creation of missing data prevention plans**
    Different individuals on clinical trial teams have access to different pieces of information, knowledge and experience. No one individual has all the expertise pertaining to missing data. Statisticians understand the impact of subject discontinuation and missing data upon trial power. Investigators may be able to identify the groups at highest risk of dropout. Project managers or monitors may have insights into the support and interventions most likely to improve subject retention. As statisticians, we should not assume that our non-statistical colleagues understand the statistical niceties of how missing data and trial discontinuations affect power, sample size and trial quality. Increasing training of trial personnel at all levels (scientific and operational staff; monitors; investigators and other site staff) and participation in the development of missing data prevention plans is a worthwhile investment for trial statisticians. It is critical, however, to ensure that training provided is simple to understand, appealing and impactful.

2.3.1   Illustrative example from HIV

The author, with colleagues, published a case study on missing data prevention (Hughes *et al.*, 2012) which outlined work done in the four areas described above. It is summarized here to illustrate the influential role which statisticians can have in the field of missing data prevention. As mentioned in Section 2.2.1, all discontinuations in HIV clinical trials are treated as failures in the primary efficacy endpoint analysis (proportion of subjects with suppressed viral load) of registrational trials, regardless of reason, using the FDA-mandated algorithm. The case study's intent was to assess the overall discontinuation rate in previous HIV clinical trials performed within the company, and to investigate the proportion of those discontinuations that were related versus unrelated to treatment. The hypothesis was that, a substantial proportion of discontinuations were for reasons unrelated to treatment and thus could potentially be avoided.

2.3.1.1   Step 1: Quantifying the amount of missing data in previous trials, and its resultant impact

In order to assess the extent of missing data created as a result of study discontin-uation due to non-treatment related reasons, data were pooled from four previous GlaxoSmithKline-sponsored HIV trials in adult subjects naïve to antiretroviral treat-ment (studies: ARIES, HEAT, KLEAN and APV109141 [Eron *et al.*, 2006; Pulido

Table 2.1   Discontinuations in ARIES, HEAT, KLEAN and APV109141.

Study:	ARIES (36 weeks)	HEAT (96 weeks)	KLEAN (96 weeks)	APV109141 (48 weeks)	Total
$N =$	515	688	875	212	2290
Completed	86%	66%	76%	85%	1738 (76%)
Adverse event[a]	3%	6%	6%	6%	125 (6%)
Protocol defined virological failure[a]	<1%	2%	2%	<1%	36 (2%)
Insufficient viral load response[a]	2%	0	<1%	0	17 (<1%)
Disease progression[a]	0	<1%	0	0	1 (<1%)
Lost to follow-up[b]	3%	14%	6%	4%	178 (8%)
Subject decision[b]	1%	5%	3%	2%	74 (3%)
Non-compliance[b]	2%	3%	3%	0	53 (2%)
Protocol violation[b]	0	<1%	<1%	<1%	9 (<1%)
Other[b]	2%	3%	3%	2%	59 (3%)

[a]Treatment-related/unavoidable discontinuation.
[b]Potentially avoidable discontinuation.

et al., 2007; Carosi et al., 2009; Smith et al., 2009; Squires et al., 2010]). Discontinuations were categorized as:

- treatment-related/"unavoidable": defined as discontinuation due to adverse event, protocol-defined virological failure, insufficient viral load response, disease progression or

- "potentially avoidable": defined as lost to follow-up, subject decision, non-compliance, protocol violation, other.

Of the 2290 HIV-positive adult subjects naïve to antiretroviral treatment, who were included in the pooled analysis, a total of 24% discontinued their clinical trial. Potentially avoidable discontinuations were observed in a total of 16% of subjects, with only 8% of subjects discontinuing for reasons more clearly related to their antiretroviral treatment (Table 2.1). Stated another way, of the trial subjects who discontinued, approximately two-thirds were potentially avoidable.

In terms of quantifying the impact of discontinuations, simple tables can often be the most effective in conveying the importance of, and value in, increasing retention efforts. Table 2.2 is one such example.

This illustrates the potential impact that reducing the number of discontinuations by small amounts can have on power and sample size. In summary, for a typical HIV Phase III non-inferiority trial, 5% fewer discontinuations could increase the trial's power from 90% to almost 95%, thus halving the risk of a type II error. Alternatively, once discontinuation rates have been consistently reduced over time, subsequent

Table 2.2   Illustrating the potential impact of increased retention in HIV non-inferiority clinical trials.

Increased retention levels	Control arm response rate[a]	Power (for fixed $N = 395$ per group)[b]	N per group (for 90% power)[b]
0%[c]	75%	90%	395
5%	80%	94%	337 (15% reduction)
10%	85%	98%	268 (32% reduction)

[a]Assuming all dropouts avoided are treatment successes.
[b]Power and sample size calculations assume a 10% non-inferiority margin and one-sided type I error of 0.025.
[c]That is, assuming historical dropout rate will not be improved upon.

sample sizes could be reduced by up to 15% while maintaining study power at 90%. It can be tempting to show power curves, which are visually appealing and show the full range of possible response rates and opportunities. However, the authors observed that not all audiences extract key information from power curves with ease and concentrating on one or two simple examples, as shown in Table 2.2, was found to be more effective.

2.3.1.2   Step 2: Identifying subgroups of subjects who require an increased level of trial retention support

Having established that the overall number, and the proportion of potentially avoidable discontinuations in HIV clinical trials was not trivial, and that the impact of reducing those discontinuations could be substantial, the question that followed was whether it was possible to identify particular subject types who were more likely to withdraw unnecessarily (i.e., potentially avoidable dropouts). Cox proportional hazards modeling was used to investigate the relationship between potentially avoidable discontinuations and demographic characteristics recorded in the database, and also trial operating characteristics. Subjects who did not discontinue for potentially avoidable reasons were censored at their last study contact date. Factors explored were those available in the clinical trial databases and were as follows: ethnicity (white/other); age (<median/≥median); gender (female/male); mode of HIV transmission (intravenous drug user vs. other/heterosexual contact vs. other/homosexual contact vs. other); country of recruitment (North America/Rest of World); trial (ARIES, HEAT, KLEAN, APV109141); and early versus late entry into a trial during recruitment period (quarters).

Cox proportional hazards modeling of these potentially avoidable discontinuations (subsequently referred to as non-treatment related discontinuations) indicated statistically significant higher rates of discontinuation in particular HIV-positive patient subgroups. Table 2.3 presents results from the multi-variable Cox proportional hazards modeling of non-treatment related discontinuation rates, for factors which were observed to be significant predictors of discontinuation. Figure 2.1 shows the Kaplan-Meier curves of time to non-treatment related discontinuation for each of those factors. Clinical trial subjects, whose mode of HIV transmission was through

Table 2.3   Cox proportional hazards modeling of non-treatment related discontinuations.[a]

Patient characteristic	Discontinuation[d] by 96 weeks	Hazard ratio (95% CI)	p-value
Ethnicity:			
White ($n = 1335$)	16%	0.61	<0.0001
vs. Other ($n = 955$)	30%	(0.49, 0.77)	
HIV transmission[b]:			
Intravenous drug use ($n = 138$)	35%	1.92	0.0004
vs. Other ($n = 2083$)	21%	(1.34, 2.74)	
HIV transmission[b]:			
Heterosexual ($n = 850$)	29%	1.43	0.0021
vs. Other ($n = 1371$)	18%	(1.14, 1.79)	
Age (years)[c]:			
<38 ($n = 1139$)	24%	1.40	0.0016
vs. ≥38 ($n = 1151$)	20%	(1.14, 1.73)	
Country:			
North America ($n = 1735$)	24%	1.31	0.048
vs. Rest of World ($n = 555$)	16%	(1.00, 1.72)	

[a]Discontinuation for reasons other than virological failure, lack of virological response, disease progression, adverse event.
[b]2221 subjects with transmission mode recorded.
[c]raw withdrawal rates by age in quartiles were <31 yr 21%; ≥31–<38 yr 17%; ≥38–<44 yr 16%; ≥44 yr 13%.
[d]Kaplan-Meier estimate.

either intravenous drug use or heterosexual contact, were at higher risk of non-treatment related discontinuation when compared to subjects whose mode of HIV transmission was through homosexual contact/other route. Likewise, non-white subjects and younger subjects were at higher risk of non-treatment related discontinuation compared to white subjects and older subjects, respectively.

Figure 2.2 presents Kaplan-Meier curves of non-treatment related discontinuation rates, for factors that were not observed to be significant predictors of discontinuation in multi-variable Cox proportional hazards modeling. While gender was an important factor in single-variable statistical analysis ($p = 0.0004$), with female trial subjects having a higher rate of non-treatment related discontinuation compared to males (21% vs. 15%, respectively), this factor was non-significant in the multi-variable survival analysis. This was due to substantial correlation in this dataset between gender and ethnicity. Few white subjects were female (151/1335, 11%) and many non-white subjects were female (307/955, 32%, OR = 3.7, $p < 0.001$). The point at which a trial subject was recruited during the trial's enrollment period had little effect on the likelihood of non-treatment related discontinuation; nor did the trial they were

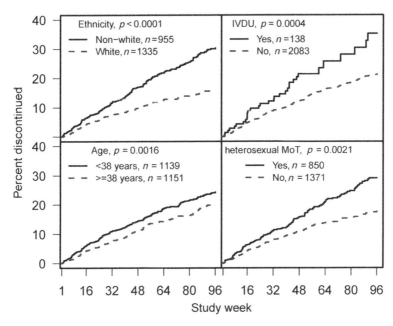

Figure 2.1   Kaplan–Meier plot of non-treatment related discontinuations: significant predictors.

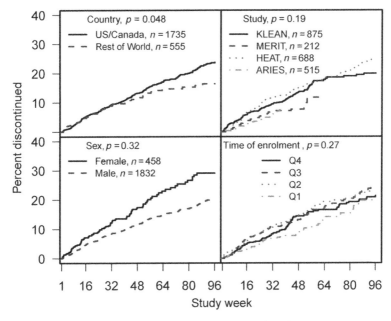

Figure 2.2   Kaplan–Meier plot of non-treatment related discontinuations: non-significant predictors.

recruited into. Country of recruitment was marginally significant ($p = 0.048$), but this was not pursued further given the inability to use this factor to identify subjects at a single site at increased risk of non-treatment related discontinuation. However, in some situations, country-based campaigns may be appropriate.

While some of the factors identified as significant may in fact have been surrogates for other factors not collected (e.g., socio-economic status), this is not expected to have impacted the utility of the analysis for informing future missing data prevention initiatives, as the analysis provided easily identifiable subject groups for increased retention focus.

2.3.1.3   Step 3: Translating statistical analysis of previous trial data into information to inform future subject care

In order to help clinical trial site staff assess the appropriate level of retention support for any given future individual trial subject, results from the multi-variable Cox proportional hazards model were translated into individual risk of a "typical" future trial subject being lost to follow-up after 1 year in a clinical trial (Table 2.4). For example, a white 35-year-old whose recorded mode of HIV transmission is heterosexual contact and intravenous drug use has an estimated 25% probability of dropping out of a trial by 1 year for reasons unrelated to treatment.

In addition, it was also observed when looking at the pattern of missed visits in another, later trial – the ASSERT study (Post *et al.*, 2010) – that only 10 out of a total of 385 subjects had any missed visits prior to either study completion or withdrawal. Of those 10 subjects with missed visits, only one subject's was an intermittent missed visit; the other nine subjects were subsequently lost to follow-up. This data indicated that in this trial at least, a single missed visit was also a strong risk factor for subsequent discontinuation and provided site staff in subsequent trials with an early warning sign to act upon. Anecdotal evidence from later trials indicates that this early warning sign has been effective in preventing subsequent withdrawal.

Table 2.4   Translating population results into individual risk.

		One-year risk of non-treatment related discontinuation			
		Not intravenous drug use		Intravenous drug use	
	Age (yrs)	Homosexual	Heterosexual	Homosexual	Heterosexual
Non-white	≤38	18%	24%	21%	28%
	39–44	12%	16%	15%	20%
	44	9%	12%	11%	14%
White	≤31	10%	13%	24%	31%
	32–44	8%	10%	19%	25%
	>44	7%	10%	18%	24%

2.3.1.4   Step 4: Education of the clinical trial team and participation in the creation of missing data prevention plans

The next step in this case study was a substantial educational effort by the statisticians to work with internal clinical, operational and monitoring staff plus external investigators and other site staff to increase their level of understanding regarding (i) the concept of statistical noise in an HIV setting and the number and nature of discontinuations typically observed; (ii) the type of clinical trial subjects more likely to discontinue; and (iii) the effect the discontinuations have on data quality, power and sample sizes required.

As mentioned above, in terms of conveying the impact of discontinuations, very simple tables such as Table 2.2 were observed to be most effective in conveying the importance and value of increasing retention efforts. Figures 2.1 and 2.2 were very effective visual aids during discussions of factors associated with a higher risk of discontinuation, but were less useful for communicating the size of the risk increases, and took no account of correlation between risk factors. Multi-variable analyses showing adjusted hazard ratios, confidence intervals and p-values were included in early versions of educational presentations but were replaced by Table 2.4. This table presented information in a way suited to clinicians or site staff, who are most interested in the absolute risk for an individual subject with a complete set of risk factors. In fact, this presentation breaks a basic rule of statistics by making no allowance for the uncertainty associated with the estimates shown: there are no confidence intervals. Technical correctness was sacrificed in order to make the key information easier to absorb by non-statistical site staff, who were seeing this slide as one of over 400 during a 2-day investigator meeting, or downloading the training materials from the study website to review on their own. In particular, a color version (using red, orange and green to denote high to medium to low risk of dropout) of Table 2.4 was found to be most helpful in understanding future risk of discontinuation – and this table was a key slide subsequently used by monitors to give their own retention presentations to the site staff at site initiation visits, once having been trained themselves by the statistics group.

These educational efforts were followed by workshops at investigator and monitor meetings to brainstorm global and country-specific proactive retention plans, targeted at subjects most at risk of dropping out of trials for avoidable reasons, and ultimately led to the creation of a variety of activities within subsequent HIV clinical trials aimed at increasing subject retention.

Within this case study, the willingness by trial personnel to work towards improved retention as a result of the educational work described – as evidenced by new initiatives and increased retention efforts within trial teams – indicated that it should not be assumed historic levels of missing data cannot be improved upon, and that perhaps we, as statisticians, are too quick to rely on using a variety of statistical methods to address missing data during analysis rather than attempting to reduce the level of missing data at source. This message is reinforced in the report on missing data from the NRC, where – as mentioned above – considerable emphasis is given to prevention as well as handling of missing data (National Research Council, 2010).

2.4   Methods for increasing subject retention

The illustrative example described above demonstrates the need to initiate missing data prevention planning as soon as the general planning for a clinical trial commences. In order to declare the intent to implement methods to maximize subject retention, and to secure the focus of all clinical trial staff on this planning, it is appropriate to highlight this in the clinical trial protocol. Some example text for the protocol is provided in Appendix 2.A.

The choice of which methods to use for increasing subject retention in clinical trials (and therefore reducing missing data) will be specific to the disease being studied, and should be made (i) using the insights of trial staff who interact with likely trial participants; and (ii) where possible by using previous trial data to select the most effective retention mechanisms. Below is a list of some suggested methods.

- Selection of trial sites with an excellent retention track record

- Pre-trial retention training and workshops

- Creation of country- and site-specific retention plans – and when appropriate, targeting these to subjects at highest risk of being lost to follow-up

- Education of study subjects regarding trial requirements and the importance of full participation (to occur during the consent process)

- Minimization of trial burden for individual subjects (e.g., number of visits and assessments, widest acceptable size of visit windows)

- Provision of financial support (travel/meal reimbursements) to participants, in countries where this is possible

- Collection of contact information at entry which is regularly reviewed and updated

- Subject reminders for appointments, with immediate follow-up after missed appointments

- Opt-in text-messaging for clinic visit reminders

- Telephone contacts and home visits in case of missed clinic visits

- Study-branded gifts

- Payment schedules to investigators that emphasize excellent follow-up (e.g., payments on a per-visit basis)

- Target setting for "acceptable" rates of missing data and (when the size and duration of trial, and speed of recruitment allows) provision of performance feedback during trial conduct, with prompt escalation if significant numbers of preventable discontinuations are observed, in order to investigate and address root causes

- Use of a specialist retention company

- Incorporation of trial retention rates into the measures used to identify the sites that make the most significant contribution to data generation and therefore meet one of the International Committee of Medical Journal Editors (ICMJE) criteria for authorship (ICMJE, 2010).

Statisticians have a role to play in several of these areas. For example, pre-trial retention training is part of the required education of the study team as described above, and statisticians are best placed to provide this training. Likewise statisticians should be heavily involved in the setting of targets for missing data levels, which can then be tracked during the course of the trial, with regular summary data on performance provided to the study team.

2.5   Improving understanding of reasons for subject withdrawal

Having a clear understanding of whether a subject's withdrawal from a clinical trial was treatment-related or not is critical for two reasons. First, it provides information on the extent of potentially avoidable dropouts in a disease area, which in turn aids understanding of whether increased efforts around subject retention are needed. Secondly, this information can then be used to derive more appropriate imputation methods for missing data. However, clinical trial Case Record Forms (CRFs) do not always capture this differentiation clearly enough, and in the case of multiple reasons for withdrawal, investigators may not always prioritize selection of a treatment-related reason above a treatment-unrelated reason. Therefore, CRF pages collecting data on reason for withdrawal should be redesigned in order to allow a clearer identification of treatment-related versus treatment-unrelated discontinuation. This topic is picked up again in Chapter 4 where it is discussed in more detail (Section 4.2.1).

Acknowledgments

The author would like to acknowledge her co-authors on the paper which was summarized here to provide the illustrative example from HIV: Julia Harris, Nancy Flack and Robert Cuffe.

Appendix 2.A: Example protocol text for missing data prevention

Section X Subject retention

Once a subject enrolls in this trial, the site will make every effort to retain the subject for the planned duration of the trial. Clinical trial site staff are responsible for developing and implementing appropriate support and retention plans. Elements of this plan may include the following.

- Thorough explanation of the complete clinical trial visit schedule and procedural requirements during the informed consent process and re-emphasis at each clinic visit.

- A simple explanation of the key data and key time points that are critical for the trial's successful analysis, and the importance of all the treatment groups to the overall success of the trial.

- Discussion at screening, and subsequent regular review of possible barriers to clinic visit attendance and full study participation and compliance.

- Collection of contact information at screening (address, phone numbers, e-mail), which is regularly reviewed at subsequent clinic visits.

- Use of appropriate and timely study visit reminders.

- Immediate and multifaceted follow-up on missed clinic visits, including the possible use of trained staff to complete in-person contact with subjects at their homes.

In cases where the subject does not return for the rescheduled visit or cannot be reached to reschedule the missed visit, the site should make every effort to regain contact with the subject so that they can appropriately be withdrawn from the study. All contact attempts should be documented in the subject's medical record. Should the subject continue to be unreachable, then and only then will he/she be considered to have withdrawn from the study with a primary reason of "Lost to Follow-up." For all other subjects withdrawing from the study, an alternative reason for discontinuation should be recorded in the CRF. Regardless of site plans to support and retain subjects within the trial, subjects may voluntarily withdraw from the trial for any reason and at any time.

References

Cardiovascular and Renal Drugs Advisory Committee AdComm Bulletin (2012) *Supplemental New Drug Application (sNDA) 202439/S–002, XARELTO (rivaroxaban), by Janssen Pharmaceuticals, Inc, for use in combination with aspirin or with aspirin + clopidogrel or ticlopidine, to reduce risk of thrombotic cardiovascular events in patients with acute coronary syndrome (ST Elevation Myocardial Infarction [STEMI], Non-ST Elevation Myocardial Infarction [NSTEMI], or Unstable Angina [UA])*, IDRAC Thomson Reuters No. 143271. http://www.idrac.com/viewing.asp?ref=US00143271, accessed 22 March 2013.

Carosi G, Lazzarin A, Stellbrink H, Moyle G, Rugina S, Staszewski S, Givens N, Ross L, Granier C, Ait-Khaled M, Leather D, Nichols WG (2009) Study of once-daily versus twice-daily fosamprenavir plus ritonavir administered with abacavir/lamivudine one daily in antiretroviral-naïve HIV-1-infected adult subjects. *HIV Clinical Trials* **10**(6): 356–367.

Cassidy EL, Baird E, Sheikh JI (2001) Recruitment and retention of elderly patients in clinical trials. *American Journal of Geriatric Psychiatry* **9**: 136–140.

Eron J, Yeni P, Gathe Jr J, Estrada V, DeJesus E, Staszewski S, Khuong-Josses MA, Yau L, Vavro C, Lim ML (2006) The KLEAN study of fosamprenavir-ritonavir versus lopinavir-ritonavir, each in combination with abacavir-lamivudine, for initial treatment of HIV infection over 48 weeks: a randomised non-inferiority trial. *Lancet* **368**: 476–82.

European Medicines Agency (2008) *Guideline on the clinical development of medicinal products for the treatment of HIV infection. EMEA/CPMP/EWP/633/02 Rev.2.* http://www.ema europa.eu/docs/en_GB/document_library/Scientific_guideline/2009/09/WC500003460.pdf, accessed 22nd March 2013.

European Medicines Agency (2010) *Guideline on missing data in confirmatory clinical trials. EMA/CPMP/EWP/1776/99 Rev.1.* http://www.ema.europa.eu/docs/en_GB/document _library/Scientific_guideline/2010/09/WC500096793.pdf, accessed 23 June 2013.

Hughes S, Harris J, Flack N, Cuffe RL (2012) The statistician's role in the prevention of missing data. *Pharmaceutical Statistics* **11**: 410–416.

International Committee of Medical Journal Editors (2010) *Uniform requirements for manuscripts submitted to biomedical journals.* http://www.icmje.org/urm_full.pdf, accessed 22 March 2013.

Magruder KM, Ouyang B, Miller S, Tilley BC (2009) Retention of under-represented minorities in drug abuse treatment studies. *Clinical Trials* **6**: 252–260.

Medpage Today Bulletin (2012) *Acute Coronary Syndrome: FDA panel narrowly rejects Xarelto for ACS.* http://www.medpagetoday.com/Cardiology/AcuteCoronarySyndrome/ 32888, accessed 16 July 2013.

Moreno-Black G, Shor-Posner G, Miguez MJ, Burbano X, O'Mellan S, Yovanoff P (2004) "I will miss the study, God bless you all": participation in a nutritional chemoprevention trial. *Ethnicity and Disease* **14**: 469–475.

National Research Council. Panel on Handling Missing Data in Clinical Trials. Committee on National Statistics, Division of Behavioral and Social Sciences and Education (2010) *The Prevention and Treatment of Missing Data in Clinical Trials.* The National Academies Press, Washington, DC, available at http://www.nap.edu/catalog.php?record_id=12955, accessed 16 July 2013.

Post FA, Moyle G, Stellbrink H, Domingo P, Podzamczer D, Fisher M, Norden AG, Cavassini M, Rieger A, Khuong-Josses MA, Branco T, Pearce HC, Givens N, Vavro C, Lim ML (2010) Randomized comparison of renal effects, efficacy, and safety with once-daily abacavir/lamivudine versus tenofovir/emtricitabine, administered with efavirenz, in antiretroviral-naïve, HIV-1-infected adults: 48-week results from the ASSERT study. *Journal of Acquired Immune Deficiency Syndromes* **55**(1): 49–57.

Pulido F, Baril JG, Staszewski S, Khuong-Josses MA, Yau L, Vavro C, Lim ML (2007) Long-term efficacy and safety of fosamprenavir + ritonavir (FPV/r) versus lopinavir/ritonavir (LPV/r) over 96 weeks. *47th Annual Interscience Conference on Antimicrobial Agents and Chemotherapy,* Chicago, IL. Abstract H-361.

Robinson KA, Dennison CR, Wayman DM, Pronovost PJ, Needham DM (2007) Systematic review identifies number of strategies important for retaining study participants. *Journal of Clinical Epidemiology* **60**: 757–765.

Seed M, Juarez M, Alnatour R (2009) Improving recruitment and retention rates in preventive longitudinal research with adolescent mothers. *Journal of Child and Adolescent Psychiatric Nursing* **22**: 150–153.

Senturia YD, McNiff MK, Baker D, Gergen P, Mitchell H, Joseph C, Wedner HJ (1998) Successful techniques for retention of study participants in an inner-city population. *Controlled Clinical Trials* **19**: 544–554.

Smith K, Patel P, Fine D, Bellos N, Sloan L, Lackey P, Kumar PN, Sutherland-Phillips DH, Vavro C, Yau L, Wannamaker P, Shaefer MS, for the HEAT Study Team (2009) Randomized, double-blind, placebo-matched, multicentre trial of abacavir/lamivudine or tenofovir/emtricitabine with lopinavir/ritonavir for initial HIV treatment. *AIDS* **23**(12): 1547–1556.

Squires K, Young B, DeJesus E, Bellos N, Murphy D, Sutherland-Phillips DH, Zhao HH, Patel LG, Ross LL, Wannamaker PG, Shaefer MS, ARIES Study Team (2010) Safety and efficacy of a 36-week induction regimen of abacavir/lamivudine and ritonavir-boosted atazanavir in HIV-infected patients. *HIV Clinical Trials* **11**(2): 69–79.

U.S. Food and Drug Administration, Center for Drug Evaluation and Research (2004) *Approval package for application number 21-446.* http://www.accessdata.fda.gov/drugsatfda_docs/nda/2004/021446_Lyrica%20Capsules_medr.PDF, accessed 16 July 2013.

Villacorta V, Kegeles S, Galea J, Konda KA, Cuba JP, Palacios CF, Coates TJ, for the NIMH Collaborative HIV/STD Prevention Trial Group (2007) Innovative approaches to cohort retention in a community-based HIV/STI prevention trial for socially marginalized Peruvian young adults. *Clinical Trials* **4**: 32–41.

Walter M, Hart S (2001) Methods employed to retain an urban population: experience of the Inner-City Asthma Study (ICAS). *Controlled Clinical Trials* **22**: 35S.

Zook PM, Jordan C, Adams B, Visness CM, Walter M, Pollenz K, Logan J, Tesson E, Smartt E, Chen A, D'Agostino J, Gern JE (2010) Retention strategies and predictors of attrition in an urban pediatric asthma study. *Clinical Trials* **7**: 400–410.

3

Regulatory guidance – a quick tour

Michael O'Kelly

Key points

- The ICH E9 guideline issued in 1998 covers many of the important points to be considered with regard to missing data. The ICH guideline has the advantage that it is widely accepted by Japan and other countries outside the United States and Europe that use the results of clinical trials.

- Current positions of the European Union (EU) and US regulatory agencies regarding handling of missing data can be found in an official European Medicines Agency (EMA) Guideline and in a U.S. Food and Drug Administration (FDA) sponsored report by a U.S. National Research Council (NRC) panel.

- The EU guideline and the US NRC report (which hereafter may be referred to in this chapter as "the regulatory documents") agree in most important areas.

- Regulators agree that methods of handling missing data are important in interpreting study results; that missing data should be prevented; that no single method will "cure" the missing data problem; that a primary analysis will need sensitivity analyses to assess its robustness to assumptions about missing data; that methods for handling missing data should be described and justified in the protocol; and that better use should be made of post-withdrawal data.

Clinical Trials with Missing Data: A Guide for Practitioners, First Edition. Michael O'Kelly and Bohdana Ratitch.
© 2014 John Wiley & Sons, Ltd. Published 2014 by John Wiley & Sons, Ltd.

- There are differences in emphasis between the NRC report and the EU guidance document regarding last observation carried forward (LOCF); regarding the importance of a "conservative" approach; regarding post hoc analyses; and regarding intermediate or non-monotone missing data.

- The NRC report emphasizes that it is important that the assumptions made about missing data be described in terms that can be understood by clinicians.

- The regulatory documents have some useful comments on classes of methods for handling missing data, including the use of available cases; the assumption of missing at random (MAR); and methods where it is assumed that data are missing not at random (MNAR).

- In practice, the latest regulatory documents are not always adhered to by the regulator, but there is a growing tendency for regulators to treat the handling of missing data as important, and to apply the principles used in the regulatory documents.

3.1   International conference on harmonization guideline: Statistical principles for clinical trials: E9

Interestingly, the International Conference on Harmonization (ICH) guideline *Statistical principles for clinical trials* (1998) covers many of the important points that form the core of the two more recent NRC and EU regulatory documents on missing data (European Medicines Agency, 2010; National Research Council, 2010), 12 years before those documents were issued. The ICH guideline has the advantage that it is widely accepted by Japan and other countries outside the United States and Europe that use the results of clinical trials. Here are the points of overlap (page references are to the ICH guideline; overlaps with the NRC report and EU guidance):

- Missing data should be **prevented** where possible (pp. 8, 22, 24)

- "**No universally applicable methods** of handling missing data" (p. 22)

- Investigate "**sensitivity** of the results ... to the method of handling missing data" (p. 24)

- "Methods of dealing with missing data ... **pre-defined in the protocol**" (p. 24)

- **Make a record of reasons for withdrawal**: "frequency and type of ... missing values should be documented" (p. 22)

Like the recent EU guidance, ICH E9 specifically recommends that the study report describe the extent of missing data and reasons for discontinuation (ICH E9, p. 30).

The ICH E9 guideline differs from the two more recent regulatory documents with regard to single imputation. In contrast to the more recent documents, it mentions the use of last observation carried forward (LOCF) without disapproval: "Imputation techniques, ranging from the carrying forward of the last observation to the use of complex mathematical models, may also be used in an attempt to compensate for missing data" (ICH E9, p. 23). Apart from this sentence, the E9 guideline does not comment on the acceptability of any particular assumptions about missing data. This contrasts with the more recent guidelines where, we will see, the strengths and weaknesses of common assumptions about missing data discussed in detail.

3.2   The US and EU regulatory documents

The two most recent regulatory documents on missing data for the United States and EU regions were issued almost simultaneously in July 2010. They agree on most important issues, but differ in character. The US document is a report commissioned by the FDA, while the EU document is an official regulatory guideline.

The FDA-commissioned report, "The Prevention and Treatment of Missing Data in Clinical Trials," (National Research Council, 2010), as expected contains recommendations on the missing data problem, but also includes fairly detailed descriptions of the statistical basis of many approaches to the analysis of missing data. It thus acts partly as a tutorial in methods for missing data. This report was written by a panel of the NRC, and sometimes reads like an academic paper – it includes more than seven pages of references to the literature on missing data. The European Medicines Agency "Guideline on Missing Data in Confirmatory Clinical Trials" (2010) is compact (12 pages vs. the NRC report's 145 pages). In contrast to the NRC report, the EMA guideline tends to comment on the statistical basis of an approach to missing data only insofar as this might be needed to discuss regulatory acceptability of the approach; and the EMA guideline has just two references to other documents, both also guidance documents.

At present, there is no official general FDA guideline on missing data. Although the NRC report is not an official regulatory guidance, we have found that US regulators sometimes quote the report in their reviews and encourage industry practitioners to follow its recommendations during their presentations at public forums. The NRC report notes that some guidelines are available and we will describe these briefly later.

3.3   Key points in the regulatory documents on missing data

Both the NRC report and EU guideline have a straightforward logical line of reasoning about missing data. Its key points are as follows:

- **Missing data are important and affect the validity, bias and interpretation of clinical trial results.** Implied is that missing data have not in the past always been handled adequately. The EU document uses its status as an official guidance to indicate that regulatory review of missing data will in the future be more rigorous. It notes that "just ignoring missing data is not an acceptable option" and notifies the reader that "This guideline … provides an insight into regulatory standards that will be used to assess confirmatory clinical trials."

- **Missing data should be prevented as far as possible.** The NRC report particularly emphasizes this, devoting 26 pages to it. Both documents cover how the study design and execution can help to reduce missing data. Chapter 2 of this book discusses this aspect of the guidance.

- **Because missing data are missing, we cannot verify our assumptions about them. Therefore, no single method can be counted on to give a comprehensive treatment of missing data.** A single primary analysis alone is not adequate when a study has missing data.

- **Sensitivity analyses are needed** to test the robustness of study results to the assumptions of the primary analysis.

- **A study's approach to missing data should be pre-specified in the protocol and justified scientifically.** The EU document is notable for recognizing that, since we cannot be sure about missing data, no planned approach to missing data will be perfect. The EMA criterion for the adequacy of an approach takes account of this: the handling of missing data should be "unlikely to be biased in favor of the experimental treatment to an important degree (under reasonable assumptions)" with "a confidence interval that does not underestimate … variability" (p. 3). This criterion may be regarded as achievable, even given a team's uncertainties about likely patterns of missing data in a planned study. The EMA guideline again recognizes the difficulty in specifying missing data analyses in advance by allowing for the possibility of post hoc analyses: "If unexpected missing data patterns are found in the data, it will be necessary to conduct some post hoc sensitivity analyses in addition to those pre-defined in the statistical analysis plan" (p. 7). The important proviso is that "It is not envisaged that these post hoc analyses can be used to rescue a trial which otherwise fails."

- **Most approaches to missing data have limitations and weaknesses** which the guidance documents describe. As noted, the NRC report has more detail on the statistical basis of approaches, and covers a wider variety of statistical methods. We will summarize these regulatory comments on methods in the next section.

- **Post-withdrawal data may be helpful in estimating treatment effect or in sensitivity analyses, but will need to be put in context.** Sponsors are "strongly encouraged" to collect post-withdrawal data (EU guideline, p. 6, and see NRC Recommendation 3, p. 3). Such data could be used to provide a true intent-to-treat (ITT) analysis. However, both documents note that if "participants are offered an alternative treatment that is not part of the study following discontinuation … subsequent data collection may be considered to uninformative" (NRC report, p. 9). Therefore, such "retrieved dropout" information will need "to be put in context" (EU guideline, p. 6).

- **Reasons for withdrawal are important** in handling missing data and should be recorded carefully.

In discussions with planners, or when writing a protocol or statistical analysis plan (SAP), it may be useful to quote the guidance documents on particular aspects the study's approach to missing data. Table 3.1 can be used to find references to key points on which the NRC and EU documents agree. Despite the difference in character of the two documents, they have remarkably similar wording in their treatment of many key issues to do with missing data.

3.4 Regulatory guidance on particular statistical approaches

3.4.1 Available cases

Both the EU guidance and NRC report discourage the use of available cases for a primary analysis. The NRC report notes (p. 55) that deleting incomplete cases provides valid inference only under the assumption that data are missing completely at random (MCAR) and adds that "this method is generally inappropriate for a regulatory setting." The EMA guidance notes that "(if) patients are excluded from the analysis this may affect the comparability of the treatment groups … (and) the representativeness of the study sample in relation to the target population (external validity)" – in other words, the findings of the study may only apply to the type of subject who is likely to complete the study – a perhaps elite subset of the population.

3.4.2 Single imputation methods

Methods such as LOCF and baseline observation carried forward (BOCF) replace a missing data point by a single value. Analyses are then carried out as if all the data were observed. The EU document points out that single imputation "risks biasing the standard error (of the estimate of treatment effect) downwards by ignoring the uncertainty of imputed values" (p. 9). The NRC report agrees: "statistical precision is overstated because the imputed values are assumed to be true" (p. 65). The EU document points out that, for conditions that are expected to deteriorate over time, LOCF can favor the treatment group with earlier withdrawals. We have seen a mild example of this in Chapter 1. However, the EMA guideline concedes that "where the condition is expected to improve … LOCF … might be conservative … where patients in the experimental group tend to withdraw earlier." If LOCF can be shown to be conservative, then an LOCF approach, despite its "suboptimal statistical properties," would provide "compelling evidence of efficacy from a regulatory perspective." Similarly, BOCF "may be appropriate in, for example, a chronic pain trial" as a

Table 3.1   Key points of agreement in the NRC and EU regulatory documents on missing data.

Key point in document	
FDA commissioned NRC report	EMA guideline
Importance of missing data	
"crucial ... should have higher priority" (p. 114)	"critical" (p. 3)
Prevent missing data	
"minimizing dropouts" (pp. 21–46)	"avoid ... unobserved measurements" (p. 6)
Cannot verify assumptions about missing data	
"assumptions unverifiable" (p. 52)	"assumptions ... cannot be verified" (p. 3)
There is no universal method for missing data	
"no universal method" (p. 48)	"no single method will provide a ... solution" (p. 8)
Sensitivity analyses are needed	
"should (conduct) sensitivity analysis" (p. 49)	"sensitivity analyses should be presented" (p. 11)
Pre-specify the approach to missing data	
"should be specified ... in study protocols" (p. 110)	"essential to pre-specify methods" (p. 6)
Pre-specify sensitivity analyses	
"prospective definition of sensitivity analyses" (p. 17)	"sensitivity analysis should be ... in the protocol" (p. 12)
Not acceptable to use only observed data	
"generally inappropriate" (p. 55)	"a consequence ... may be a bias" (p. 5)
Treat the MAR assumption with caution	
"not ... valid estimator of intention-to-treat effect" (p. 55)	"(provides) estimate (had) patients continued on treatment" (p. 10)
Post-withdrawal data may give limited help	
"may be ... uninformative" (p. 9)	"'retrieved dropout' information ... put in context" (p. 6)
Important to record reasons for withdrawal	
"reasons for missing data must be documented" (p. 49)	"reasons for discontinuation should be given" (p. 7)

quantitative representation of the fact that "the patient does not … derive benefit from treatment." In the final analysis, the EU guidance does not rule out the use of LOCF and BOCF. The NRC report simply provides the arguments against LOCF: LOCF "is not necessarily (conservative), since, for example, LOCF is anti-conservative in situations where participants off study treatment generally do worse over time" (p. 66).

3.4.3   Methods that generally assume MAR

Both the NRC and EU documents are blunt about a weakness of methods that assume MAR, that is, assume that missing values can be adequately predicted on the basis of observed values of patients with similar previous outcomes. The EMA declares that "the MAR assumption (provides) an unbiased estimate of the treatment effect that would have been observed if all patients had continued on treatment for the full study duration" and is thus "likely to overestimate the size of the treatment effect likely to be seen in practice" (EMA guidance, p. 10). The FDA-commissioned report agrees: "any method that relies on MAR is estimating the mean on the condition that everyone had remained on treatment. This generally will not provide a valid estimator of the intention-to-treat effect" (NRC report, p. 55). The NRC report also reminds us that where the mean of the response is non-linear in the explanatory variables (e.g., where the response is binary and logistic regression is used) the protocol or SAP must be clear as to whether the between-subject (population-averaged) or within-subject (subject-specific) treatment effect is being estimated. These are identical for some variables, for example, normally distributed, but may be different for others, for example, binary variables.

The EMA guideline is also cautious about the danger of data dredging when arriving at a model for the most frequent implementations of MAR – mixed models with repeated measures (MMRM), multiple imputation (MI) and weighted generalized estimating equations (GEE). The guideline emphasizes the need to pre-specify the model used and, in the case of MI, the random seed used. The NRC report (p. 64) notes the need to be cautious about MMRM because of its dependence on the correctness of its parametric model. This also applies to MI (NRC report, p. 69). The estimation of the variance–covariance matrix in MMRM may involve assumptions that are difficult to verify, such as the assumption of normality (NRC report, p. 64 again).

As noted in Chapter 1, an improved version of weighted GEE has been proposed recently, which has the attribute of being doubly robust. That is, its estimates will be valid if either the model for missingness or the model for the responses is correct. The NRC report opines that "With more published applications to real data and carefully designed simulation studies, the use of doubly robust estimators could become more (common) in the near future. However, at present, the operating characteristics of this method in applied settings with finite samples need to become more completely understood" (NRC report, p. 59). Chapter 8 of this book gives an account of doubly robust estimation.

The NRC report gives a list of possible estimands (pp. 22–29) formulated so as to be interpretable when a trial has missing data. (An "estimand" is that which is to be estimated in the trial analysis). We note that among these estimands, the only ITT-like one "Outcome Improvement for All Randomized Participants" requires that post-withdrawal efficacy be available and included in the analysis. The report itself notes that this particular estimand pertains to the effect of treatment policy, rather than the effect due to the experimental treatment. (See Section 4.2.1 on post-withdrawal data for a further discussion). Perhaps because of the weakness of the other approaches, the use of MAR is not ruled out, despite the reservations clearly expressed in both guidance documents. "In many cases, the primary assumption can be missing at random" (NRC report, p. 49). The EU guidance does not make this kind of explicit concession to the MAR approach. Nevertheless, its criterion that the analysis should be "unlikely to be biased in favor of the experimental treatment to an important degree (under reasonable assumptions)" may allow the justification of MAR for the primary analysis in some cases, and even perhaps in the majority of cases. An important proviso is that, given the weaknesses pointed out above, any MAR analysis will need to be supplemented by sensitivity analyses that test the robustness of results to the MAR assumption. Recommendation 11 of the NRC report states "random effects models in particular, should be used with caution, with all their assumptions clearly spelled out and justified" (NRC report, p. 77).

3.4.4   Methods that are used assuming MNAR

Methods used to handle missing data under the MNAR assumption include pattern-mixture models (PMMs), selection models (SEM), and shared parameter models. We present a non-technical overview here, with a more technical overview of PMMs in Chapter 7 as well as a technical summary of SEMs and shared parameter models in an appendix to that chapter. We note that most of the methods below can be used with binary as well as with continuous responses, although the theory on the validity of some of the methods is not as clear as in the binary case.

With PMMs one can specify a variety of assumptions, including MNAR assumptions, and the assumptions may differ by pattern of missingness. The subjects allotted to each pattern are often determined by treatment group and time of discontinuation, but can also be determined by reason for discontinuation, or in other clinically justifiable ways. The pattern-mixture approach requires clearly defined assumptions about clearly defined types or patterns of missingness. In other words, PMMs facilitate transparent pre-specification of assumptions tailored to each pattern of withdrawal, which is helpful to clinicians reviewing the study plan and eventually the clinical study report. As an example of an MNAR assumption, subjects who withdrew early because of lack of efficacy might be assumed to worsen over time until the protocol-defined end of the study (even if their previous efficacy gives no evidence for this); while subjects who withdrew for administrative reasons might be assumed to follow the MAR assumption. The EMA guideline sees merit in presenting results under such a mixture of assumptions: "It may be appropriate to treat data missing for different reasons in different ways" (p. 11). The NRC report states that "Many pattern mixture formulations are well suited to sensitivity analyses because they explicitly separate the observed data distribution from the predictive distribution of missing data given observed data." It adds "The models are transparent with respect to how missing observations are being imputed because the within-pattern models specify the predictive distribution directly" (p. 74). The report's Recommendation 9 states that "assumptions (should be) stated in a way that can be understood by clinicians" (p. 76). As noted, PMMs suit this requirement.

SEMs assume a single distribution for the "full" data – both the observed and missing values – and model this jointly with the missingness indicator. The NRC report notes in favor of SEMs that "it may seem natural to assume the combined distribution ... over observed and missing cases follows a single distribution" (p. 74). Sensitivity analyses can be implemented in SEMs by estimating the dependence of missingness on the unobserved values via a model parameter. However, the NRC report acknowledges that there is in fact no information about that very parameter, and that the model can only be fit "because of the parametric and structural assumptions being imposed on the full-data distribution." While the full-data approach may be seen as an advantage, the authors of the report state that the dependence of SEMs on parametric assumptions is "a reason to exercise extreme caution (because) none of the assumptions underlying this parametric model can be checked from the observed data." As Carpenter and Kenward (2007, p. 120) put it "the relationship between response and the unseen data can only be estimated subject to uncheckable modeling and distributional assumptions." See Section 4.2.4.2 and appendix for a further discussion of limitations of SEMs as an approach for sensitivity analysis. Semi-parametric SEMs may offer a way of using the selection model approach that is more robust. However, semi-parametric SEMs are challenging to implement, and software is not readily available. Furthermore, there remains the difficulty of interpreting the results of a selection model in terms that clinician or a patient can understand. The NRC report notes that "it may not be intuitive to specify the relationship between non-response probability and the outcome of interest, which typically has to be done in the logit or probit scale."

Shared parameter models attempt to model the relationship between missingness and outcome by positing a latent variable common to both. One may generate sensitivity analyses by estimating this variable and then artificially altering it to posit scenarios that are closer or farther away from MAR. As with SEMs, the NRC report notes the difficulty of interpreting the results: "Although these models can be enormously useful for complex data structures, they need to be used with extreme caution in a regulatory setting because of the many layers of assumptions needed to fit the models to data" (p. 76).

Given all the advantages and disadvantages outlined in the report (p. 103) for these three approaches, PMMs would seem to be most suitable for transparent interpretation.

We note that the above reasoning applies mostly to monotone missingness, and that the NRC report identifies dealing with non-monotone missingness as one of the key areas for future research, arguing that it is not always appropriate to treat it as MAR.

The EMA guideline in its Introduction states that "This document is not an extensive review of all the available methods" (p. 4), and later simply notes that "approaches that investigate different MNAR scenarios such as a PMM, SEM and a shared parameter model (SPM) may be useful" (p. 10).

Even where a trial is planned to have a primary efficacy parameter that is continuous, we briefly note here that a responder analysis can sometimes be useful as a potentially conservative sensitivity or MNAR analysis. In a typical responder analysis, a success/failure endpoint is calculated from a value or combination of values in a subject's data, while a subject with values missing for the endpoint is treated as a failure. For such an analysis to be potentially conservative, a greater proportion of missings must be expected in the experimental arm. The EMA guideline includes responder analysis as a possible supportive or sensitivity analysis, notably "where the ... missing data is so substantial that no imputation or modeling strategies can be considered reliable." The NRC report does not assess responder analysis.

3.5   Guidance about how to plan for missing data in a study

The NRC report gives six principles for handling missing data (p. 48–49):

1. Examine the response to determine the nature of the missingness and its meaning. Example: a missing CD4 count after the subject died requires a certain subset of approaches, and could not easily, for example, be handled using the MAR assumption.

2. Define an estimand that is as robust as possible to missing data. As noted above, the NRC report suggests a number of such estimands (pp. 22–27) but it is difficult to see clinicians, patients or regulators accepting easily any of those mooted, except where the planned objective of the study is quite restricted.

3. Document the reasons for missing data.

4. Decide on a set of primary assumptions about missing data that are transparent and accessible to clinicians.

5. Conduct an analysis that is valid under those assumptions.

6. Perform sensitivity analyses that capture departures from the primary missing data assumptions.

The EU guideline emphasizes throughout the importance of pre-specification of analyses (the NRC report mentions the need for pre-specification but does no more than that). The EU guideline (p. 6) suggests using data from previous studies to help define assumptions with regard to missing data for future studies. The guideline suggests that the following factors could help the study team to decide a reasonable primary analysis and a set of sensitivity analyses (EU guidance, p. 8):

– Likely proportion and timing of patient withdrawals in each treatment group;

– Likely differences in reason for withdrawal between treatment groups;

– Likely trajectory of the primary response over time.

3.6   Differences in emphasis between the NRC report and EU guidance documents

We noted at the beginning of this chapter that the NRC report and the EU guidance document agree on most important issues. The previous section covered some comments from the NRC report on the detail of statistical methods, and we have noted that the EU guidance does not go into the same level of detail about statistical bases of approaches. Table 3.2 presents other key differences in emphasis, complete with page numbers so that the reader can view the context. However, we shall see that even here there are almost no real conflicts between the documents.

3.6.1   The term "conservative"

The NRC report has the academic's preference for a more technical term of an approach that aims to minimize bias as opposed to a general notion of a "conservative" approach. The frequent use of the term "conservative" in the EU guidance is tempered by frequent qualification of this word as meaning "unlikely to be biased in favor of the experimental treatment." Such a qualified meaning for the term brings the EU guidance reasonably close to the NRC report in its recommendations for minimizing the bias of estimators.

3.6.2   Last observation carried forward

While we have seen that both NRC report and the EU guideline agree that single imputation methods like LOCF risk underestimating the variance of the estimate of treatment effect, the NRC report expresses only the down side of LOCF as an estimator. The EU guidance describes a limited potential use for LOCF. The NRC highlights important and widespread misconceptions about the alleged conservatism of the LOCF approach (pp. 65–66).

3.6.3   Post hoc analyses

As with LOCF, the NRC report describes only the disadvantages of post hoc analyses. In contrast, the EU guidance allows a place in the study report for post hoc sensitivity analyses, if missing data patterns are not as expected. This is consistent with the general awareness in the EU guidance that perfect planning for missing data is not always going to be possible.

3.6.4   Non-monotone or intermittently missing data

This rather technical item seems to be the only one on which the NRC and EU documents truly disagree. Recall from Chapter 1 that intermittently missing data typically occur when a subject who completes a clinical trial fails to turn up for some visits in the middle of the trial. The EU guidance only mentions intermittently

Table 3.2   Items where the NRC report and EU regulatory guidance document differ in emphasis.

Where emphasis differs between the documents	
FDA commissioned NRC report	EMA guideline
Conservative approach	
"the need for conservative methods receives too much emphasis in … guidelines" (p. 19)	"important that … the method can be considered 'conservative'" (p. 4)
LOCF	
"LOCF is anticonservative … where participants … do worse over time" (p. 66)	"LOCF … might be conservative … where the condition (improves) over time" (p. 9)
Post hoc analyses	
"secondary and sensitivity analyses … are certainly more valuable than post-hoc exploratory analyses" (p. 17)	"If unexpected missing data patterns are found in the data, it will be necessary to conduct some post hoc sensitivity analyses" (p. 7)
Non-monotone or interval missing data	
"non-monotone dropouts may require more specialized methods (than simple MAR-based ones)" (p. 103)	"(MAR) could lead to biased results especially when data are missing due to withdrawal (rather than data for an interim visit being missing)" (p. 10)
Assumptions should be understood by clinicians	
"assumptions (should be) stated in a way that can be understood by clinicians" (p. 76)	Not mentioned in the document
Study report	
"sensitivity analyses should be part of the primary reporting" (p. 106) "more standardized documentation of missing data" (p. 112)	Section 5.3 (p. 7) describes items required for the final study report
Training	
"(FDA) and … companies that sponsor clinical trials should carry out continued training (in) missing data analysis" (p. 113)	Not mentioned in the document

missing data in passing, and implies (EU guidance, p. 7) that it is not as important a consideration as data missing due to early discontinuation (i.e., monotone missing data). It seems that the NRC report is aware of controversy raised by Robins and Gill (1997), regarding apparent difficulties in applying MAR assumptions to intermittently missing data. The arguments of Robins and Gill are quite complex, but in essence the reasoning seems to be that intermittently missing data are MAR only if their missingness is not dependent on the missingness of the previous observation – they argue that this assumption is not plausible. (See also Daniel and Kenward (2012), for a discussion of the Robins and Gill argument).

The NRC report states that uncertainty about how to handle non-monotone missing data "raises concern among members of the panel that non-monotone dropouts may require more specialized methods for modeling the missing data mechanism, and accounting for departures from MAR." In practice, the amount of non-monotone data is not usually large in clinical trials, so this conflict between the two regions in regulatory tone is may not cause difficulties in implementing future development plans.

3.6.5 Assumptions should be readily interpretable

The NRC report emphasizes how important it is that the assumptions made in a clinical trial about missing data should be understood by non-statisticians and specifically, by clinicians. This is a criterion that is not covered by the EU guidance, and is a useful point to bear in mind when planning a study, especially when choosing sensitivity analyses. We saw above that the NRC report applied this criterion of interpretability to two methods for sensitivity analysis (SEMs and PMMs) and gave a more favorable "review" to PMMs as a result.

3.6.6 Study report

In line with its concern with the everyday practice of clinical trials, the EU guidance describes items it would expect in a final study report. In particular, the EU guidance recommends a "critical discussion of the number, timing, pattern, reason for and possible implications of missing values ... in the clinical report" (p. 3). The NRC notes that "Systematic investigations of factors related to treatment dropout and withdrawal and to missing data more generally are needed," recommends better standard reporting of information about missing data, and discusses options for deciding whether a trial result overturns the null hypothesis. However, it does not give detailed recommendations about the contents of an individual study report. See Section 4.6 for a more detailed discussion of the NRC suggestions for methods whereby it might be decided whether a trial result overturns the null hypothesis.

3.6.7 Training

The NRC report in its Recommendation 17 recommends "continued training ... to keep abreast of up-to-date techniques for missing data analysis" for analysts both

in industry and in FDA, and recommends also that FDA clinical reviewers should
receive training.

3.7   Other technical points from the NRC report

3.7.1   Time-to-event analyses

On time-to-event analyses with missing data, the NRC report notes that ideally the
statistical model should distinguish between administrative censoring (due to the
subject reaching the scheduled end of the trial) and informative censoring. The key
reference is to Scharfstein and Robins (2002). However, the Scharfstein and Robins
paper is quite complex and no implementation of their method is publicly available
at the moment. See Section 3.8.1 below for recommendations about missing data in
time-to-event analyses from the EU.

3.7.2   Tipping point sensitivity analyses

It is noteworthy that in the chapter on sensitivity analyses in the NRC report, all the
suggested sensitivity analyses involve adding an amount Δ to some parameter so as
to shift the assumption of the primary analysis and make the result less favorable
to the experimental treatment. The report suggests that inference about the primary
result can be tested as follows: "one can proceed by generating an estimate of m
(the treatment effect) for each value of Δ that is thought to be plausible … $\Delta = 0$
(might correspond) to MAR … .examining inferences about m over a set or range
for Δ that includes $\Delta = 0$ will summarize the effects of departures from MAR on
inferences" (NRC report, p. 89). The NRC report shows how such an approach could
be implemented using the selection model or PMM method. This kind of stress-test
of a primary analysis is sometimes referred to as a "tipping point" test. The idea is
described in a paper by Yan *et al.* (2009) from FDA: "Tipping points are outcomes
that result in a change of study conclusion. Such outcomes can be conveyed to clinical
reviewers to determine if they are implausibly unfavorable. The analysis aids clinical
reviewers in making judgment regarding treatment effect in the study." We shall
describe straightforward methods to implement such tipping point analyses in SAS
in Chapter 7.

3.8   Other US/EU/international guidance documents that refer to missing data

3.8.1   Committee for medicinal products for human use guideline on anti-cancer products, recommendations on survival analysis

The Committee for Medicinal Products for Human Use (CHMP) guideline on the
evaluation of anti-cancer medicinal products in man (European Medicines Agency,

2008), provides some recommendations for handling missing data in survival analysis. Key points in its line of reasoning are consistent with those in the recent US and EU regulatory documents on missing data: "There is no way to handle this problem that is optimal for all anti-cancer studies" (p. 2 of the Appendix), so any primary analysis should be accompanied by sensitivity analyses. "Outcome data should be collected ... for all randomized patients," so it is not generally acceptable to include only available cases. For survival data in particular, the Appendix suggests predefining and justifying rules of censoring. Censoring rules might, for example, "consider withdrawal or change of therapy prior to adjudicated progression/recurrence as events in an analysis of (progression free survival or disease free survival)." Regarding sensitivity analyses, the Appendix states only that they "should be sufficient to demonstrate that the trial results are robust and will depend on the clinical situation and nature of the trial data observed (e.g., patterns of patient withdrawals)."

3.8.2   US guidance on considerations when research supported by office of human research protections is discontinued

The US Office of Human Research Protections (OHRP, 2008) in the Department of Health and Human Services (DHHS) has issued a draft "Guidance on Important Considerations for when Participation of Human Subjects in Research is Discontinued." This guidance is aimed at studies funded by or supported by the OHRP, and covers the basics (i.e., ensuring that the reason for discontinuation is documented and allowing for the use of data from discontinued subjects in a final study report.)

3.8.3   FDA guidance on data retention

In 2008, the FDA issued a "Guidance for Sponsors, Clinical Investigators, and IRBs: Data Retention when Subjects Withdraw from FDA-regulated Clinical Trials" (U.S. Food and Drug Administration, 2008). As with the OHRP guidance, the objective of this short guidance is to ensure that data from subjects who discontinued are retained. It also provides for continued collection of data after a subject withdraws, if permission is given by the subject (p. 6 of the data retention guidance).

3.9   And in practice?

The following anecdotal evidence gives a picture of regulators in the US and EU coming gradually to treat missing data as more important in their reviews, and beginning to apply the principles described in the US NRC report and the EU guidance.

Some regulators still recommend or approve LOCF, even for diseases whose symptoms worsen over time. We have seen a regulator approve LOCF as a primary analysis for Parkinson's disease, whose symptoms do worsen with time.

BOCF is regarded by some regulators as justifiable or required as a way of penalizing treatments that are not tolerated, particularly in studies of pain.

During a visit to regulators in EU countries recently, the potential inadequacy of single imputation methods was raised by the regulatory groups at three of the five meetings. The three groups that raised question of valid methods for missing data had a statistician among the regulators.

At a discussion on missing data at a meeting of the European Federation of Statisticians in the Pharmaceutical Industry (EFSPI) on Advances in the Treatment of Missing Data in 2011, a number of speakers noted that they had encountered regulators who required LOCF for the primary analysis. However, other speakers stated that they had encountered regulators who referred to the new regulatory documents and took into account those documents' deprecation of single imputation methods such as LOCF.

In a review of a SAP in 2011, FDA quoted the NRC report and, after discussion, approved a sensitivity analysis that used a PMM approach to implement control-based imputation, using the method described by Ratitch and O'Kelly (2011) and Ratitch et al. (2013). Control-based imputation models post-withdrawal data from the experimental treatment arm as if they were from the control arm (see Chapter 7 for a description of how to implement this method in SAS, with example code.) The regulator required a justification that the control-based imputation did in fact constitute a true and "conservative" stress-test of the primary study result. To do this, it was required to show from historic data evidence that in fact subjects who discontinued early from the experimental arm usually tended to continue to have symptoms that compared favorably to the control group, and that therefore the scenario with control-based imputation was rather less favorable to the experimental arm than would be likely to happen in clinical practice. The cautious nature of FDA's acceptance of control-based approaches is evident in a briefing document for a meeting of the Pulmonary Allergy Drugs advisory committee (U.S. Food and Drug Administration, 2013). The briefing document carefully notes the shortcomings of MAR and LOCF approaches (as might be expected); but the document also critiques the control-based analysis. The control-based analysis in this case was called copy difference from control (CDC), and is now better known as Copy Increment from Reference (see Section 7.3.5 for a full description). The critique in the briefing document echoes a criticism of control-based assumptions made during at least one conference by an FDA statistician, that the control subjects who remain in the study are themselves an "elite" group whose symptoms may be unrepresentatively good; and that therefore control-based assumptions are not as conservative as they appear to be, and perhaps not conservative enough. This argument is noted later in this book, in Section 4.2.2.3. Despite the critique, though, the conclusion in this case was "Nonetheless, it is reassuring that the results of the LOCF, MAR and the CDC MI analyses (applying various missing data assumptions) conducted by the applicant were all consistent in magnitude and direction to the primary analysis (MMRM)." Thus evidence from sensitivity analyses may be accepted, even when their assumptions are critiqued by the regulator.

Reviewing a protocol for a study to test for equivalence, the EMA pointed out that counting subjects with missing data as failures in a responder analysis would tend to bias towards a conclusion of equivalence – the more early discontinuations, the more equivalent the two treatment groups would appear. Instead, the regulator accepted an MAR approach, but also required sensitivity analyses to test the study result for robustness to the MAR assumptions.

Awareness among regulators of the importance of missing data is also applied in areas other than the planning and conduct of clinical trials. At an EMA-International Federation of Pharmaceutical Manufacturers Associations (IFPIA) workshop on Modeling and Simulation in London in November, 2011, regulators pointed out the importance of including a variety of assumptions about missingness in a specifi cation of a simulation exercise, so that the robustness of a new method to plausible patterns of missingness could be assessed.

Finally, Section 2.2.2 includes an example showing that FDA may refuse to accept the results of a study with unwarranted proportions of missing data, when there is not an adequate plan in the protocol to prevent missing data and to deal with that missing data, when it occurs.

References

Carpenter JR, Kenward MG (2007) *Missing Data in Randomised Controlled Trials – A Practical Guide*. National Health Service Co-ordinating Center for Research Methodology, Birmingham, UK, http://www.hta.nhs.uk/nihrmethodology/reports/1589.pdf, accessed 18 June 2013.

Daniel R, Kenward MG (2012) A method for increasing the robustness of multiple imputation. *Computational Statistics and Data Analysis* **56**: 1624–1643.

European Medicines Agency (2008) *Appendix to the guideline on the evaluation of anticancer medicinal products in man (CHMP/EWP/205/95 REV. 3): methodological considerations for using progression-free survival (PFS) as primary endpoint in confirmatory trials for registration, EMEA/CHMP/EWP/27994/2008.* http://www.ema.europa.eu/docs/en_GB/document_library/Other/2009/12/WC500017749.pdf, accessed 23 June 2013.

European Medicines Agency (2010) *Guideline on Missing Data in Confirmatory Clinical Trials. EMA/CPMP/EWP/1776/99 Rev.1.* http://www.ema.europa.eu/docs/en_GB/document_library/Scientific_guideline/2010/09/WC500096793.pdf, accessed 23 June 2013.

International Conference on Harmonisation of Technical Requirements for Registration of Pharmaceuticals for Human Use (1998) *Statistical principles for clinical trials: E9.* http://www.emea.europa.eu/docs/en_GB/document_library/Scientific_guideline/2009/09/WC500002928.pdf, accessed 23 June 2013.

National Research Council. Panel on Handling Missing Data in Clinical Trials. Committee on National Statistics, Division of Behavioral and Social Sciences and Education (2010) *The Prevention and Treatment of Missing Data in Clinical Trials.* The National Academies Press, Washington, DC, available at http://www.nap.edu/catalog.php?record_id=12955, accessed 16 July 2013.

Office of Human Research Protections (2008) *Guidance on important considerations for when participation of human subjects in research is discontinued.* Washington DC. http://www.hhs.gov/ohrp/documents/200811guidance.pdf, accessed 23 June 2013.

Ratitch B, O'Kelly M (2011) Implementation of Pattern-mixture models using standard SAS/STAT procedures. In *Proceedings of Pharmaceutical Industry SAS User Group*,

Nashville. http://pharmasug.org/proceedings/2011/SP/PharmaSUG-2011-SP04.pdf, accessed 23 June 2013.

Ratitch B, O'Kelly M, Tosiello R (2013) Missing data in clinical trials: from clinical assumptions to statistical analysis using pattern mixture models. *Pharmaceutical Statistics*, **12**: 337-347, available at http://onlinelibrary.wiley.com/doi/10.1002/pst.1549/pdf, accessed 20 June 2013.

Robins J, Gill, R (1997) Non-response models for the analysis of non-monotone ignorable missing data. *Statistics in Medicine* **16**: 39–56.

Scharfstein D, Robins J (2002) Estimation of the failure time distribution in the presence of informative censoring. *Biometrika* **89**: 617–634, available at http://www.jstor.org/stable/4140606, accessed 23 June 2013.

U.S. Food and Drug Administration (2008) *Guidance for sponsors, clinical investigators, and IRBs: data retention when subjects withdraw from FDA-regulated clinical trials*. Rockville. www.fda.gov/downloads/RegulatoryInformation/Guidances/UCM126489.pdf, accessed 23 June 2013.

U.S. Food and Drug Administration (2013) *Briefing document, Pulmonary Allergy Drugs Advisory Committee Meeting: NDA 204-275: fluticasone furoate and vilanterol inhalation powder for the long-term, maintenance treatment of airflow obstruction and for reducing exacerbations in patients with chronic obstructive pulmonary disease (COPD)*. http://www.fda.gov/downloads/AdvisoryCommittees/CommitteesMeetingMaterials/Drugs/Pulmonary-AllergyDrugsAdvisoryCommittee/UCM347929.pdf, accessed 23 June 2013.

Yan X, Lee S, Li N (2009) Missing data handling methods in medical device clinical trials. *Journal of Biopharmaceutical Statistics* **19**: 1085–1098, available at http://www.tandfonline.com/doi/pdf/10.1080/10543400903243009, accessed 23 June 2013.

4

A guide to planning for missing data

Michael O'Kelly and Bohdana Ratitch

Key points

- Those who use reports of clinical trials for decision-making have a growing concern with whether a trial result is robust to missing data: this is an additional motive to adopt a scientific approach to handle missing data and to incorporate a description of the approach clearly in trial protocols and statistical analysis plans.

- Trialists and statisticians can alleviate the problem of missing data via the design of the trial, including the decision as to what data to collect and when.

- Historic data and its patterns of missingness can be used to eliminate inappropriate statistical analyses, and may suggest some methods as justifiable.

- A missing at random (MAR) approach is often justifiable as a primary analysis, although likely biased to some degree.

- Multiple imputation (MI) can be used in the framework of pattern-mixture models (PMMs) to implement a variety of sensitivity analyses that are useful across many indications and treatments in stress testing the primary analysis.

Clinical Trials with Missing Data: A Guide for Practitioners, First Edition. Michael O'Kelly and Bohdana Ratitch.
© 2014 John Wiley & Sons, Ltd. Published 2014 by John Wiley & Sons, Ltd.

- At the core of any analysis of missing data will be plots of the probability of discontinuing over time, and plots of the outcome over time for selected subjects, for example, for subjects discontinuing at a range of time points and/or discontinuing for a variety of different reasons.

4.1   Introduction

Although it does refer to other parts of the book, this chapter may be read on its own by a trialist beginning a study with missing data. As with the rest of this book, the actions described here are those that the statistician will usually take, but we have attempted to make the exposition readable by all trialists.

Missing data can *bias* the results of a trial or make it difficult to generalize results from a trial. In this regard, the trialist's primary objective should be to preserve and enhance as far as possible the *credibility and applicability* of the study results in the face of potential missing data. To do so requires clear logical reasoning about the threats that missing data may pose to the credibility of results. This logical reasoning should be presented in the protocol, should take account of the trial objective, and the protocol should describe clearly the trial's strategies for missing data. The chosen design should be justified based on historic data about the treatment, the indication, and on data about the likely health of subjects who discontinue early. In the last several decades, a number of useful new statistical techniques have been described for analyzing outcomes in the presence of missing data. The growing awareness of how missing data can affect trial results, plus the availability of these new statistical methods, has led to regulators' *demand for better practice* in pharmaceutical trials with regard to missing data.

4.1.1   Missing data may bias trial results or make them more difficult to generalize to subjects outside the trial

A trial result gains breadth and security of inference when the analysis is performed according to the intention-to-treat (ITT) principle. To follow the ITT principle, one includes in the primary analysis of a trial all randomized subjects, regardless of adherence to the treatment. At least in theory, inclusion of all randomized subjects in the analysis increases one's freedom to make inferences about subjects similar to those randomized to the trial. (Of course, the conduct of the study and the choice of countries and investigator sites may limit inference, even if the ITT principle is followed in other ways).

For ITT to hold, trial subjects do not have to adhere to the treatment regimen to which they are assigned. The ITT approach usually includes in the estimate of treatment effect subjects who did not take the study treatment correctly, or sometimes even those who did not take study treatment at all. This allows the result to take into account any notable difficulties in actually administering (or receiving) the treatment.

As Little and Yau (1996) put it, "If, for example, a potent and effective drug is avoided by the majority of subjects because of unpleasant side effects, then this negative feature is taken into account in the ITT analysis, but it is ignored in an 'as treated' analysis focused on effects for those who took the treatment." The International Conference on Harmonization (ICH) E9 Guideline "Statistical Principles for Clinical Trials" (1998) states that the ITT principle also "implies that the primary analysis should include all randomized subjects," but recognizes that complete follow-up "may be difficult to achieve" and states that the full analysis set should be "as complete as possible."

In addition to increasing breadth of applicability, inclusion of data from all randomized subjects helps to limit bias in the use of trial results. Applicability and bias are related. This can be seen if we consider a study with a rather restrictive primary estimand such as "Outcome improvement during adherence to treatment" ("estimand" means "that which is to be estimated"). Post-treatment data from subjects who discontinued treatment would be excluded from this primary analysis – the estimate of efficacy in subjects adhering to treatment would not be biased by this exclusion. However, inference from that same estimate of treatment effect would be biased if an attempt were made to apply it to all subjects with the indication, or even just all subjects similar to those enrolled in the study. The narrower the applicability of an estimand, the more difficult it is to avoid drawing biased conclusions from it, even if these are inadvertently biased. Narrowly defined estimands are also of less interest to regulators deciding whether to approve a treatment. In general, furthermore, if the characteristics of dropouts are not well understood, or if the reasons for early discontinuation are not explicitly taken into account in the trial result and inference from this result, the study may be biased in ways that the reader of the study report cannot quantify or be sure about.

If we include data from subjects who withdrew, we help to ensure a rounded view of efficacy – the treatment effect is estimated not just based on the "elite" subjects who completed the trial but also on those who for one reason or another – perhaps side effects – did not make it to the end of the trial. One way of including subjects who withdrew is to collect post-discontinuation data. The question of how post-discontinuation data may be used in estimating treatment effect will be discussed under the heading "Protocol/Case Report Form/Statistical analysis plan considerations" below. However, post-withdrawal data are not often available in current clinical trials, and indeed we shall see (in Section 4.2.1) that it is not always clear whether post-withdrawal data should be included in the analysis, because the effect of the post-study treatment may mask the effect of the study drug, or may make the analysis biased in favor of the experimental treatment.

As noted, in practice regulators have not, in the past at least, regarded a restricted estimand such as "Outcome improvement during adherence to treatment" as useful in deciding whether to approve a new treatment. Usually, it will not be possible to find a useful primary estimand that is completely immune to the missing data in a study. As a rule, the inference from an estimand will need to be fairly widely applicable, and will need to take into account or adjust for subjects who withdrew early.

4.1.2   Credibility of trial results when there is missing data

As a first step towards maintaining credibility of trial results, the trial team must plan to prevent missing data as far as possible. See Chapter 2 for suggestions on how this may be done. Given that some missing data is unavoidable, the statistician must then find a way to render the trial result credible, even with the resulting missing data. Results could be undermined by missing data, for example,

- when there is a very high rate of dropout in a trial with an indication that did not historically show high rates in other trials;

- when last observation carried forward (LOCF) is used for degenerative/progressive disease and inferences are made about the condition of the subjects at the end of the trial;

- in symptomatic trials (chronic conditions) when subjects respond to treatment, but cannot tolerate it and discontinue; (the credibility would be compromised if these subjects are still assigned a favorable outcome at the end of the trial).

The statistician can minimize the risk to credibility by planning a primary analysis that is not likely to be biased to an important degree in favor of the experimental treatment arm when there are missing data, and by planning sensitivity analyses that stress test the assumptions about missing data used in the primary analysis. These sensitivity analyses should implement a set of assumptions that challenge those of the primary analysis, and preferably are likely to be less favorable to the experimental arm. The statistician should plan sensitivity analyses so as to satisfy the regulator, the clinical expert and the patient that under a range of plausible alternatives, especially alternatives unfavorable to the experimental arm, the primary study result would still hold.

To maintain the credibility of the study in the face of missing data, the statistician must not only present appropriate primary analysis and sensitivity analyses but must also be able to state the assumptions of these analyses in a way that makes clinical sense, and that a non-statistician can understand. An analysis will be credible in the face of missing data only if that analysis is clinically credible. We emphasize that the dialogue between statistician and clinical expert is essential to achieve this.

4.1.3   Demand for better practice with regard to missing data

The new regulatory documents have urged that clinical trials be designed and executed so as to prevent missing data as far as possible. However, the writers of the regulatory guidances are aware that it is not possible to plan so as to completely prevent certain types of missing data: subjects have a right to withdraw both from the randomized treatment and the trial, and do not have to agree to provide follow-up data. It is not surprising that the bulk of the new regulatory documents are devoted to handling the missing data that does occur in trials.

Until recently, single imputation methods were dominant in clinical trials. Other methods were often regarded as too complex, not understood by clinicians and/or implementations were not readily available. Because of this, people opted for simpler approaches and sometimes mistakenly considered them to be universally conservative. For some time, there was a gap between the methodological research (quite advanced) and practical use (basic).

A crescendo of research on missing data can perhaps be thought of as beginning with Rubin (1976). The research since Rubin has provided methods for modeling missing values based on observed trial values. These methods include multiple imputation (MI); and direct likelihood, particularly in the form of the use of mixed models for repeated measures with a categorical time effect (MMRM). The research has also provided a framework called pattern-mixture models (PMMs), which breaks the problem of missing data in a trial into distinct strands of missingness. Another method has been devised, which models simultaneously the probability of missingness and the probability distribution of the outcome – the method known as selection modeling. Yet another option suggested is known as shared parameter modeling: here, missingness and outcomes are linked by a posited random variable which can be thought of as a latent variable. Inverse probability weighting (IPW) – regression weighted by the inverse of the probability of being observed – has also been shown to be a useful way of taking account of missing data; a development of this is weighted augmented estimation, sometimes using generalized estimating equations (GEEs), also known as the doubly robust approach (Molenberghs and Kenward, 2007). During this period, the literature has also provided hundreds of examples of the application of variants of these and other approaches. Many of the papers on missing data have shown how conclusions from a study could vary depending on how missing data was handled (see, e.g., Siddiqui *et al.* (2009) on LOCF vs. MMRM). In the face of these developments, it is not surprising that regulators and others have made missing data a more important aspect of their reviews of new drug applications (NDAs) and have provided new guidance documents on missing data. The ICH E9 guideline on statistical principles for clinical trials mentions missing data frequently and has a brief non-technical section on missing data. In 2001, European Agency for the Evaluation of Medicinal Products issued a guideline *Points to Consider on Missing Data* (Committee for Proprietary Medicinal Products, 2001), and more recently in 2010, European Medicines Agency (EMA) replaced it with a new *Guideline on Missing Data in Confirmatory Clinical Trials* (European Medicines Agency, 2010). In United States, Food and Drug Administration (FDA) sponsored a National Research Council (NRC) panel which issued a report *The Prevention and Treatment of Missing Data in Clinical Trials* (National Research Council, 2010). (In this and in other chapters, we sometimes, for convenience, refer to these two latest documents as "regulatory documents.") In regulators' reviews of new protocols and statistical analysis plans (SAPs), trialists have found that advice with regard to missing data is changing to match the guidance documents, although not in a uniform or completely consistent manner. In particular, there is an increasing tendency to require that protocols and SAPs give a scientific justification for the methods used to handle missing data in a trial. In practice, some trialists continue using traditional methods – one justification being that these still need to be used to allow comparison with previous trials. Among regulators, too, some are more open to the ideas of the new guidance documents than others. Again, we have encountered a growing tendency for regulators to encourage trialists to break this pattern and use only methods that are appropriate to the trial at hand.

4.2   Planning for missing data

As well as contributing to the planning process in purely quantitative matters, the statistician can help by advocating a development that takes missing data into account both for studies currently being planned and for future studies. We will first look at this more general contribution a statistician can make to a development and its studies. Then we will describe the statistician's contribution to the statistical sections of the protocol and to the SAP.

4.2.1   The case report form and non-statistical sections of the protocol

The following paragraphs cover some actions that the trial statistician may take to improve the design and running of a trial with respect to missing data. See also Chapter 2 on the prevention of missing data.

Objective and estimand: The trial statistician should review the objective and estimand to ensure that, insofar as is consistent with the objective, the estimand will be estimable given the kind of missing data expected in the study. For example, the estimand "Outcome improvement during adherence to treatment" (posited by the NRC report) might sometimes the objective of a study, and would be estimable in the presence of even a large proportion of early discontinuations. On the other hand, if an estimate for a degenerative disease after 52 weeks is needed, but the trial does not have adequate retention strategies, the estimand will not be estimable unless such strategies are introduced.

When the objective allows for a control or reference treatment, the trial statistician may want to advocate including a control or reference arm that is as close as possible to the "standard of care" for the trial indication and population, if this is consistent with the objective of the trial. There are two advantages in including a treatment arm that is close to the standard of care. First, subjects and investigators will be less likely to opt for withdrawal from the control or reference arm if it is a treatment that is generally agreed to be acceptable for the indication. Second, a control arm close to the standard of care can facilitate a range of useful sensitivity analyses. With such a control arm, for example, it would be possible to use study data to implement an assumption that withdrawals from the experimental treatment arm receive standard of care – a clinically realistic assumption. We discuss this later in the chapter under the heading "Control- or reference-based imputation." However, a control arm close to the "standard of care" may not always be consistent with the objective of the trial (e.g., when a placebo control will give acceptable evidence of efficacy in a non-serious indication).

Enriching the study population: The trial statistician may suggest, and may also critically review, an attempt to prevent missing data by selecting a population less likely to discontinue. Subjects likely to be compliant, likely to benefit from study treatments or likely not to have side effects could be selected via a run-in period. This "enriched" population could be less likely to discontinue early from the trial. The disadvantage of this strategy is that the trial result will not be as generalizable as a result from a standard ITT population (Burzykowski *et al.*, 2009). Nevertheless, in some therapeutic areas, such as pain, and some psychiatric indications, it is common to enrich the study population in this way. This may make sense in indications where an initial "trial" period is possible in clinical practice, which can be the case in chronic conditions. For such a design, efficacy and safety must be capable of being ascertained quickly (during the enrichment period); the study objective will be to assess whether treatment then gives a sustained effect for a longer duration.

Amount and frequency of data collected: The trial statistician should review the level of data collected, balancing the advantage of frequent visits and full data versus the burden for the subject, a burden which may contribute to the withdrawal from the trial.

Endpoints with inherent probability of being missing: If appropriate, the trial statistician should keep the team conscious of the possibilities for missing data inherent in candidate primary parameters. Here are some examples:

- a compound endpoint where a problem with the calculation of any component could lead to a missing result for the endpoint;

- endpoints such as the 6-min walk test for pulmonary indications, where a proportion of subjects on the trial are likely not to be able to perform the test;

- a lab parameter on its own as the primary endpoint, if the indication is such that a significant proportion of subjects are expected to die while participating in the study – for example, CD4 count on its own as primary parameter in a study of HIV.

Protocol violations leading to discontinuation from treatment: the trial statistician should consider whether data should be collected after protocol violations that lead to discontinuation. If the decision is made not to collect the data, the trial statistician should establish whether the data would be suitable for analysis and ensure that the study team discusses the credibility and generalizability of the analysis without data from such subjects. If data are to be collected after discontinuation, consider how they may impact the analysis/conclusions (see more on this below).

Measures to reduce attrition: the trial statistician should encourage the team to consider how to reduce attrition via, for example, visit scheduling, transportation, childcare, reminder calls, keeping burdensome measurements to a minimum (e.g., pharmacokinetic (PK) measurements involving hours or overnights in hospital) and managing expected side effects with acceptable concomitant medications. If available, summaries from historic data of concomitant medications for subjects who completed versus subjects who discontinued previous studies could help in planning for this last strategy. See Section 2.4 for a full discussion of measures to increase subject retention.

Reasons for withdrawal: with the growing awareness of how missing data affect results, the withdrawal page of the Case Report Form (CRF) is becoming very important to the statistician in her efforts to handle missing data credibly. Consider the following points with regard to collecting the reason for withdrawal:

- What reasons would be most helpful for our analysis (the ones we could really incorporate into imputation mechanism/sensitivity analysis)? For example, a subject discontinued with reason "Lack of efficacy" could for certain analyses reasonably be assumed to have values MAR; knowledge that a subject discontinued for safety or tolerability reasons could be useful as suggesting that his/her values are missing not at random (MNAR), that is, discontinuation might not be predictable via the usual MAR models; knowledge that a subject discontinued for administrative reasons is useful because it can justify the assumption of values missing completely at random (MCAR) for the subject. (See Chapter 1 for definitions of MCAR, MAR and MNAR mechanisms.)

- Consider the risks and benefits of collecting just one primary reason, as opposed to allowing a number of reasons to be given for withdrawal. Using a single main reason for discontinuation has many advantages; but is the study such that we are losing some good information if just one primary reason for discontinuation is collected?

- If at all appropriate, allow for discontinuation due to lack of efficacy, and due to a positive outcome (cure or relief of symptoms).

- Consider the commonly used reason "withdrawal of consent." This reason could mean many different things. Consider whether it would be possible to collect more details, such as whether the withdrawal of consent was due to perception of efficacy, lack of tolerability of the study treatment or inability to comply with study visit requirements.

- If a subject may be withdrawn due to protocol violation, in collecting the reason for withdrawal consider how to allow the investigator to indicate the principal underlying cause of the violation, if any; the underlying cause could be an efficacy issue (e.g., if violation was the taking of forbidden efficacy treatment) or a safety issue (e.g., if violation was an action to alleviate side effects). Make sure that as far as possible the reason is unambiguous and withdrawal can be clearly attributed to issues with efficacy or safety if this is indeed the case, and if necessary, collect additional information. Summaries of adverse events (AEs) for completers versus withdrawals, whether or not withdrawal was recorded as due to AE, may be useful to investigate the recorded reasons.

- Collect cause-specific death (related or not related to the disease under study) or collect information that would facilitate this categorizing of death in some objective way. This would be especially useful in long-term trials in an elderly population where subjects are likely to die from unrelated causes.

- The reason "lost to follow-up" may be related to the outcome (e.g., if a person's health deteriorates so that the person needs to move to be cared for by a relative). Consider means of capturing that, and of distinguishing from a subject with whom contact was simply lost for reasons unknown.

- Consider how to measure and communicate any positive impact of changes in the design of the CRF for entry of reasons for discontinuation.

Collecting post-withdrawal data: the repeated mention by the NRC report of the importance of collecting post-withdrawal data has prompted much discussion about whether such post-withdrawal data are really useful. If good treatments for the indication are available outside the trial, will post-withdrawal treatment "contaminate" efficacy scores, giving a falsely positive outcome for early withdrawals? The apparently rigorous strategy of strict ITT collection of data for all subjects, including post-withdrawal data for early withdrawers, could favor a dangerous treatment, if numerous early withdrawals gain access to a more tolerable alternative treatment. In fact, however, while they state the importance of post-withdrawal data, both the NRC report and European Union (EU) guidance documents are careful to point out just this kind of difficulty (see also Section 3.2). The guidance documents expect that any post-withdrawal data contributing to the primary efficacy test would need to be put in context – one important piece of context would be the concomitant treatment that the withdrawn subject was receiving after withdrawal. The use of post-withdrawal data is still going to be a problem, though. We can talk about putting it in context, but there is no simple way to include that context quantitatively in the summary statistic that will determine whether the experimental treatment is approved. For the adventurous, Carpenter and Kenward (2007) suggest eliciting prior beliefs from clinicians about likely outcomes when trial subjects withdraw early, and incorporating these priors in a Bayesian framework in the primary analysis. Carpenter and Kenward include WinBUGS code for a sample application of this idea in their online monograph. In what has proved a very influential contribution, Little and Yau (1996) looked at a trial where it was plausible to assume that subjects who discontinued from the experimental arm might subsequently receive treatment equivalent to that of the control arm. Little and Yau in this case proposed imputing post-discontinuation values for the experimental arm based on outcomes from the control arm. We shall see below and in Chapter 7 how useful this idea has turned out to be in handling missing data. More generally, where data are available about post-withdrawal treatment but not about post-withdrawal outcomes, Little and Yau note that it would be possible to use a variety of in-study treatment arms quite flexibly to impute appropriate outcomes, depending on the actual treatment taken post withdrawal.

However, Keene (2010) notes how difficult it is to avoid a dilution of the estimate of treatment effect when good alternative treatments are known to be available, and a less-than-optimal control group is for one reason or another required. He describes how a significant proportion of subjects in the control arm in a chronic obstructive pulmonary disease (COPD) trial withdrew and went on alternative treatment. The ratio of the rate of exacerbations in an on-treatment analysis was 0.75 in favor of the experimental arm (95% CI: 0.55–1.01, $p = 0.06$); but in the strict ITT analysis, the ratio was only 0.85 in favor (95% CI: 0.65–1.11, $p = 0.23$).

It is difficult to make good use of post-withdrawal outcomes in a straightforward manner, unless the objective of the trial is to study a treatment regime, as opposed to the effect of an experimental treatment. However, collecting post-withdrawal outcomes is undoubtedly valuable for planning and justifying future strategies for missing data. A notable feature of regulatory reviews of strategies for missing data is the tendency for the regulator to request scientific justification of assumptions about outcomes of subjects who withdraw. For this, obviously, one needs post-withdrawal data, but these are scarce in the literature. Only by collecting outcomes post withdrawal in current studies, will trialists give themselves a basis in the future for justifying objectively and logically the assumptions of primary and of sensitivity analyses for missing data, whatever those assumptions might be. Such data would give a historic mean post-withdrawal outcome for the experimental arm or a similar treatment. Such a mean might be used in assumptions about missing data of withdrawals for future studies. If some of the historic data are not appropriate because the post-withdrawal treatments had been "too good," it might be possible to select just those subjects that received standard of care. Armed with such information the statistician may then have a scientific basis to justify assumptions for the primary analysis or for the sensitivity analyses.

To see the value of collecting post-withdrawal data for planning purposes, suppose post-withdrawal data are collected. Suppose further that subjects discontinuing from the experimental treatment group tend to revert rapidly back to their baseline value. This could suggest imputing baseline-like values to subjects who discontinue from the experimental treatment group, and would provide a justification for such a strategy. Suppose, in contrast, post-withdrawal data for subjects in the experimental treatment group who switch to "standard of care" show that they tend to fare close to, but somewhat better than, completers in the control group. A credible strategy could then be justified that would impute missing data for the experimental treatment group using observed data from the control group as suggested by Little and Yau (1996). For withdrawals who switched to the standard of care used in the control group, this imputing would in this case, if anything, underestimate any efficacy attributable to the experimental treatment. Note that in both of these illustrations, subjects who after discontinuation received treatment that was better than the "standard of care" might well in truth have efficacy better than either of the treatment groups in the study, but this better efficacy would be ignored, and efficacy for withdrawals would universally be assumed to be only as good as efficacy on "standard of care." The regulatory documents acknowledge that superior alternative treatments received by trial subjects could make post-discontinuation data difficult to use, because the efficacy of the alternative treatment could be credited to the study treatment. If we artificially assume for all discontinuations only the efficacy associated with the "standard of care," we eliminate this difficulty by assuming a clinically plausible scenario for all withdrawals that is not likely to favor the experimental treatment group. The estimand we get by imputing to all withdrawals, no matter what their subsequent treatment, is the kind of efficacy they *would have had* under the "standard of care" or under the control treatment. Such an estimand can be called "the effect attributable to the randomized treatment" (Mallinckrodt, 2013). This kind of estimand has, on occasion, been accepted by regulators both in the United States and EU, provided data are available about what happens to withdrawals on the experimental treatment, and that data supports the imputation strategy for withdrawals from the experimental treatment group.

4.2.2 The statistical sections of the protocol and the statistical analysis plan

4.2.2.1 Summary of what the protocol should say about missing data in its statistical sections

The statistical section of the protocol should include a detailed discussion on the following points, each of which we will explore below:

- how missing data are handled in the primary analysis and why the selected method may be appropriate;

- the implication from the clinical point of view of the assumptions with regard to missing data made by the primary test on the conclusions;

- what deviations from the primary assumptions regarding the missingness mechanism will be tested in the sensitivity analyses; the protocol should state the motivation for these sensitivity tests from a clinical perspective first, and then translate the sensitivity tests into statistical terms (i.e., then the different statistical models to be used, and their assumptions);

- how the observed missing data patterns will be explored (e.g., Kaplan–Meier analysis for time to discontinuation based on different reasons; plots over time of the primary outcome measure for completers and for withdrawals, and by treatment group and reason for discontinuation; logistic regression to identify factors or covariates that predict withdrawal, etc.), and how these findings may affect sensitivity analyses (e.g., additional sensitivity analyses may be allowed for, based on these explorations of the observed missing data patterns);

- distributional assumptions of statistical models, and their ability to model outcomes adequately; if appropriate, it may be proposed to assess the sensitivity of the primary result to distributional assumptions.

4.2.2.2 Pre-specification and flexibility in planning for missing data

The trialist must pre-specify the handling of missing data. The protocol should pre-specify "a detailed description of the selected methods and a justification of why the methods to be applied are expected to be an appropriate way of summarizing the results of the study and allow assessment without an important degree of bias in favor of experimental treatment. The sensitivity analyses envisaged should also be prespecified" (European Medicines Agency, 2010). However, the trialist may adjust the handling of missing data based on the actual data in the study. "It may be acceptable to allow in the study protocol the possibility of updating the strategy at a later point (e.g., during a blind data review)" (European Medicines Agency, 2010). For example, if the blind data review revealed that the proportion of missing data was unexpectedly high and often due to AEs, an alternative primary or an additional secondary analysis might be proposed (if not already proposed), with a binary success/failure outcome, treating subjects with missing data as failures. In this case, a protocol amendment could be required, and of course the change should be recorded in the SAP and signed off before the unblinding of the study.

The EMA guideline even allows for post hoc sensitivity analyses, but never to rescue a study by "improving on" the statistical significance of results from the planned analyses. A post hoc sensitivity analysis might be justified, for example, if after database lock unblinded results showed that the experimental treatment group had an expectedly high rate of loss to follow-up. A useful extra sensitivity analysis in that case might assume a very poor outcome for subjects who were lost to follow-up, in case such missingness stemmed in some way from the effects of the treatment itself.

Statisticians who are faced with a protocol that is a *fait accompli* may still address missing data adequately in the SAP. If the primary analysis cannot be changed, the statistician can generally add sensitivity analyses to test the assumptions of the primary analysis sufficiently to give adequate credibility to the results.

4.2.2.3 Sources of bias in analyses of missing data

As a preliminary to describing how one might choose and justify a primary analysis, we note some of the potential biases in the commonly used approaches to missing data. No method is without potential bias. Both NRC report and EU guidance documents recognize this, and emphasize that a primary analysis alone will not be sufficient when there are missing data – sensitivity analyses will also be needed. We note that the statistician can use previous studies and the literature to form a scientific view of likely patterns of relationship in missingness and efficacy, and thus choose and justify a primary analysis. In later sections, we will demonstrate this process in a variety of examples. We will then give general guidance for a variety of strategies as to when to use and when to avoid them.

Here are some typical sources of bias for common approaches to handle missing data.

Available data: This method estimates the treatment effect using only observed data at the primary time point. Subjects who complete a trial are likely to be healthier than those who discontinue early (see Section 1.3). If a higher proportion of subjects in the experimental arm complete the study, compared to the control arm, then available data will tend to overestimate the treatment effect, if an ITT approach is intended. If a higher proportion of subjects in the control arm complete the trial, using available data may decrease the power of the trial to detect superior efficacy in the experimental arm. However, an analysis using only available data does provide very useful background information with which to judge the primary and the sensitivity analyses, and an available cases analysis should almost always be planned in the protocol or SAP for this purpose.

Single imputation approaches: Single imputation methods replace an unknown missing value with a single imputed value, and then treat the imputed value as if it had been actually observed. Examples of single imputation include LOCF; baseline observation carried forward (BOCF) and worst-case imputation. With the exception of the rare case of LOCF when the estimand of interest actually is the last observed value, these and similar single imputation methods have the disadvantage of depriving the analysis of any element of uncertainty due to missingness – in effect they artificially increase the sample size for the primary statistical test. In general, therefore, these methods will tend to bias the variability of the estimate of treatment effect downward. This in turn will tend to lead to false positive claims for the experimental arm. (We note, though, that we have encountered at least one trial where the LOCF values were so different from the observed values that the variance of the treatment effect was actually markedly higher than that from other approaches, but this is unusual). However, we anticipate our discussion of MI here to note that the use of last observed data as a basis for imputing later values can be implemented in more sophisticated ways, which circumvent the poor estimation of variance that we get with single imputation. Roger (2012) and Carpenter *et al.* (2013) has made available software that uses MI to impute to withdrawals the *distribution* of the last observed visit with either the subject's own last mean carried forward (OLMCF) or the study average last mean carried forward (ALMCF). (For convenience for the rest of this chapter, we will refer to LOCF, OLMCF and ALMCF as "LOCF-like"). We show in Chapter 7 how standard SAS code can also implement LOCF-like imputations with reasonable variability. In the OLMCF and ALMCF versions of LOCF, the uncertainty due to the missing data is adequately reflected, and an important objection to the LOCF-like approach is thus overcome. The same objection has been similarly overcome for BOCF: Ratitch and O'Kelly (2011) and Ratitch *et al.* (2013) show that it is straightforward to use observed baseline values in MI to impute to missing values the appropriate distribution of the study baseline, if desired. This approach may be called average baseline carried forward (ABCF). For the rest of this chapter, we will refer to it as a BOCF-like approach. As with LOCF, then, one can thus implement the BOCF assumption while allowing for the uncertainty due to the missing data. Both methods are described in Chapter 7.

The above methods overcome the objection about underestimated variance in LOCF and BOCF, but other problems of potential bias remain with such approaches.

In Chapter 1, we noted that, for a progressive disease, LOCF-like approaches will impute better values, the earlier a subject discontinues. For progressive diseases, therefore, LOCF-like approaches will tend to overestimate the treatment effect, if subjects in the experimental arm discontinue earlier or more frequently than those in the control arm. On the other hand, LOCF-type imputation could also lead to false negative findings. Consider a progressive disease, where the experimental arm has a safety advantage. LOCF would tend to miss the disease progression in the control arm because subjects in the control arm discontinued earlier and hence the potential false negative result. Similar risks of bias apply in indications such as insomnia and depression, which tend to improve spontaneously over time. With such an indication, the treatment effect will be overestimated if subjects in the control treatment group tend to discontinue earlier than subjects in the experimental treatment group, because LOCF-like assumptions will deny to early discontinuations the improvement that can be expected over time in the indication.

BOCF is often recommended by the regulator for trials where symptoms are the focus, for example, where chronic pain is the endpoint. It may be argued that BOCF is clinically plausible because subjects off medication are likely to revert to the pre-trial level of pain. In favor of BOCF, regulators have argued also that, for subjects who discontinue a treatment due to side effects, it would be inappropriate to attribute any efficacy to that treatment, even if the subject did benefit prior to discontinuation. It could be said that such an approach is using efficacy as a surrogate for a combined risk–benefit score. Whether this is the case, and whether it is a good thing or not, it seems likely that BOCF-like approaches will continue to be recommended for certain indications in the future, especially, by tradition, for indications related to pain. Despite this, one could envisage bias under BOCF in a pain study. Consider the case where: (1) in reality there is no clinically significant treatment effect compared to placebo, but there is some "placebo" effect at the primary time point (both groups improve somewhat compared to baseline); and (2) the study treatment has some transient effect that makes subjects stay on study longer than those on placebo. In this case, the proportion of subjects imputed to a zero change from baseline will be larger in the placebo group, and thus treatment difference between active and placebo groups will be overestimated and lead to a false positive conclusion. In general, also, in symptomatic trials single-imputation BOCF will be likely to underestimate the variance of the treatment effect. Thus, there are a number of situations and uses where BOCF could be anti-conservative.

Although they have the merit of an assumption that clearly works against treatment groups with a high rate of withdrawal, worst-case approaches have some unattractive features, especially when the outcome is continuous. We note that the term "worst case" has two uses in the literature. "Worst-case *imputation*" often means the practice of imputing the worst possible or worst observed value where data are missing, - see, for example, European Medicines Agency (2010, p. 9) and Kelleher *et al.* (2001). "Worst-case *analysis*" often means imputing the worst outcome for the experimental treatment arm but imputing the best outcome for the control treatment arm - see, for example, European Medicines Agency (2010, p. 12) and Myers (2000). The worst-case assumption is rarely clinically plausible. We see "worst-case analysis" as more clinically implausible than "worst-case imputation," and for this reason emphasize "worst-case imputation" in this book. When the term "worst case" is used hereafter, we refer to "worst-case imputation" as defined above unless otherwise stated. Worst-case approaches tend to result in imputations that lack the variability that is appropriate when there is missing data. By definition, there are usually no ways to impute worst case with some variability, as there now are for LOCF and BOCF approaches. Finally, when the outcome is continuous, it is often difficult to identify a worst case. Typically, the worst observed value in the study is used, but this seems unsatisfactory because of the heavy influence of this single extreme value on the result. Given an infinitely bad efficacy score, a single missing observation could overturn any result. Following Carpenter and Kenward (2007), we will not include worst-case analysis as an option for continuous outcomes. (Much of this paragraph is based on Carpenter and Kenward (2007, pp. 13, 27, 121). We note, though, that "poor case" imputation is feasible, and could be done preserving variability, using methods similar to the LOCF-like analyses described in Chapter 7. A "poor case" could be imputed by sampling from "poor" percentiles of the distribution of the outcome, or from earlier visits in a study where study treatment is not expected to have attained its full effect.

In particular, in trials where the objective is to prove non-inferiority or superiority, BOCF and worst-case imputation can lead to false positive findings. It is true that, if the proportion of dropouts differs by treatment group, the BOCF or worst-case assumptions may tend to favor one treatment group or the other. But if the proportion of dropouts is about the same in each treatment group, any method that imputes a similar outcome for missing data across treatment groups has a likelihood of biasing the study conclusion in favor of equivalence or non-inferiority – the more missings, the more the treatment groups will look the same. For example, there has been a strong tradition in trials of rheumatoid arthritis (RA) of using a binary endpoint, such as ACR20, or 20% improvement in aspects of the American College of Rheumatology (ACR) score, and imputing treatment failure to subjects with missing data at the primary endpoint. The regulators now routinely advise against using this approach in non-inferiority and equivalence trials for RA, because of the bias towards the conclusion that the treatment groups are similar. Note that ACR20 is an example of a responder (success/failure) endpoint. When subjects with missing data are counted as failures, a responder analysis in effect uses worst-case imputation, although one can also view it as a BOCF analysis, with withdrawals assumed to have no change from baseline.

Time-to-event analysis has also been used to take account of withdrawals, with discontinuation being counted as an unfavorable "event." Again, because the worst is assumed for early withdrawals in the context of the primary hypothesis, this can be thought of as worst-case imputation. As with other worst-case and LOCF-like approaches, the treatment effect may be overestimated here if a greater proportion of subjects discontinue from the control arm.

Approaches assuming MAR: any approach that assumes missing at random assumes that missing values are similar to those observed, given the study data (see Section 1.5). Thus, for a subject who discontinued early and has missing data, MAR assumes a value for the endpoint based on the observed data of subjects whose baseline covariables and symptoms up to withdrawal are similar to that of the discontinued subject. Suppose no post-withdrawal data are collected, as is still common in clinical trials. In these circumstances, MAR's estimate of efficacy for the discontinued subject will be based on subjects who remained on study treatment. Such subjects are likely to be an "elite" group of stronger or healthier subjects, and of course also have remained on treatment, while the withdrawal has ceased study treatment. In some cases, MAR is likely then to overestimate the efficacy for that subject, in the context of an ITT analysis. For subjects who withdraw for drug intolerability reasons but who positively responded to treatment in terms of the primary outcome prior to discontinuation, MAR is likely to impute rather more favorable symptoms than might be clinically plausible, especially given that the subject may no longer be receiving treatment for the indication. However, as against this, MAR takes into account a withdrawal's previous outcomes in imputing; for withdrawals, previous outcomes tend to be poor; so outcomes for withdrawals will tend to be imputed based on poorly performing completers, and the imputed outcome will tend to be relatively poor, compared to the mean observed outcome for the subject's treatment group. Thus, insofar as, prior to withdrawal, the average symptoms of subjects who discontinue tends to be relatively poor, MAR will tend in the main to impute less favorable values for discontinuations, based on other subjects with poor outcomes. Because MAR will in practice, in the main, base imputations on completers with relatively poor results, any overestimation of treatment effect due to the use of completers in the model will tend to be modest, and will be smaller than a simple assumption that "withdrawals are similar to those who remain on treatment."

The overall effect of MAR versus other assumptions on the estimate of treatment effect will depend on the relative proportions of dropouts in each treatment group, and on the timing of dropouts.

Multiple imputation and direct likelihood methods such as MMRM can be used to implement the MAR assumption. As noted in Chapter 1, MI can include ancillary variables, including post-baseline variables, to help model missing values of the outcome, which is not possible when using MMRM, and thus may model missing values better than MMRM. Inverse probability weighted estimation, including doubly robust estimation, can also be used, although it is so rather more rarely in pharmaceutical trials; when selection models are used, it is generally to model MNAR assumptions. (These methodologies are all briefly described in Chapter 1. Chapters 5 and 6 describe MMRM and MI in detail, with example SAS code to implement them. Appendices 7.I and 7.J describe selection models and shared parameter models, respectively. Chapter 8 describes weighted regression and doubly robust estimation, and includes SAS code to implement doubly robust estimation.) MAR assumes independence of missingness from unobserved values *conditional on the model used*, but since data are missing it is not possible to test satisfactorily whether the model is correct. This makes MAR vulnerable to model misspecification (National Research Council, 2010, p. 70). This is another potential source of bias in MAR approaches. If there is doubt about the model, a semi-parametric MAR approach such as GEE with IPW may be preferred. The clear disadvantage is that the weighting of the GEE makes it inefficient, compared to parametric approaches. The efficiency of IPW is improved in doubly robust estimation, which augments the modeled estimate with a function of the observed data that can model the missing data.

We saw in Chapter 1 that MCAR assumes that missingness is independent of observed and unobserved outcomes, given the statistical model; given the statistical model and the observed outcomes, MAR assumes that missingness is independent of unobserved outcomes; and MNAR assumes that missingness is dependent on the unobserved outcomes. If there are clinical grounds for believing that efficacy for discontinued subjects will differ from efficacy for similar subjects who continued in the trial, then the MAR assumption does not hold, and we must consider adopting some MNAR assumption for the primary analysis of the trial. The practical problems believed to be associated with MNAR approaches have led some to recommend avoiding MNAR for the primary analysis: "MNAR methods are not well suited for the primary analyses in confirmatory clinical trials wherein a dependable, pre-specified method is needed" (Mallinckrodt *et al.*, 2008) "... no individual MNAR analysis can be considered definitive." However, Little and Yau's (1996) idea of using results from selected trial arms to impute missing values for other trial arms gives rise to a convenient and intuitively appealing set of MNAR approaches, and software is now becoming available to implement these (see Chapter 7). MNAR methods stemming from Little and Yau's paper are sometimes referred to as using control- or reference-based imputation.

Control- or reference-based imputation: If a particular set of MNAR assumptions seems most clinically plausible for the trial, this set can and should be chosen as the basis for primary analysis (rather than, say, MAR), and then sensitivity analyses could implement some other MNAR assumptions, or indeed the MAR assumption. An MNAR assumption that can sometimes be justified is that withdrawals from the experimental treatment group have efficacy like that observed in similar subjects in some reference group, usually the control treatment group, after withdrawal. An advantage of this strategy is that it is straightforward to describe to clinicians, and it can be easily vetted for clinical plausibility. It has been argued that a source of bias here is that the subjects in the control group who stay in the study are likely to be themselves an elite subset, with outcomes better than those subjects from the control group who discontinued. The reasoning then is that if we use the control arm to impute data for subjects from the experimental arm, we are assuming too favorable an outcome. Against that we note that relatively poor outcomes from partially observed control subjects who withdraw are included in the control-based imputation model. If, despite this, imputations based on the control group are somewhat optimistic, we note also that the imputed values will be used for both control and experimental treatment groups. This does not palliate the bias, if it exists, in the estimate of efficacy score for each treatment, but should make that bias less serious for an estimate of treatment effect, where the potentially elite group of control completers would have been used to impute missings for both the experimental treatment group and the control group with which it is contrasted. Finally, we note that, if it is deemed clinically plausible, it is possible in some varieties of control-based imputation to reflect the fact that withdrawals tend to have poor outcomes relative to others in *their own treatment group*, by imputing outcomes that are relatively poor compared *to the control group*. See Section 7.3.5 for more detailed discussion of varieties of control-based assumption.

Other MNAR approaches: As noted, the variety of MNAR assumptions is of its nature infinite, and so it is difficult to discuss the bias that could be inherent in MNAR. If the MNAR assumption is implemented via MI, then the variance of the estimate of treatment effect is likely to be sensible. It will remain for the statistician, clinician and perhaps also the regulator to work together to find MNAR assumptions that are plausible for missing data for each study, indication and treatment, and that will thus give rise to estimates of treatment effect that can be accepted as "unlikely to be biased in favor of the experimental treatment to an important degree" (European Medicines Agency, 2010). For example, we have seen an MNAR primary analysis that, after considerable consultation with the regulator, implemented the assumption that a subject who discontinued due to AE or lack of efficacy subsequently had efficacy distributed like baseline, while for subjects who discontinued for other reasons, efficacy was distributed similarly to two mid-study visits.

4.2.3   Using historic data to narrow the choice of primary analysis and sensitivity analyses

In choosing and justifying a primary analysis and sensitivity analyses, the statistician will need to take account of the following:

- objective of the study (superiority, non-inferiority, equivalence);
- the type of the primary outcome measure (continuous, categorical, composite measures, co-primary endpoints);
- the expected spontaneous changes over time in the primary outcome – natural course of disease, whether treated with the control treatment, the experimental treatment, standard of care or (if applicable) with no treatment; for example, expected to improve, expected to deteriorate or remain stable; and the rate of changes, if any;
- potential relationship between missingness, treatment assignment and outcome:
  - difference between treatment groups in proportion of dropouts;
  - difference between treatment groups in timing of dropouts;
  - reason for subject dropout (efficacy/safety/other by treatment group);
  - relationship of the observed outcome to dropout;
  - planned dropout, for example, specific AEs or forbidden medications that are expected to trigger the decision to withdraw;
  - combinations of the above;
  - likely outcome for subjects who discontinue from the experimental treatment.

Evidence about the following relationships, if they exist, can also help to improve the planned approach:

- relationship of secondary endpoints to dropout;
- relationship of baseline characteristics to dropout.

The statistician should gather as much information as possible in terms of what is the most likely pattern of missing data with respect to the above aspects for a given trial. This information can be gathered from other statisticians, clinicians and project managers (if a clinical research organization (CRO) is involved, both sponsor and CRO can contribute), results of previous studies and the literature. The statistician should then include in the protocol or SAP a discussion on how the selected analysis method uses or is influenced by the above information (e.g., in the explicit imputation or implicit assumptions in direct likelihood approaches such as MMRM) and why it is appropriate in terms of bias and effect on variance of the treatment effect estimate, based on each aspect of the missing data pattern. In the remainder of this chapter, we will provide examples of such discussions for several clinical trials. For three illustrative datasets, the feasibility of options for handling missing data will be examined. We believe that there will often be a number of feasible and justifiable options for handling missing data in a study. The final set of primary and sensitivity analyses should be a well-defined subset of these. In Chapter 7, we will take each indication in turn, and choose a subset of analyses for each such as might be chosen in a real clinical trial. We will then show in detail how the analyses may be implemented in SAS; we also discuss the results of these analyses in the three illustrative datasets.

4.2.3.1 Using historic data, example 1: Parkinson's disease

To illustrate how historic data can inform the process of finding feasible approaches to missing data, we take the planning of a study in early Parkinson's disease (PD), using the illustrative dataset that features in Chapter 1 and that will also be used in Chapters 5–7. Our illustrative study has the objective of showing superiority of a new treatment over a control that is close to standard of care. The primary test is based on change in a standard measure of efficacy, a sub-score of UPDRS, measured at Week 24. For PD, as for many diseases, data are available for expected spontaneous changes over time. Figures 4.1–4.3 show efficacy results for three longitudinal studies in early PD, two of which we have already cited in Chapter 1:

For all studies, a low efficacy score is better, a high score is worse. All three studies show an initial improvement (even in the placebo groups) followed at some time before Week 20 with a reversion to the progression associated with PD. Thus although PD is a progressive disease, simple progression is not to be expected in a clinical trial of PD, in any treatment group.

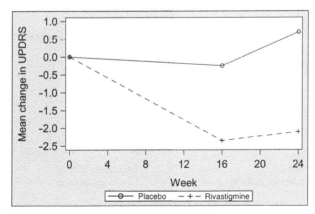

Figure 4.1   Efficacy scores in early Parkinson's disease, rivastigmine study (Emre et al., 2004).

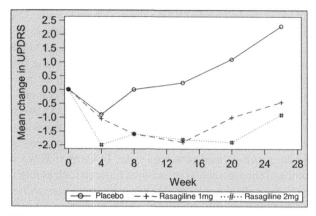

Figure 4.2   Efficacy scores in early Parkinson's disease, rasagiline study (Parkinson Study Group, 2004a).

The papers referenced also give some data regarding proportions of subjects discontinuing in the studies and their reasons for discontinuation. These are presented in Table 4.1.

For the newer treatments rivastigmine and rasagiline, rates of discontinuation are considerably higher than for their respective control treatment groups (27.3% vs. 17.9% and 6.4% vs. 3.6%). In the rivastigmine study, a higher proportion of subjects in the control group withdraw due to lack of efficacy, compared to the experimental treatment group; but the largest source of withdrawal is AE/death in the experimental arm. In the levodopa study, in contrast, the rate of withdrawals is higher in the

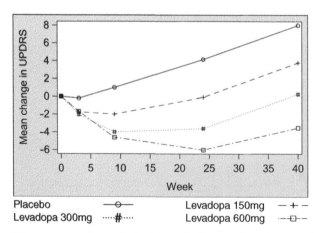

Figure 4.3   Efficacy scores in early Parkinson's disease, levodopa study (Parkinson Study Group, 2004a).

Table 4.1   Discontinuation from Parkinson's disease studies, by treatment group and reason.

	Rivastigmine study		Rasagiline study		Levadopa study	
	Active	Control	Active	Control	Active	Control
N	362	179	266	138	271	90
Reason discontinued						
Lack of efficacy, %	0.6	2.2	N/A	N/A	3.0	14.4
AE/death, %	18.2	11.7	N/A	N/A	1.8	3.3
Other, %	8.9	5.1	N/A	N/A	6.2	4.5
Overall, %	27.3	17.9	6.4	3.6	11.0	22.2

control arm (again due to lack of efficacy) and AE/death is a relatively infrequent reason for discontinuation.

For this study, as for all, an important part of the planning will be to decide on a subject retention plan. This will be a task for the entire study team, including the statistician (refer to Chapter 2 for suggestions).

A second task will be to arrive at primary assumptions about missingness and missing values that are considered most plausible for this trial. This stage will be a collaborative effort between clinicians and statisticians. Historic data such as we present above provides considerable evidence to help with this. Let us suppose that our treatment is thought to be similar in its safety profile to rivastigmine. If this is the case, it may be thought reasonable in the new study to expect more discontinuations in the experimental arm, with a relatively high proportion of these due to AE, while discontinuations in the control arm are likely to be due to lack of efficacy. An initial improvement can be expected in all treatment arms, followed by disease progression at about mid-study.

This next stage – identifying a reasonable set of approaches for the primary and sensitivity analyses – is mainly the responsibility of the statistician.

Inasmuch as there is historic evidence, the statistician should postulate plausible deviations from the assumption made about missing data by the primary analysis. For our illustrative PD data, evidence is lacking about the likely outcome of subjects who discontinue treatment, especially in the case of the experimental treatment. Unfortunately, such evidence will often be lacking, until more studies collect post-withdrawal data. The uncertainty about outcomes after withdrawal should here motivate the statistician to posit a suitably wide variety of scenarios for subjects who discontinue, when planning sensitivity analyses for this trial.

In this first example, to help illustrate the reasoning in detail, we will start by eliminating approaches that are unsuitable, given the assumptions that we have derived from historic data and our knowledge of the experimental treatment. As noted, we will then identify a set of reasonable approaches.

LOCF-like approaches: We know from the historic data that in studies such as the one we are planning, the indication is expected to worsen, albeit after a short period of improvement. We have seen that, for such progressive diseases such as Parkinson's disease, LOCF tends to favor the treatment with more or earlier withdrawals. Despite initial improvement, the generally progressive nature of PD suggests that LOCF is not a sensible approach here. In addition, we see that in a treatment similar to the experimental arm (rivastigmine) there were considerably more withdrawals in the experimental treatment group, compared with the control. It would be reasonable to suppose therefore that, in the study being planned, a greater proportion of subjects would discontinue from the experimental arm than the control arm, and that therefore LOCF would tend to be biased in favor of the experimental arm, especially if withdrawals were in the later part of the study when subjects' efficacy score is expected to revert to the gradual worsening that is typical of PD. This is further reason that LOCF-like approaches are not sensible for this study.

BOCF-like approaches: The progressive nature of Parkinson's also means that by the end of the study, for a significant proportion of subjects, efficacy score could be expected to be worse than baseline. This would likely rule out BOCF as a sensible approach, since the baseline score imputed to withdrawals by BOCF could be quite a favorable outcome, and could therefore bias the estimate of efficacy in favor of treatments with more withdrawals. So the statistician would likely rule out BOCF-like approaches also.

Armed with the historic data the statistician, having eliminated some options, can assess a set of options for missing data that could be justified for the study.

Worst-case approaches: What about a worst-case approach? We have given objections to the worst-case approach for continuous outcomes. However, a responder analysis, counting subjects with a missing value as a non-responder, could help interpret the study. As noted earlier, such an analysis uses a variety of worst-case imputation. Given the poor sensitivity of binary responses, compared with continuous ones, a responder analysis is not usually the optimal choice, from the statistical point of view, for a primary analysis. Nevertheless, responder analysis could be useful when a significantly greater proportion of discontinuations are expected in the experimental arm compared with the control arm, and an unambiguously negative interpretation is desired for the withdrawals. Such a worst-case imputation may be particularly appropriate if a high proportion of withdrawals due to side effects are anticipated in the experimental arm. We have seen some evidence in Table 4.1 that a rivastigmine-like treatment might indeed have significant withdrawals due to side effects.

Assuming MAR: An approach that uses study data to model missing outcomes – an MAR approach – has the advantage that it will impute missing values taking into account the trajectory of symptoms of the trial indication (as it does in Figure 1.6). For a progressive disease such as PD, MAR will tend to reflect the general worsening, and will be less likely than LOCF-like approaches to benefit a treatment group with a higher proportion of withdrawals. The objection of the NRC report and EU guidance documents remains, that MAR may attribute treatment benefit to withdrawals even though they are no longer taking the treatment. Despite this objection, MAR has been accepted in many indications as a primary analysis. We have noted also that MAR will reflect the poor post-baseline symptoms that are typically observed prior to withdrawal; and that this may tend to counteract the fact that under MAR withdrawals are modeled on patients who remain on treatment. But more and more frequently, if MAR is assumed, sensitivity analyses are required to ascertain that the result from the primary analysis holds when less or no effect from the study treatment is assumed in withdrawals. Depending on clinical opinion and evidence from historic data (if any) regarding the outcome of subjects who discontinue the experimental treatment, MAR may be a choice for the primary analysis in this case. That is, it may be justified as "not biased to an important degree in favor of the experimental treatment." For implementation, see Chapters 5 (MMRM) and 6 (MI), and also in some cases Chapter 8 (weighted and doubly robust estimation).

Control-based imputation: Control-based imputation uses a reference study arm to impute the missing values of the experimental treatment arm. This is an MNAR approach, in that it imputes missing values in a way that is not directly modeled from the relationships observed in the study. If it is reasonable to assume that subjects who withdraw from the experimental arm have symptoms whose trajectory is like that of subjects observed in the control arm, then the statistician can justify using such control- or reference-based imputation in the primary analysis. Further, as noted above, control-based imputation could be acceptable, even when withdrawals are taking an alternative treatment that is better than the control. In that case, the primary analysis will be based on scores that do not necessarily reflect what actually happened to subjects, but assign a poor outcome for the subjects with missing data, giving an estimated mean efficacy score that could be used to estimate the effect *attributable to* study treatment. For implementation via a pattern-mixture approach using MI, see Chapter 7.

Other MNAR approaches: Depending again on clinical opinion and evidence from historic data, particularly about the likely outcomes of subjects who discontinue treatment, other MNAR assumptions may be justified for the primary analysis. Many useful MNAR options can be implemented using variations on reference-based imputation. For example, as noted earlier it could be judged clinically reasonable for some indications to assume a BOCF-like outcome for withdrawals due to side effects, and a mid-study own-treatment value for other withdrawals. Alternatively, it may be judged reasonable to assume that certain withdrawals are worse than modeled by MAR, by some chosen amount delta. Both these sets of assumptions use in-study values in a flexible way to impute missings. Chapter 7 indicates how such options can be implemented similarly to the more commonly discussed reference-based imputation.

The choice of sensitivity analyses for this study in PD should stress test the assumptions adopted by the primary analysis, and should do so in a way that either is not likely to favor the experimental treatment group, or indeed is likely to be unfavorable to it. Then if the results of sensitivity analyses are consistent with those of the primary analysis, readers of the trial report will have reason to be confident of the conclusions from the primary analysis, despite missing data. Thus, if a MAR approach is taken for the primary analysis, a suitable sensitivity analysis could be an MNAR approach that assumes withdrawals from the experimental treatment arm had efficacy worse than similar subjects who remained in the study – just how much worse will depend on evidence from the literature regarding withdrawals, and on what the team decide is clinically reasonable for withdrawals. If the protocol is discussed with the regulator, this can be a source of helpful advice also. For PD, there are a number of useful options for sensitivity analyses among those mentioned above, all using the idea of reference-based imputation. Options include assuming that withdrawals from the experimental treatment arm have efficacy

- as bad as the control arm (i.e., control-based imputation, using one of the varieties discussed in 7.3.5);

- worse than other subjects in the experimental arm by some clinically-selected delta (here the reference treatment is the subject's own treatment group, modified by the delta); or

- worse than subjects in the control arm by some clinically-selected delta (i.e., control-based imputation, again modified by a chosen delta).

An additional option for a sensitivity analysis that is applicable to most indications, including Parkinson's disease, is to make a variety of different assumptions for outcome in the experimental arm, depending on the subject's reason for withdrawal. Any of the above three assumptions in the bullet points above, and the MAR assumption, may be suitable. For example, MAR may be assumed for subjects who discontinued for administrative reasons; it may be assumed that subjects who discontinued for lack of efficacy have missing outcomes that can be modeled on the control arm; and that subjects who discontinued for safety reasons have missing outcomes that can be modeled on the control arm, worsened by some delta.

A second option for sensitivity analysis that is generally applicable, of which there are a number of examples in the NRC report (National Research Council, 2010) is the tipping point approach (see also Chapter 3 and Chapter 7). This approach simply extends the delta-adjusting approach, by repeatedly adding more extreme deltas, until the conclusion of the primary analysis could no longer be made. Clinicians can then assess the plausibility of the delta that resulted in the change of conclusion. If that delta is plausible, then the conclusion from primary analysis may be doubted. If the delta is not plausible, then the conclusion of the primary analysis may be regarded as resistant to that particular stress test.

We note that delta adjustment and "tipping point" analyses for missing binary responses are discussed separately in Section 4.2.3.3.

Implementation of all the above sensitivity analyses is described in Chapter 7.

Summary: The following approaches could be suitable for primary analyses for the PD study, depending on clinical input regarding likely outcomes for withdrawals:

- MAR approach implementable either via MI or via direct likelihood approaches such as MMRM;

- Control-based imputation for the experimental arm.

The following could be useful sensitivity analyses in this case:

• Control-based imputation for the experimental arm (if not used as primary);

• Assume a variety of outcomes for missing values, depending on reason for discontinuation;

• Tipping point analysis, using delta adjustment for subjects on experimental arm, increasing delta until primary conclusion is nullified.

If the experimental arm has notably more discontinuations than the control arm due to side effects, then the following analysis could be considered:

• Responder analysis imputing treatment failure for subjects with missing data.

An available cases analysis should also be included to provide background information with which to assess the primary and sensitivity analyses. Furthermore, if a direct likelihood approach such as MMRM is used for the primary analysis, and sensitivity analyses use MI, it is helpful to include as background an MI analysis that follows the direct likelihood model and assumptions as closely as possible. The results of the MI and direct likelihood analyses would be expected to be very similar. Such an MI analysis, not strictly speaking a sensitivity analysis itself, will reassure the reader of the study report that any change in the estimate of treatment effect in the "real" sensitivity analyses is due only to the change in assumptions, and not to the change from using MMRM to using MI.

As noted above, MI can include post-baseline auxiliary or ancillary variables to help model missing values of the outcome, which is not possible when using MMRM, and thus may model of missing values better than MMRM. If the primary analysis uses MMRM it will be useful, therefore, to include not only a matching MI but also, as a kind of sensitivity analysis of the MMRM model, a "full" MI. By a "full" MI we mean an MI that includes extra variables (e.g., likely post-baseline variables other than the primary outcome) that seem to be associated with missingness. If the sensitivity analyses are planned to use other variables additional to those used in the primary analysis (e.g., additional demographic variables or additional interactions with visit), these additional variables should also be included in the "full" MI analysis.

If the primary analysis used a direct likelihood approach such as MMRM, the statistician then has a choice with regard to the MI model to be used as a basis in sensitivity analyses.

1. The statistician may choose the MI model that matches the MMRM analysis. Results from such an MI will be easy to interpret – changes in the estimate of treatment effect should be due solely to changes in assumptions about missing data modeled in the MI sensitivity analysis.

2. The statistician may choose the "full" MI model as a basis for the sensitivity analyses. Results based on the "full" MI may model missing values better, compared to the primary analysis. But the sensitivity analysis from a "full" MI cannot be compared directly to an MMRM analysis to give a verdict

about robustness. The reader of the study report will need to compare such sensitivity analyses with the MAR "full" MI, and assess robustness to the MAR assumption in this indirect way.

3. The statistician can always perform the sensitivity analyses twice – once using as a basis the model that matches MMRM, and once with the "full" MI model.

See Appendix 4.A for sample protocol/SAP text that might be used for this planned study. (Protocol text describing a subject retention plan is included in the Appendix to Chapter 2).

In Chapter 7 we will attempt to make a reasonable selection from the justifiable primary and sensitivity analyses above, and implement them for our illustrative PD dataset.

We shall see that there are a cluster of options for primary and secondary analyses, many of which appear above, that will turn out to be sensible across most indications, albeit with details of the assumptions needing to be adjusted, depending on clinical expectation of outcomes for subjects who discontinue early. It should also be noted that the actual primary and sensitivity analyses that make it into the protocol will depend not just on scientific arguments. In practice, the following factors will also influence the final decision about the approaches to missing data:

- precedent in studies already performed: the wish of the team developing a new treatment to match approaches in previous studies in the development program and/or in the therapeutic area will sometimes lead to the choice of a primary analysis known to be suboptimal with regard to missing data; precedent in regulatory decisions: although it is known that regulatory practice with regard to missing data is beginning to change, the development team may feel it is safer to propose an approach to missing data that has previously been accepted by the regulator, even if historic data suggests the approach is biased; we note that prominent FDA statisticians have themselves encouraged new thinking on missing data (O'Neill, 2011; Permutt, 2011), so adherence to precedent may become less attractive over time;

- particular regulatory advice may encourage an approach to missing data that is not optimal and even not in accordance with the regulatory guidance documents – we have seen instances of regulators encouraging the use of LOCF in progressive disease, for example, even though regulatory guidance discourages this; we have seen regulators accept an available cases analysis as primary, stating that this would be acceptable provided the proportion of missings was not high.

Nevertheless, the statistician can and should in such cases put the argument for an evidence-based approach to missing data that takes account of likely patterns of outcome and of missingness.

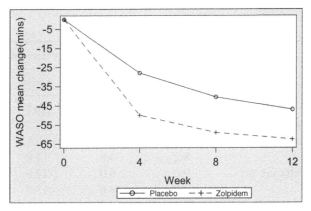

Figure 4.4   Change in WASO, zolpidem study (Krystal et al., 2008).

4.2.3.2   Using historic data, example 2: Insomnia

As a second illustration of using historic data to identify a set of justifiable options for a primary analysis, when missing data are a concern, we look at a trial of a treatment for insomnia. We will take the points made in discussing example 1 as read, and so our description of the process for this example and the following one will be briefer than for the PD example.

The objective in this insomnia study is to show superiority to a control treatment, this time a placebo control. We will suppose that the primary efficacy parameter is to be median minutes wake time after sleep onset (WASO) at 3 months.

As with PD, historic data are available regarding expected spontaneous changes in symptoms over time. Figures 4.4 and 4.5 are fairly typical examples from the literature.

The measure for both studies is WASO, where a low score is better, a high score is worse. We see from the historic data that subjects with this indication tend to improve

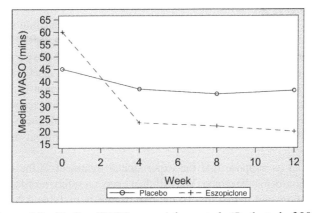

Figure 4.5   Median WASO, eszopiclone study (Roth et al., 2005).

Table 4.2   Discontinuation from example studies of insomnia, by treatment group and reason.

	Zolpidem study		Eszopiclone study	
	Active	Control	Active	Control
N	669	349	593	195
Reason discontinued				
Lack of efficacy, %	4.8	23.5	N/A	N/A
AE/death, %	8.2	4.6	12.8	7.1
Voluntary withdrawal, %[a]	9.6	6.0	13.8	26.0
Other, %	13.0	18.6	12.9	10.3
Overall, %	35.6	52.7	39.5	43.4

[a]Includes "patient/investigator request."

over time, although the rate of improvement may be slower for the placebo group. This contrasts with the Parkinson's subjects, whose efficacy scores improved but then worsened. It seems reasonable, therefore, to expect in the planned illustrative study a pattern of improvement over time in efficacy scores in both treatment arms, similar to that which we see in the historic data.

The papers referenced in the figure captions give summaries of proportions of subjects discontinuing in the studies, and their reasons for discontinuation. These are presented in Table 4.2.

In the two studies we have taken as examples, a higher proportion of subjects tends to discontinue from the control arm, compared to the active arm. However, other studies from the same period (see, e.g., in www.clinicaltrials.gov NCT00784875 and NCT466193 (Purdue Pharma LP, 2007; Eli Lilly and Company, 2008) with similar experimental arms show a variety of patterns, so there is substantial uncertainty in the case of insomnia as to the relative rates of dropouts that may be expected in experimental and control arms.

In the two example studies, the main reasons for discontinuation in the control arm are lack of efficacy in the zolpidem study (23.5% vs. 4.8% for the experimental arm) and patient/investigator Request (26.0% vs. 13.8% for the experimental arm). However, there is some evidence of a greater proportion of discontinuations due to AD in the experimental arm, compared with the control arm (8.2% vs. 4.6% and 12.8% vs. 7.1% in the zolpidem and eszopiclone studies, respectively). We note that in other studies of zolpidem and eszopiclone, including the NCT00784875 and NCT466193 studies just cited, differences in rates of dropout due to AE are very small.

However, let us suppose that the experimental treatment in the study we are planning is a non-benzodiazepine. We will then expect a safety profile and a pattern of discontinuations not unlike that of the two examples in Table 4.2. That is, it is reasonable to expect a higher proportion of withdrawals in the control arm, compared to the experimental arm, but with the experimental arm having a somewhat higher proportion of dropouts due to AE. As always, the entire study team should collaborate on a subject retention plan, making use of historic data such as we have presented here and of information from previous studies in the development plan for the treatment. Refer to Chapter 2 for examples of other relevant information that may be gathered and suggestions for potential preventive actions.

As with PD, evidence about the likely outcome of subjects who discontinue the experimental treatment is sparse. Holm and Goa (2000) state that "there is little evidence of . . . rebound insomnia or withdrawal symptoms after discontinuation of the drug when it is given as recommended." Blumer *et al.* (2009) in a study of pediatrics with attention-deficit/hyperactivity disorder, stated that "both (zolpidem and placebo) groups experienced worsening from baseline in latency to persistent sleep (LPS) on post-discontinuation nights 1 and 2, (and) the difference was not significant . . . Similarly, total sleep time (TST) on post-discontinuation night 1 was lower than baseline values for both groups. The effect was not observed on night 2." Thus such evidence as is available suggests that symptoms worsen only for a short period after discontinuation for both placebo and experimental treatment groups.

In summary, historic data suggests that it would be reasonable to assume general monotone improvement in efficacy scores in all subjects while they are in the study. Figures 4.4–4.5 suggest that efficacy scores for the control group are often worse than for experimental arms; and the overall trajectory of the control group (i.e., the slope of the plot of mean efficacy score) tends to be shallower, although Figure 4.4 suggests that this may not always be the case for later visits; this suggests that a control-based approach is not likely to favor the experimental arm, and could encourage its use as a primary or sensitivity analysis (though see 7.5.2 for further discussion about this). We may expect a higher proportion of dropouts in the control arm, but more dropouts due to AE in the experimental arm. There is some uncertainty about likely efficacy scores after discontinuation, but "rebound," if it occurs after discontinuation of treatment, is likely to be short-lived. It will be the responsibility of the clinical expert and the statistician to agree on likely patterns of efficacy, safety and discontinuation such as we have just summarized.

The statistician will then be responsible for identifying a primary analysis with assumptions for missing data that can, given the above information from historic data, be justified as not being biased in favor of the experimental arm to an important degree. The statistician will also be responsible for finding sensitivity analyses that stress test the chosen primary analysis in a clinically interpretable and plausible way.

We can quickly run through some options for primary and sensitivity analyses as we did for the hypothetical PD study:

LOCF-like approaches: These are likely to penalize the treatment arm that has earlier or more frequent discontinuations, and so to that extent appealing, even though probably not clinically plausible. But the historic data suggests that there will be more frequent discontinuations in the control group, so LOCF will likely penalize the control arm more than the experimental arm. Therefore, LOCF-like approaches could be said to be likely to favor the experimental arm. This makes LOCF unattractive as a primary analysis, and not very useful as a stress-testing sensitivity analysis. However, a hybrid approach could be considered, where MAR is assumed for the control arm an LOCF-like for the experimental arm. While such an approach would be seen as likely to avoid favoring the experimental arm, like standard LOCF it may be difficult to justify as plausible in clinical terms.

BOCF-like and worst-case approaches: These have the same advantages and disadvantages as LOCF-like approaches.

Assuming MAR: As with PD, it may be regarded as an advantage that MAR will capture the general efficacy trend over time and apply it to withdrawals. In this case, however, the trend is for efficacy scores to improve. Clinicians, regulators and sufferers from insomnia may baulk at MAR's assumption that even subjects who cease to take medication will improve in their symptoms over time. They may point out that such evidence as we have suggests that after discontinuation from treatment, even placebo treatment, symptoms worsen temporarily. Against this, it can be argued that symptoms in the placebo treatment group improved in past studies, so subjects discontinuing treatment may do so as well, in the medium and longer term. Some additional justification of MAR can be made by noting its inherently sophisticated use of a subject's observed data to model missing data. Subjects who discontinue tend to have observed efficacy scores somewhat worse than the mean for their treatment group. MAR will generally reflect this by imputing values at the primary time point that are likewise somewhat worse than the mean for the treatment group. In summary, MAR is a potential assumption for the primary analysis in this case, but a careful justification would be needed.

Control-based imputation: The statistician will need to consult with clinicians and check the literature further regarding likely outcomes of subjects who discontinue study treatment. If it is reasonable to assume for insomnia that enrolled subjects treated with the experimental treatment who withdraw from the experimental arm have symptoms whose trajectory is like that of subjects observed in the control arm, then the statistician can justify using such control- or reference-based imputation in the primary analysis. We have noted that the overall trajectory of the control group (i.e., the slope of the plot of mean efficacy score) can be shallower than that of the experimental arm in insomnia studies, so there is at least some evidence that control-based imputation will be likely to impute worse scores for dropouts from the experimental arm, compared with MAR. We shall, however, see a surprising result from control-based imputation in the insomnia dataset in Section 7.5.2.

Other MNAR approaches: If there is evidence that outcomes could be poor after discontinuing treatment, and moving to standard therapy, then consider an MNAR approach that attributes a suitably poor result to withdrawals from the experimental arm. There is some evidence that at least an initial worsening is associated with discontinuing treatment in insomnia, so there may be case for such an MNAR assumption here. If not deployed in the primary analysis, then such an approach could well be useful as a sensitivity analysis. As with the PD study, another MNAR option that could be useful with insomnia would be to make a variety of different assumptions for outcome in the experimental arm, depending on the subject's reason for withdrawal. As noted in our discussion of Table 4.2, in the historic data, side effects (AEs) and withdrawal of consent seem to be relatively common reasons for withdrawal in the experimental arm, with lack of efficacy more prominent common in the control arm. An analysis delta-adjusting the efficacy of those who withdraw with a reason of AE or consent withdrawn could be plausible.

Summary: The following approaches could be suitable for the primary analysis for the illustrative study in insomnia, depending on clinical input regarding likely outcomes for withdrawals:

- MAR approach implementable either via MI or a direct likelihood approach such as MMRM;

- Control-based imputation for the experimental arm;

- Delta adjustment of MAR outcome for subjects in the experimental arm who discontinued for lack of efficacy, AEs or through personal choice.

The following could be useful sensitivity analyses:

- Control-based imputation for the experimental arm (if not used as primary);

- Responder analysis imputing treatment failure for subjects with missing data;

- LOCF-like assumption for experimental arm with MAR assumption for control arm;

- Assume a variety of outcomes for missing values, depending on reason for discontinuation, perhaps as in the third option for primary analysis above;

- Tipping point analysis, using delta adjustment for subjects on experimental arm, increasing delta until the primary conclusion is nullified.

As with the previous example, an available cases analysis should also be included to provide background information with which to assess the primary and sensitivity analyses. Again, if MMRM is used for the primary analysis, a matching MI should be provided to assure the reader of the study report of the similarity of the two methodologies; a "full" MI, with all useful post-baseline explanatory variables, should also be included; and the statistician will need to choose which of the MI models to use as a basis for the sensitivity analyses, or whether to perform the sensitivity analyses twice, once with the model that matches MMRM, and once with a "full" model as a basis.

As with the PD case, Chapter 7 will attempt to select a realistic subset of the above possible primary analyses and stress-testing sensitivity analyses, and show the results in our illustrative insomnia dataset.

We can see that the array of viable options is close to that for the study inPD, even though subjects with PD are expected to worsen while subjects with insomnia are expected to improve over time; and despite the fact that a greater proportion of subjects were expected to discontinue in the experimental arm for PD, while the control arm were expected to have a greater proportion of discontinuations in the case of insomnia.

See Appendix 4.A for a sample protocol/SAP text many of whose elements apply to this planned study.

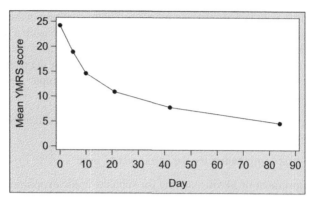

Figure 4.6   Young mania rating scale (YMRS) in subjects treated with valproate (Bowden et al., *2010). The profile for subjects treated with lithium in this study is very similar.*

4.2.3.3   Using historic data, example 3: Mania

In the third example, we are planning a study in mania of a treatment similar to valproate, with efficacy that is hoped to be somewhat better than lithium. The objective is to show superiority to the lithium control. In this case the planned primary efficacy parameter is a binary responder variable derived from the Young Mania Rating Scale (YMRS). For the YMRS scale, lower scores are better. The primary test of the null hypothesis of no treatment difference in proportion of responders is planned to be at the Week 6 visit.

For mania, the available evidence about the trajectory of symptoms is more complex than for PD or insomnia. Mean YMRS scores in Bowden *et al.* (2010) presented in Figure 4.6 suggest that for the majority of subjects on treatment the symptoms will improve.

However, the symptoms of mania are often cyclical in nature. There is evidence that a subset of subjects with mania may relapse or fail to respond (Lipkovich *et al.*, 2008 – see Figure 4.7).

Post *et al.* (2005) also present YMRS scores for non-responders and early discontinuations (Figure 4.8). Again, the data suggest that a rapid worsening may occur in a subset of subjects with mania, even while treated. While neither Post *et al.* nor Lipkovich *et al.* present direct data about YMRS scores after the subject has discontinued, the trajectories of symptoms they present could provide a basis for some clinically plausible pessimistic scenarios that could be used for early discontinuations in sensitivity analyses.

Thus the historic data suggests that subjects in studies of mania such as we are planning can overall be expected to improve over time; but a significant proportion of subjects may relapse and change from improvement to worsening efficacy scores.

From the literature, Table 4.3 summarizes proportions of subjects discontinuing in two studies of mania, and their reasons for discontinuation.

Table 4.3   Discontinuation from studies of mania, by treatment group and reason.

	Valproate study (double blind, 12-month follow-up)		Olanzapine study (open label, 12-week follow-up)	
	Active	Lithium	Active	Lithium
N	132	138	217	214
Reason discontinued				
Lack of efficacy, %	9.8	9.4	18.9	25.7
AE/death, %	6.1	6.5	14.3	15.9
Withdrawal of consent, %	5.3	5.1	12.9	15.9
Lost to follow-up, %	8.3	6.5	0.9	0.5
Other, %	2.3	1.4	6.5	9.3
Overall, %	25.8	20.7	53.5	67.3

Note: Valproate study data from Bowden *et al.* (2010), in subjects with a manic or mixed episode); Olanzepine study in subjects with remission, from Tohen *et al.* (2005).

The two studies in Table 4.3 had different objectives and accordingly featured subjects with different expected symptom trajectories. This is reflected in differing rates of withdrawal. However, there does not appear to be significant differences between experimental and control arms in rates of withdrawal within each study. Nor are there obvious imbalances in reasons for withdrawal between the groups within a study, except perhaps for the case of lack of efficacy for subjects in the lithium arm in the olanzapine study, which was an open label study. However, the rate of withdrawal in both studies is relatively high. This means that the issue of missing data will be an important one for the study that we are planning, and the credibility of its results will likely depend quite heavily on the choice of primary and sensitivity analyses. There was no strong or definite pattern of differences in reasons for discontinuation in experimental versus control groups over the studies surveyed.

Thus previous studies in mania where lithium is the control treatment lead one to expect a relatively high proportion of discontinuations in the planned study, but one would expect the proportions in experimental and control arms to be similar. To put the rates of withdrawal in perspective, Table 4.4 presents proportions of

Table 4.4   Percentage of subjects with mania relapsed and responding in three example studies.

Study	N	% relapsing	% responding
Tohen *et al.*, 2004	68	49.2	
Bowden *et al.*, 2010	255		54.1
Lipkovich *et al.*, 2008	222	45.0	55.0

Note: Some authors report only relapsing subjects, some report only responders.

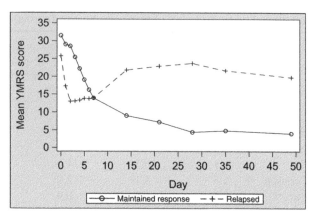

Figure 4.7   YMRS in subjects treated with olanzapine or divalproex: a group of subjects who did not maintain a response (N = 36) and a group who responded slowly and maintained response (N = 30) (Lipkovich et al., 2008). Lipkovich et al. also identified a group of rapid responders who maintained response (N = 92) and a group of rapid responders who did not maintain response (N = 36). These latter two groups are not plotted here.

responders and responders for the three trials we mention. The trials had just over 50% responders.

In summary, from the historic data for mania in settings similar to that of the planned study, the clinician and statistician might assume a mean improvement in symptoms over time, but with some examples – perhaps many – of relapses. We do not have strong historic evidence of the superiority to the control arm of treatments similar to the experimental treatment, so control-based assumptions may not be attractive here. Despite the availability of differing trajectories in the historic data in Figures 4.7 and 4.8, there is actually little evidence about symptoms after study withdrawal in this indication. Since sudden changes often seem to occur in individual efficacy

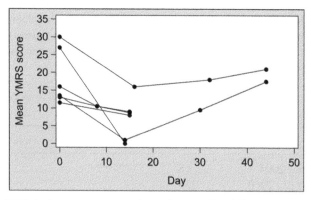

Figure 4.8   YMRS of two non-responders (data to day 44) and four early dropouts (Post et al., 2005).

scores, one may need to assume that post-withdrawal efficacy scores will not always be well modeled by scores before withdrawal. On the other hand, the rather smooth curve of Figure 4.6 suggests that relapsers and responders may to some extent cancel out. All this suggests that if MAR is assumed by the primary analysis, a sensitivity analysis positing poor outcomes for a significant proportion of withdrawals will be needed to stress test the MAR result. An assumption of 50–75% completers seems reasonable, but there is no evidence of differences in reasons for discontinuation between treatment groups, when the treatment groups are similar to those planned in the illustrative study.

Evidence such as the historic data above and evidence from previous studies in the development plan should be assessed by the study team as a whole. As with the other examples, the entire study team should also collaborate on a subject retention plan.

We again run through options for primary and sensitivity analyses for this illustrative case, showing how what we have learned from historic data allows us definitely to reject some assumptions, while helping us make an informed judgment – which may still be tentative – on the suitability of other assumptions.

LOCF-like approaches: For indications with an uncertain or varying trajectory such as we see for mania in Figures 4.7 and 4.8, it would not be possible to be sure about whether LOCF would under- or overestimate efficacy for the experimental arm. Therefore LOCF-like approaches have little to recommend them for this indication.

BOCF-like and worst-case approaches: Data from the small sample of studies we have identified give no evidence that rates of discontinuation are likely to differ as between experimental and control arms. If the planned study has similarly balanced rates of withdrawal, a worst-case imputation for withdrawals is not likely to be biased in favor of the experimental arm to an important degree. Therefore, a BOCF-like approach could be an option for this study. However, the worst-case assumption may be somewhat pessimistic clinically, given that it is unlikely that all withdrawals will relapse. This option should be viewed with caution, given that we expect high rates of withdrawal in both arms. The pessimistic assumption of BOCF could end up biasing the result slightly in favor of the experimental arm, if that arm had a small safety advantage over the control arm. Overall, a BOCF-like approach could be considered as an option for a sensitivity analysis, but probably not the primary analysis.

Assuming MAR: Given the likely mixed trend in efficacy, MAR has the attraction that it will make use of any worsening of symptoms immediately prior to discontinuation in its modeling of later post-withdrawal efficacy. Against the use of MAR is the possibility that sudden worsening in symptoms may occur (as seen in Figures 4.7 and 4.8) and be unrecorded and thus not reflected in imputations that assume MAR. As with the previous insomnia study, MAR is a potential assumption for the primary analysis in this case, but a careful justification would be needed. Note that it is straightforward to implement an MAR analysis of a binary variable using MI – the implementation will be described in Chapters 6 and 7.

Control-based imputation: The attractions of control-based imputation are not clear in the case of this indication and study. The control treatment, lithium, is quite effective, and as yet the evidence for the superiority of the experimental arm is mainly from animal studies. Therefore the assumption that withdrawals from the experimental arm will be similar to the control arm may not be particularly unfavorable to the experimental arm, and could possibly even bias the study in favor of that arm. Control-based imputation could perhaps be used as one of several sensitivity analyses.

Other MNAR approaches: For this indication, the data suggests that some subjects may have sudden shifts in the trajectory of symptoms. Where a subject's symptoms suddenly worsen change after withdrawal, and this is not recorded, it will of course be difficult to impute that worsening from study symptom data. The investigator's view of the reason for discontinuation may be valuable for this kind of subject. It will make sense to include as a sensitivity analysis the option of making a variety of different assumptions for outcome in the experimental arm, depending on the subject's reason for withdrawal.

Because of the evidence that relapses may occur, the statistician could also include a MNAR sensitivity analysis that simply attributes a poor result to all withdrawals from the experimental arm. For this indication, we have some quantitative data on the likely trajectory of treatment failures or relapsers. If the primary efficacy parameter were continuous, a delta-adjustment approach could give credibly pessimistic results – we could worsen the MAR result for the experimental arm by a delta estimated from, say, Figure 4.7 or 4.8. We could extend this approach by repeating it with successively more extreme deltas, to perform a "tipping point" analysis. It will be recalled that the "tipping point" analysis was considered an option for the two previous examples also. However, when the number of discontinuations is expected to be relatively high (as with this indication), it should be borne in mind that even a mild delta, when applied *to the entire set of withdrawals*, may be clinically implausible; furthermore, unless the evidence for the primary statistical test is very strong indeed, even a mild delta, if applied to all withdrawals, is likely to overturn any conclusion of the primary analysis. It will often be more clinically plausible to apply a delta or succession of deltas to a pre-planned subset of withdrawals, perhaps based on reason for withdrawal (e.g., those withdrew due to side effect or lack of efficacy, if such reasons are available).

If there is an underlying continuous variable from which the binary response is calculated, then delta and tipping point analyses can be performed on the continuous variable (perhaps along with other associated variables), as described in Section 4.2.3.1 above, and the binary response calculated from the imputed, delta-adjusted continuous variable (see Bunouf *et al.* (2012) for an example).

If it is desired to delta-adjust the binary response directly, perhaps because it is not derived from any other variable, a variety of delta and tipping point analyses are possible. In the case of our illustrative trial, the primary analysis is to be a binary (success/failure) variable that is not directly associated with any continuous variable. One tipping point analysis for this case has been described by Yan *et al.* of the U.S. Food and Drug Administration (2008), and has been submitted to the FDA (U.S. Food and Drug Administration, 2010). It consists of performing the primary analysis on the binary endpoint repeatedly for every possible scenario with regard to the missing endpoints. This could be called "tipping point analysis via exhaustive scenarios." In a simple example, if there were three missing endpoints in the experimental arm and two in the control arm, the primary analysis would be repeated assuming each of the following scenarios:

- three failures in the experimental arm with two successes in the control arm;
- three failures in the experimental arm with one success and one failure in the control arm;
- three failures in the experimental arm with two failures in the control arm;
- two failures and one success in the experimental arm with two successes in the control arm;
- two failures and one success in the experimental arm with one success and one failure in the control arm;
  and so on, up to
- three successes in the experimental arm with two failures in the control arm.

Those scenarios that have a p-value <0.05 are then indicated in a plot. The robustness of the primary result may be judged by the plausibility of the scenarios that render the p-value non-significant.

We note that if the number of missing responses is relatively large, a very large number of combinations of possible successes/failures exist in the treatment groups, of course. This will be less of a problem if one plans to implement the delta adjustment only on a subset of the discontinuing subjects. We have mentioned that that delta-adjusting a subset can often be more plausible clinically than applying the delta indiscriminately to all withdrawals.

An alternative tipping point analysis that uses a subset of the scenarios above is straightforward to implement when the primary analysis uses MI or can be approximated by MI. The procedure, which could be called "tipping point analysis via deviation from imputed success," can be as follows. Suppose m_i subjects in the experimental arm are imputed as responders. Repeat the primary analysis for each imputed dataset with $1, \ldots, m_i$ subjects in the experimental arm that were imputed as responders changed to non-responders.

Similarly, instead of changing $1, \ldots, m_i$ subjects, the experimental arm subjects could be changed randomly with a probability p; again, p could be increased until the p-value from the primary analysis is non-significant. We refer to this as "tipping point analysis via deviation from imputed probability of success."

Each of the above methods of implementing delta adjustment could be useful for the illustrative mania dataset.

Summary: The following approaches could be suitable for primary analyses for the study in mania:

- MAR approach using MI;
- worst-case imputation, that is, a subject with missing response is assumed to be a treatment failure (responder = N).

Whichever of the options above that was not selected for the primary analysis should be included as a sensitivity analysis. Other possible sensitivity analyses in this case include:

- Assume a variety of outcomes for missing values, depending on reason for discontinuation;

- Tipping point analyses, using successively more extreme scenarios until the primary conclusion is nullified, for subjects with a reason for discontinuation that suggests the possibility of relapse, side effect or treatment failure (note that this sensitivity analysis is a development of the previous one):

    o tipping point analysis via deviation from imputed probability of success;

    o tipping point analysis via deviation from imputed success.

We note that if the outcome were continuous, as opposed to binary, an option for sensitivity analysis would be delta adjustment of MAR outcome for selected subjects in the experimental arm, based on profile of "relapsers" from historic data.

Again, an available cases analysis should also be included to provide background information with which to assess the primary and sensitivity analyses.

Two factors in this example lead to a rather more restricted set of options for handling missing data, compared to the previous examples:

1. It is considered a possibility that the efficacy of the planned experimental treatment may not be as good as that of the control treatment (although of course there is some evidence from animal studies that it may be), so control-based approaches may not be appropriate.

2. The trajectory of the symptoms for the indication is unpredictable, so that any LOCF-like approach would not be suitable because it would run the risk of biasing the result in favor of the experimental arm.

See Appendix 4.A for a sample protocol/SAP text many of whose elements apply to this planned study.

4.2.3.4   Using historic data, general conclusions from examples

We can note that an MAR primary analysis, a delta-adjusting sensitivity analysis and a sensitivity analysis that assumes different outcomes depending on the reason for discontinuation are methods that may suit all three of the above examples, even though those examples differ as to efficacy trajectory; as to expected balance in discontinuation; as to expected balance in reasons for discontinuation; and as to type of primary efficacy parameter (binary vs. continuous).

4.2.4   Key points in choosing an approach for missing data

Use information from previous studies in the experimental treatment and in similar treatments to justify primary and secondary analyses.

The following recommendations are largely abstracted from points raised by three previous examples.

4.2.4.1 Assumptions for missing data: When to consider, when to avoid

MAR

Consider using where subjects who discontinue are likely to have post-withdrawal efficacy that could be imputed reasonably well from study data. Because it assumes that treatment differences observed in the study pertain also to post-withdrawal missing data, MAR is particularly suitable for studies where the objective is to assess equivalence or non-inferiority – it is unlikely that missing data will bias the conclusion in favor of equivalence or non-inferiority under the assumption of MAR, because any observed treatment differences are likely to be honored in inference about missing values.

Avoid using if there is evidence that the outcomes of subjects who withdraw early will tend to have post-discontinuation outcomes that could not be modeled from the study data, that is, if MNAR pertains, particularly if there is evidence that subjects who discontinue may have efficacy worse than observed in similar subjects who remain in the study.

LOCF-like approaches

Consider using when the indication is expected to improve over time, and the experimental treatment group is expected to have a higher rate of withdrawal than the control group. Use preferably as a sensitivity analysis rather than as a primary analysis. Under these rather restrictive conditions, LOCF-like methods are likely to underestimate the treatment effect, and so may be regarded as desirable by regulators, and perhaps by clinicians and subjects. However, it should be borne in mind that the lack of change in efficacy post-withdrawal that is assumed by LOCF will rarely be clinically plausible, so LOCF would need to be carefully justified if used. The absolute values of post-withdrawal efficacy imputed by LOCF-like approaches are difficult to be sure of in advance, because under- or over-estimation of efficacy with LOCF-like imputation depends both on the timing of withdrawals and the efficacy trajectory over time in each treatment group.

Avoid using

(a) if efficacy is expected to worsen during the time of the study, because for such indications LOCF has the unappealing effect of underestimating the progression of the disease in each arm;

(b) if efficacy is expected to improve during the time of the study, but earlier discontinuation, or a higher rate of discontinuations, is expected in the control group – in this case the missingness may underestimate the efficacy of the control group;

(c) if the likely efficacy trajectory is unknown, because the bias of the LOCF-like approach will likewise be unknown;

(d) if the objective of the study is to show non-inferiority or equivalence: LOCF-like approaches have some sensitivity to treatment differences when imputing, but the MAR assumption uses more data to inform imputation and should reflect in-study differences between treatment groups more accurately, in its inferences about missing post-withdrawal data; MAR will therefore be more likely to avoid a "false positive" finding of equivalence than LOCF, in the presence of missing data where the objective is to assess equivalence or non-inferiority.

BOCF-like and worst-case approaches

Consider using BOCF if historic data or expert opinion lead to the conclusion that symptoms of subjects who withdraw from a study are likely to revert to pre-study levels. A "poor case" approach may also be considered if justified by historic data, with discontinuations assumed to have outcomes that can be represented by samples from a pre-defined, relatively unfavorable region of the distribution of the outcome variable, such as from early visits where treatment has not had its full effect. A BOCF-like approach is sometimes required by the regulator, independent of the expected outcome for withdrawals, if it is felt that for the indication concerned it is simply incorrect to attribute any benefit to a treatment where the subject withdrew, or where a subject withdrew for reasons such as side effects. Studies in pain are an example where for this reason the regulator often requires a BOCF-like approach for the primary analysis. Alternatively, a mixture of BOCF and LOCF is sometimes favored by the regulator for pain studies, for subjects who discontinue due to AEs and for other reasons, respectively. If the primary endpoint is binary, then an approach that considers discontinuations as "failures" or non-responders may be useful, but only if a higher rate of discontinuation is expected in the experimental arm.

Avoid using where the objective of the study is to show non-inferiority or equivalence. BOCF-like and worst-case imputation tends to impute similar values to missing data in the reference and in the experimental arms. Such approaches will tend to bias the estimate of treatment effect towards the conclusion of similarity. For studies where the primary parameter is continuous, worst-case imputation is generally clinically implausible, and should be avoided; for a continuous primary parameter, "poor case" imputation may be useful. If we define a worst-case analysis in the special sense of imputing the worst case for the experimental arm and best case for control, then this analysis should be avoided unless there is some clinical evidence that withdrawals from the control arm are likely to have better outcomes than withdrawals from the experimental arm (a condition not often fulfilled in clinical trials).

Control- or reference-based imputation

Consider using if it is regarded as clinically plausible to attribute control-like efficacy to subjects who discontinued. Note that it may be valid to attribute control-like efficacy even for subjects who switched to a treatment more effective than control, if the estimand is "effect attributable to the study treatment" (see the discussion towards the end of 4.2.1 under the heading **Collecting post-withdrawal data**). If not used for the primary analysis, control-based imputation is often useful as a sensitivity analysis. Control-based imputation is particularly attractive if the control treatment is "standard of care," or close to it, because in this case the trajectory of efficacy attributed to withdrawals from the experimental arm can often be argued to be clinically neither too favorable nor too unfavorable.

Avoid using if there is some possibility that the experimental arm is not superior to the control or reference arm, or indeed if there is some evidence that withdrawals from the experimental arm have efficacy worse than that observed in the control treatment.

Assuming a variety of outcomes for missing values, depending on reason for discontinuation

Consider using almost always. If used as a primary analysis, each assumption should be justified from historic data. If used as a sensitivity analysis, it may suffice to make the case that the assumptions are unlikely to overestimate the treatment effect to an important degree, given what is known from historic data.

4.2.4.2 Methods of implementing assumptions: When to consider, when to avoid

Likelihood-based analysis of continuous outcome variables

Consider using a direct likelihood approach such as MMRM for MAR analyses where the outcome is continuous. A direct likelihood approach may be attractive if the stochastic nature of MI is thought to be an obstacle to acceptance of MI by the potential audience of the study report. A direct likelihood approach will also be attractive (compared to MI) when there are no ancillary post-baseline variables considered to be reasonably important to ensure MAR (i.e., no ancillary variables strongly related to dropout or missing outcome).

Avoid using where there are post-baseline ancillary data that could be used to help estimate missing values. Such augmenting data may be used in MI approaches, but not in approaches such as MMRM. Avoid using MMRM also directly to implement control-based PMMs, for example, using SAS PROC MIXED, because it is not clear how to estimate the variance of the treatment effect with the MMRM version of PMMs so as to allow a statistical test of the effect of the experimental treatment. (This warning does not apply to the joint modeling version of MI described in Chapter 7, which makes use of an MMRM-like model).

Likelihood-based analysis of binary response variables using longitudinal generalized linear mixed models

Consider using to implement MAR assumptions – the equivalent of MMRM for the whole exponential family of distributions – where there are good grounds to believe that the GLMM will converge, for example, where

- the model will be relatively simple with few or no categorical variables, or

- the observed data are not expected to be sparse for any combination of model variables

GLMM may also be preferred for practical reasons when implementing MAR assumptions (e.g., perhaps for a Poisson outcome that cannot be well modeled via MI in software that is available to the team). There is still discussion as to whether MI converges to a unique distribution when the response is binary (see further discussion and references in Section 4.5 below); this may encourage some to prefer GLMM to MI where GLMM is feasible.

Avoid using where the model or the data are such that convergence difficulties are expected. When MAR is assumed, one may also wish to avoid GLMM when it is desired to estimate population-averaged effects and there are grounds to believe that these cannot be well approximated from the GLMM subject-specific estimates. Inference from p-values and confidence intervals in GLMM where MAR is assumed are subject specific; whereas the broader confidence intervals and larger p-values associated with population-averaged inference are usually what are required in clinical trials. Although it is possible to approximate population-averaged inference from subject-specific estimates, and/or calculate population-averaged estimates that are "close to" MAR (see Chapter 5), the lack of direct population-averaged inference for MAR may be regarded as an obstacle to using GLMM by some.

Doubly robust estimation

Consider using as a supportive analysis for the primary MAR analysis when there are doubts about the statistical model for imputing missing data in the study, or when there is uncertainty about how to predict missingness from study data. Note that doubly robust methods remain unbiased when the model for efficacy is incorrect or the model of missingness is incorrect, but not when both models are incorrect. A doubly robust implementation of the primary analysis may frequently be worth considering as a sensitivity analysis. However, results from doubly robust estimation should be viewed with caution because the method is not guaranteed to be as powerful as parametric MI or MMRM.

Avoid using if there is evidence that efficacy and missingness is likely to be estimated in a reasonably unbiased manner by the other statistical models. As noted, doubly robust estimation is not guaranteed to be as powerful as estimation from a parametric model, hence if assuming MAR, MI or a direct likelihood approach such as MMRM may be preferred, especially for a primary analysis. Doubly robust requires that the probability of missingness be estimated at each visit. This, in turn, requires the model for the binary missingness variable to converge at each visit. If a study has many visits, the probability of at least one of these visits failing to converge is quite high. Therefore, avoid doubly robust estimation if there are many visits in the study and it is desired to include all visits in the modeling of missing data.

Multiple imputation.

Consider using for binary and normally-distributed variables, especially if post-baseline ancillary variables are available that could help model missing values. Consider MI for implementing PMMs also. MI allows a wide variety of assumptions about missing data to be implemented in a relatively straightforward manner.

Avoid using for outcomes that are not binary or normally distributed, unless software is available to the team to implement MI for such outcomes. (Stata®,[1] for example, allows for MI of Poisson and probit, while SAS does not support these distributions.)

---

[1] Stata® is a registered trademark of StataCorp LP.

Pattern-mixture models.
Consider using to implement sensitivity analyses for most studies.

Selection models and shared parameter models.
Consider using as sensitivity analyses if there is a requirement to model assumptions for the distribution of the observed and missing data as a whole, (as opposed to the subset-by-subset assumptions implemented by PMMs). Use selection models and shared parameter models only if confident that the modeled parameters can be interpreted clearly by a non-statistician. See Appendices 7.I and 7.J for a description of example selection and shared parameter models, and code to implement them.

Avoid using unless there is a good reason to use these approaches. This is probably controversial advice. However, we find the results from selection models difficult to interpret and difficult to explain to clinicians. Little (1993) noted with regard to PMMs that "some have argued that by modeling the distribution of $X_1, \ldots, X_V$ separately for each missing data pattern, problems of identifiability are made explicit that are obscured in the selection modeling approach." Little's view is stated in more rigorous terms by Daniels and Hogan (2008, pp. 168–169). Daniels and Hogan argue that selection models make assumptions about the missingness mechanism in a way that is inextricably linked to assumptions about the distribution of the outcomes, and so are not even in theory suited to be used as sensitivity analyses. They also propose an elegant definition of what is required of a sensitivity analysis, and show that selection models do not meet this definition. See Appendix 4.B for a fuller account of their argument.

Although it is understood that shared parameter models can sometimes usefully test for an association between the distribution of the outcome and the missingness, these shared parameter models too we find difficult to interpret and explain to non-statisticians, and even to statisticians, and for this reason we do not recommend the shared parameter model as a sensitivity analysis unless specifically required for good reason.

4.3   Exploring and presenting missingness

In addition to the usual tables of disposition and counts by reason for discontinuation, a Kaplan–Meier plot by treatment group of the probability of remaining in the study over time will be useful in supporting the assessment of the patterns and effect of missing data. Consider also presenting Kaplan–Meier plots by reason for discontinuation. If subject numbers are small, it may be useful for plotting purposes to group withdrawals according to reasons definitely unfavorable to the treatment (e.g., AE and Lack of Efficacy) versus other reasons.

Apart from sensitivity analyses, probably the most important tool for making sense of missing data is the plot of the mean outcome over time by selected categories of discontinuation (including completers, of course). This kind of plot may, for example, show that subjects who withdraw from a study have a mean efficacy profile worse than completers – this is usually, but not always, the case. If it is the case, then this is evidence that some of the missingness may be predictable from prior outcomes – that is, that some of the missingness is MAR. Note, however, that this cannot be used to infer that the study as a whole is MAR for the primary analysis, because (we believe) it is likely that at least some missingness will be MNAR in every study. Plots may reveal differences in efficacy profile between those who withdraw very early and those who withdraw towards the end of the study. This may help us to improve the model that we use to impute missing data, visit by visit, or may lead us to look for ancillary data that could explain the changes over time. Chapter 6 shows examples of how this can help to inform the strategy for missing data. In addition to plotting the outcome, consider plotting other, related variables (e.g., subscore(s) of the primary score; secondary measure(s) related to the outcome). These plots may be helpful to clinicians who may be able to advise the team on likely variables that distinguish patterns in the outcome value related to missingness.

The above plots may be planned to be blinded to treatment, and used prior to database lock to refine the statistical model used in the primary analysis. Recall also that, at least in the EU guidance, post hoc analyses related to missingness are recognized as useful, though not to "rescue" a failed primary analysis. It is possible, and may be advisable, to make use of information from unblinded plots in supportive post hoc analyses with better-informed models of missingness. We recommend allowing for this possibility in the protocol and SAP. If the reader is well informed in this way about patterns of values related to missingness, she/he will feel more confident to assess the study conclusion and its credibility. This kind of exploratory work is also very important in Phase 2 trials to gather information that can be used to plan a Phase 3 trial.

Spaghetti plots – plots of outcome over time with one line plotted per subject – are often useful, and may be presented for selected subjects (e.g., a random selection or, say, completers vs. those who withdrew due to AEs).

Logistic regression, with the missingness indicator at final visit as a response, is a useful tool to investigate study variables that may explain missingness. It may be used either to explore for variables related to missingness or to confirm observations from plots. Chapter 6 includes examples of methods to explore missingness.

4.4 Model checking

It would be outside the scope of this book to cover the process of checking the models of missingness and the model to impute the outcome – we refer the statistician to a textbook such as Draper and Smith (1981) or Cook and Weisberg (1982). It is certainly important to perform this model checking where there is missing data but, as noted earlier, when data are missing results from model checking must be viewed with caution. We note that for the analysis of later phase clinical trials, it is not usually recommended to exclude apparent outliers from an analysis, because of the risk of being seen as "dredging" the data for a significant result in favor of the experimental arm. Therefore, this aspect of model checking is less prominent in the practice of clinical trials. However, if it is possible that certain outliers are influencing the estimate of treatment effect in favor of the experimental arm, then it is good practice to present analyses excluding such outliers, and this should provide reassurance as to the credibility of the result.

In order to serve as checks of the robustness of the primary analysis, sensitivity analyses must be, as far as possible, implemented on the same basis as the primary analysis. That is, sensitivity analyses should be implemented using a modeling technique that is as similar as possible to that of the primary analysis; and should use a model that, except for the elements modified to test sensitivity, is as similar as possible to that of the primary analysis. This is because we want to be sure that any differences between the results of primary and sensitivity analyses are due to the change in assumptions of the sensitivity analysis regarding missingness, and not to some change in methodology. In this way, we will learn the maximum about the robustness or fragility of inference from the primary statistical test with respect to missing data. Thus, the population, time points and the choice and method of calculation of the outcome and study variables should be as far as possible identical for primary and sensitivity analyses. Of course, the outcome variable for the sensitivity analysis may be a variation on a variable used in the primary analysis, (e.g., a success/failure dichotomization). In that case, if regression is being used the link function may differ, but as far as possible the explanatory variables should be those used in the primary analysis, even if those explanatory variables prove statistically non-significant in the sensitivity analysis. We have already noted the exception to the above general rule, that the imputation model in MI may use a fuller model to impute missing values compared to a direct likelihood method such as MMRM. However, the analysis model (the model applied to the imputed data) should be the same as that used in the primary analysis. To make use of an MI sensitivity analysis when the primary analysis is MMRM, the reader of the study report should be assured via a step-by-step presentation that allows the reader to distinguish changes in results due to methodology from changes in results due to a change in assumptions about missing data – we have noted this in the examples above. Thus, if using MMRM as primary, include a matching MI analysis. The results of this MI and the MMRM should be similar. This will reassure the reader that any change in the estimate of treatment effect in subsequent analyses is not due to the change from MMRM to MI methodology. A second step should then be performed, enlarging the MI model with any ancillary variables that seem associated with missingness or missing values. This should improve the imputation of missing values in MI for the sensitivity analyses. If the MI augmented with ancillary variables gives a changed estimate of treatment effect, this will then be attributable to the fuller model. Finally, subsequent sensitivity analyses may or may not then make use of these ancillary variables in the imputation model, while estimating imputed values under MNAR assumptions.

We have noted that in our experience the two MAR approaches (MI and direct likelihood implemented via MMRM) usually give results that are extremely close. However, we should also note that for missing binary responses MI can give somewhat different results than generalized linear mixed models (GLMM), the approach that is the binary equivalent of MMRM. As noted, there is still disagreement in the literature as to whether certain MI approaches should in theory lead to a unique joint distribution of binary responses (Little and Rubin, 2002; Molenberghs and Kenward, 2007,

p. 149). We shall see in Chapter 7 an example of a GLMM and a corresponding MI that give results that are similar but could not be called "extremely close." In Table 7.11 in that chapter, the estimates of the log odds ratio for the experimental arm versus control are 0.26 for both MI and logistic regression GLMM, but the standard errors differ and the p-values are 0.0666 and 0.0847, respectively, with 1000 imputations.

4.5   Interpreting model results when there is missing data

It is widely acknowledged that we lack a way, finally, of deciding on the credibility of an analysis in the face of missing data. The NRC report (2010, pp. 105–106) discusses this problem. It suggests possible options as follows:

1. estimate the treatment effect at the lower and upper bounds of the range of selected sensitivity parameters; then calculate a 95% confidence region for the treatment effect based on these bounds;

2. estimate treatment effect by averaging over values of the sensitivity parameters "in some principled fashion";

3. carry out inference under MAR and determine the set of sensitivity parameter values that would lead to overturning the conclusion from MAR; results can be viewed as equivocal if the inference about treatment effects could be overturned for values of the sensitivity parameter that are plausible.

Developers of new treatments are understandably reluctant to give hostages to fortune by taking options 1 or 2. Option 1 could tend to give a rather wide confidence interval. Option 2 also could lead to an estimate of treatment effect skewed strongly in one direction by an unexpected result from one of the sensitivity analyses, and perhaps because of this is recommended by the NRC report only for "settings in which reliable prior information about the sensitivity parameter is known in advance." Option 2 would presumably also require a confidence interval, although this is not stated by the NRC report. Both these options serve the purpose of decision-making about a study's result, in that they lead to a single estimate of the treatment effect (i.e., the less favorable bound of the confidence interval). However, they have two disadvantages: (1) their potentially wide confidence intervals would tend to be wider, the more sensitivity analyses are planned; this could inhibit developers of new treatments from planning an adequate set of sensitivity analyses (as well as potentially requiring rather large sample sizes); (2) a good set of sensitivity analyses could well test different aspects of the assumptions of the primary analysis, and each sensitivity analysis might well need a separate interpretation, and have a greater or lesser importance clinically: the yoking together of such a set of analyses in a single estimate could be an over-simplistic and perhaps mechanistic approach.

If we cannot support some such synthesis of sensitivity analyses as is suggested in options 1 and 2 above, it is likely that the least well defined of the strategies, option 3, or a version of this strategy that allows for single yes/no assumptions in addition to "parameter values," will be the one used in most clinical trials. Although not satisfactory in terms of allowing a definite decision-making rule, option 3 is scientifically appealing in that it allows for full use of other information from the study to interpret the importance or lack of importance of deviations from the primary result in the sensitivity analyses. Thus, for example, if it is planned in one sensitivity analysis to assume a poor outcome for withdrawals due to AE, then a clearly non-significant result from this sensitivity analysis, tied to a relatively high proportion of AEs in the experimental treatment arm, would on its own facilitate a fairly straightforward decision not to accept the primary result (assuming the primary result was significant).

Nevertheless, the credibility of the study will gain if some criteria for interpretation of results can be defined before database lock. Clinically important differences (CIDs) are often available for standard efficacy scores. These CID quantities may be used to calibrate "tipping point" analyses. For example, it could be stated in advance that a study result will be regarded as credible if, to nullify the result, it is necessary to apply a delta adjustment of one CID, or perhaps some proportion of or multiple of a CID, to MAR-imputed values for the experimental arm. When setting such a criterion, however, the proportion of withdrawals likely to be delta-adjusted should be borne in mind. For an indication where a large proportion of withdrawals are expected, a delta adjustment of even 25% of a CID is a severe adjustment, and may not be clinically plausible – remember that in this case the criterion is equivalent to assuming that every single withdrawal worsens by the amount of the delta, or to a mean worsening of delta amongst all withdrawals. In general, a delta adjustment will often make more sense clinically when applied to subjects withdrawing for a particular class of reason, for example, due to AEs or due to lack of efficacy (see 4.2.3.3). An alternative criterion, and one that is allied to CID for some indications, is the standard deviation (SD) of the score, or some fraction of the SD (Mergl *et al.*, 2011; Guico-Pabia *et al.*, 2012).

In summary, we do not see options 1 or 2 as viable or attractive scientifically. Variants of option 3, with definite criteria for at least some (but probably not all) of the planned sensitivity analyses, may be the best strategy for aiding the decision as to whether a study is robust to missing data. Clearly, though, as most are agreed, further work is needed on how to evaluate sensitivity analysis for missing data.

4.6   Sample size and missing data

It is a challenge to identify a set of plausible assumptions for estimating sample size, when there is missing data. The NRC report notes that in practice it is usually assumed that withdrawals will provide no information for the primary analysis – that is, it is assumed that data are MCAR. Dropouts are taken into account by "(inflating) the sample size that was initially planned to achieve a stated power by the inverse of one minus the anticipated dropout rate" (National Research Council, 2010, p. 31). The NRC report points out that the true effect of missingness on power is probably more complicated and likely would need simulations to estimate. Simulations would also need a range of assumptions, and often we do not have a lot of data on which we might base such assumptions. The NRC report notes these difficulties and suggests that the question of sample size when missing data are expected "is an area for research."

However, there are some additional albeit crude ways in which the statistician can take missing data into account when estimating power.

If a "worst-case" success/failure response is planned for the primary analysis, with missing response counted as failure, then data about discontinuations in similar studies may allow the statistician to estimate likely rates of failure, adding the expected proportion of discontinuations (from previous studies) to the expected proportion of failures (in previous studies and from clinical experts) to find a working estimate of the likely failures in the planned study. If the "worst-case" approach is used for both control and experimental arms, the same calculation of proportion counted as failures can be done for both arms.

As an example of the kind of calculation possible, we take an artificial example based on planning a study in RA. Suppose that the outcome for the planned study is success/failure based on a score such as ACR20. Suppose further that

- the overall completion rate is expected to be 60%;

- 30% and 50% of subjects are expected to discontinue early from experimental and control arms, respectively;

- the responder rate for completers will be 60% and 40% for experimental and control arms, respectively;

- 20% of subjects who discontinue had a success as their last observation, 25% on experimental treatment and 15% on control (a higher proportion of discontinuations from the experimental arm is assumed due to AEs, while more discontinuations for lack of efficacy are assumed in the control arm);

- using a per-protocol population plus LOCF would increase the responder rate over LOCF in the full analysis set by 10% for both arms.

With these assumptions we can estimate success, failure and percentage improvement of the experimental arm over the control arm for four approaches as shown in Table 4.5.

The treatment effect and the variance of its estimate drive the sample size required to achieve a given power for a given analysis. If the primary analysis assumes MAR, the statistician can when estimating sample size try to take account of the following factors that affect the variance of the estimate of treatment effect relative to that of an available cases analysis:

1. proportion of missings in the treatment groups and their timing – the higher the proportion of missings, the less information MAR has to infer missing values, and the higher the variance of its estimates of treatment effect; however, if many withdrawals occur late in the study, then to that extent MAR estimates will have relatively lower variance: available cases cannot use subjects with missing data, but for withdrawals an MAR analysis can use information from earlier visits in inference about the primary endpoint;

Table 4.5   Probable responder rates for a variety of approaches to missing data for an RA study, given assumptions.

Method	Responder, experimental arm (%)	Responder, control arm (%)	% improvement of experimental over control
Available cases	60	40	50
Worst-case imputation	42	20	110
LOCF	50	25	100
PP+LOCF	55	27	~100

Responder proportions are calculated as follows: worst-case: (1-% discontinuing) * (% responder for completers); LOCF: worst-case + (% discontinuing * % with success in last observation); PP+LOCF: LOCF + (LOCF * 10%)
Note: we thank Zoran Antonijevic for this example and its calculations.

2. correlation between visits (the stronger the expected correlation, the better use MAR can make of earlier observations to model missing values);

3. the distribution of the observed outcomes of withdrawals, compared to those subjects who remain in the study – if the distribution of observed outcomes of withdrawals is different than that of those who remain in the study, then with a continuous outcome MAR may infer relatively large disparity among outcomes at the primary study endpoint compared to an available cases analysis, resulting in relatively high variance for the estimate of treatment effect.

If some of the above three items are known from previous in-house studies, they can inform the range of likely variances that the statistician uses to estimate sample size for the future study. The items could be used to simulate scenarios and inform estimates of sample size. We have seen instances where historic data was used to create simulations, and where the results from the simulations were used in the discussion of sample size in the protocol.

Appendix 4.A: Sample protocol/SAP text for study in Parkinson's disease

Primary analysis: The primary efficacy variable will be the change from baseline in UPDRS subscore at Week 24. A mixed model will be used for the repeated measures (MMRM), with treatment group, visit and pooled country as fixed effects, and baseline as a covariate. Analyses will be implemented using SAS PROC MIXED (SAS Institute Inc., 2011). Interactions with visit will be included for treatment group and baseline. A restricted maximum likelihood (REML) approach will be used. An unstructured variance–covariance structure will be used to model the within-subject errors. This variance–covariance matrix will be estimated across treatment groups. If the model fails to converge, a heterogeneous Toeplitz structure (the TOEPH option in

SAS PROC MIXED) will be used. The Kenward–Roger approximation will be used to estimate denominator degrees of freedom and adjust standard errors. The primary comparison will be the contrast between treatments at the last visit (Week 24).

The primary analysis and its handling of missing data: The MMRM model assumes that missingness is at random (MAR). That is, MMRM assumes that, given the statistical model and given the observed values of the outcome, missingness is independent of the unobserved values. A corollary is that MAR assumes that a subject's missing values can be estimated based on similar subjects who remained in the study. This infers that withdrawals (who may not receive study medication) have similar symptoms to some who continue to be treated. The EMA guidance on missing data (European Medicines Agency, 2010, p. 3) notes that the primary analysis should be "unlikely to be biased in favor of the experimental treatment to an important degree (under reasonable assumptions)" with "a confidence interval that does not underestimate ... variability." While MAR's assumption of the similarity of withdrawals and those who stay in the study may not be realistic for all subjects, MAR can be justified as not being biased to an important degree in favor of the experimental arm in three respects:

- given that subjects tend to have poor efficacy scores just before they withdraw, MAR will model imputations for early withdrawals based on subjects with similarly poor symptoms: MAR will to that extent reflect that withdrawals are "different" from those who stay in the study;

- other studies (Emre *et al.*, 2004; Parkinson Study Group, 2004a; Parkinson Study Group, 2004b) suggest that all treatment arms will tend to have worsening symptoms from about Week 15 onwards; it is desirable to reflect such worsening in inference about missing data; because MAR assumes that missing data follows the study pattern, under MAR missing values will be faithful to the general worsening over time that is expected in this indication;

- evidence from historic data in non-levodopa studies (Emre *et al.*, 2004; Parkinson Study Group, 2004a) suggests that a higher proportion of withdrawals are to be expected in the experimental treatment arm in this indication; thus the relatively poor efficacy likely to be imputed by MAR for withdrawals would favor the control arm, rather than the experimental arm in this study.

Note: the following paragraph may be omitted, but the text may be useful if ethics committees or regulators question the choice of analyses.

Other choices for handling missing data in the primary analysis were considered but rejected as follows. With a progressive disease, analyzing the last available observation (LOCF), would tend to favor the treatment group with earlier or more frequent withdrawals, and so is clinically counter-intuitive, and unsuitable from the clinical point of view. The option of BOCF was also rejected because it would similarly favor the treatment group with higher rates of withdrawal since, given the progressive nature of PD, many subjects would be expected to have worse symptoms at the end of the study than at baseline, and would thus be advantaged by the BOCF imputation in a counter-intuitive way.

As noted, MAR may be biased to a certain degree in that it infers that subjects who left the study have symptoms pertaining to treated subjects. Therefore, as recommended by the US NRC report on missing data (National Research Council, 2010, p. 49) and the EU Guidance on missing data (European Medicines Agency, 2010, p. 12), a number of sensitivity analyses are included, to assess the robustness of the primary estimate with regard to missing data, when the MAR assumption is replaced by assumptions that are likely to be relatively less favorable to the experimental treatment.

Sensitivity Analysis: To assess the robustness of the study conclusions to missing data, models that assume MNAR will be used. The assumptions of these sensitivity analyses for the missing data "stress test" the MAR assumptions of the primary analysis. Unfortunately, evidence is lacking about the likely outcome of subjects who discontinue treatment, but the assumptions of the primary analysis can at least be stress tested by positing outcomes that, while clinically plausible, are likely to be worse for the experimental arm than the outcomes assumed by MAR.

Analyses using MI: The models for all MI analyses (both for non-monotone and monotone missing imputation) will be fully described in the SAP, including the order of imputation of variables. The SAP will be finalized and signed off before database lock, that is, before the treatment groups are unblinded. The SAP will also specify all tuning parameters used by the MI; the number of imputations to be used in analyses; any transformations applied to explanatory variables; and the value of the seeds supplied for the stochastic element of MI. If, due to convergence issues, these tuning parameters need to be modified, full details will be given in an appendix of the study report. Likewise, it may sometimes be necessary to modify or simplify the MI model when data for certain combinations of explanatory variables is sparse or when explanatory variables are highly correlated. This tends to be rare in implementing MI, but if amendment of the model is necessary for such reasons, full details will be given in an appendix of the study report. For the final pooling of analyses of the imputed datasets, the calculation of least squares mean estimates will be fully specified, and will use, as representative values of the covariables, means calculated from the observed data.

Available cases analysis, and multiple imputation analyses assuming MAR: The primary analysis will be repeated using MI assuming MAR. This analysis will verify that MI and MMRM analyses give results that are consistent with each other. This should be the case theoretically, since they both use the same information, that is, they both use the statistical model and prior outcomes to make inferences about missing outcomes. A second MI analysis will be performed that will use auxiliary data to improve the imputation of missing outcomes, and will estimate the relationship between visits in UPDRS separately for each treatment group (the equivalent in MMRM of estimating the variance–covariance matrix separately for each treatment group). Depending on exploratory analyses presented as part of the blind data review, this second MI analysis may include as explanatory variables UPDRS subscores other than the primary subscore, and/or may include individual items from the questionnaire. This analysis will provide a baseline to aid the reader in assessing the sensitivity analyses, all of which will use this second, larger MI model.

Also for reference purposes, available cases at each visit will be analyzed as for the primary analysis, but with the fixed effects only.

The UPDRS score is widely accepted to be approximately normally distributed (see, e.g., Schenkman *et al.*, (2011)); therefore a non-parametric analysis will not be included. Outcome models for UPDRS are well established; therefore a sensitivity analysis using doubly robust estimation is not judged necessary.

Control-based imputation: The first proposed MNAR sensitivity analysis, which assumes that the trajectory of withdrawals from the experimental arm is as bad as that of placebo subjects, imputes an outcome almost certainly worse than that assumed by MAR, and is thus expected to be a reasonable stress test for MAR (Little and Yau, 1996; Ratitch *et al.*, 2013). Note that this approach constitutes a PMM as defined by Molenberghs and Kenward (2007, p. 221). The "patterns" here are defined by the treatment group and the time of withdrawal. The time of withdrawal is used in the definition of the pattern to allow the estimate to take account of the worsening over time that tends to be observed in all subjects. By the end of the study earlier withdrawals are likely to have worsened somewhat more *vis-à-vis* their last observed symptoms, compared to late withdrawals. A formal definition of the assumption of this sensitivity analysis is that subjects who drop out will be assumed to have correlations with future visits similar to subjects in the placebo group. For example, where values for the placebo group are, as expected, positively correlated with future visits, subjects in the experimental treatment group who drop out after visit t will be imputed to have a mean score at visit $t + n$ close to the mean for visit t plus the difference in the means of the placebo group at visits t and $t + n$, adjusted for observed covariates and outcomes prior to withdrawal. Note that, insofar as between-visit correlations are less than unity, the imputed values for the experimental arm will to that extent drift towards the mean of the placebo group. Subsequent to imputation, the imputed datasets are then analyzed as per the standard MI analysis process. Note that in this analysis, placebo missing observations are imputed assuming MAR and here follow the pattern of observed placebo observations, while missings for the experimental arm are assumed MNAR.

The above PMMs will be implemented by MI. As a preliminary step, non-monotone or intermediate missing data (expected to be relatively infrequent) will be imputed using the MCMC option of SAS PROC MI under MAR assumptions for both arms. When non-monotone or intermediate missing data has been imputed, the values for each pattern will be then imputed via the sequential regression method, using SAS PROC MI option MONOTONE REG. The MNAR imputation is achieved by using only appropriate study data in the estimation of the imputation model in each pattern. For example, to impute for time t assuming that the experimental arm missing data has the correlations of the placebo group, include only placebo observations up to and including time t, plus only observations from subjects in the experimental arm that have observations up to but not beyond time $t - 1$. First, all missings for the first post-baseline visit are imputed, then missings for the next visit are imputed using observed data plus the missings just imputed; and so on to the final visit. See, for example, Ratitch *et al.* (2013) for SAS code to perform this procedure.

Analysis where assumptions for missing data depend on reason for discontinuation: A second sensitivity analysis will be performed identical to the control-based imputation analysis, except that for subjects who withdraw from the study with primary reason of lack of efficacy or AE, the UPDRS score would be imputed at each visit to be worse than that imputed by MAR by a constant amount delta. A delta-adjustment analysis assumes that subjects who discontinued had outcomes that were worse than otherwise similar subjects that remained in the study (Carpenter and Kenward, 2007; National Research Council, 2010). The difference (adjustment) in outcomes between dropouts and those who remain will be implemented as a shift in location (that is, a shift in mean UPDRS motor score). As with the control-based imputation above, the delta adjustment here will start by imputing all missings for the first post-baseline visit, then applying the delta adjustment for the visit; then missings for the next visit are imputed using observed data plus the missings just imputed and delta-adjusted; and so on to the final visit. Thus delta adjustments will be applied to every visit after discontinuation, resulting in an accumulation of adjustments. It should be noted that the total delta resulting at the end of the study will be less than or equal to the sum of the deltas applied at each visit, because a delta will be "passed on" to the next visit only insofar as the visits are correlated. Correlation between visits is usually positive but would rarely be very close to unity, so in practice the cumulative delta at the end of the study for a subject may be considerably less than the sum of the deltas applied. This method of applying the delta is used to mimic in a realistic fashion the actual carry-over of side effects or poor efficacy associated with the experimental arm, that might be associated with the decision to withdraw due to lack of efficacy or AE, from the point at which the subject discontinued treatment. Only the experimental treatment arm is delta-adjusted while the control arm is handled using a MAR-based approach.

It has been suggested (Shulman et al., 2010) that a minimal CID in PD might be measured as 2.3–2.7 points on the UPDRS motor subscore; Shulman et al. suggest that a large CID for the motor subscore might be 10.7–10.8 points. In the context of the total UPDRS score (the total score is not the primary parameter of the study), Hauser and Auinger (2011) argue for a slightly smaller score as CID. Using CGI-I as a benchmark, they come up with a slightly smaller minimum CID on the UPDRS total score than Shulman et al.'s: 3.5, versus Shulman et al.'s 4.1–4.5. We follow Shulman et al.'s suggestion for a minimal CID for a subscore, and impose a delta of 2 points per visit for subjects who discontinue with primary reason of lack of efficacy or AE. This corresponds to just less than a minimally CID for each month the subject remains in the study.

MAR imputation with successively more severe delta adjustment: The method of delta adjustment will be used also in a further sensitivity analysis. Sensitivity will in this analysis be assessed by repeatedly adjusting MAR imputations to provide a progressively more severe stress test to assess how extreme departures from MAR would need to be to overturn the primary result. The delta that overturns the primary result is known as the "tipping point" (Yan et al., 2008; U.S. Food and Drug Administration, 2010). The successive delta adjustments will be implemented as described in the previous section.

To cover a range somewhat wider than the minimal CID suggested by Schulman *et al.*, a tipping point will be identified by repeating the entire imputation process using successively increased deltas from 1 to 5 in steps of 1. A judgement as to the credibility of the primary study result can then be informed from a clinical point of view, by assessing the plausibility of the value of the delta that was needed to nullify the primary result – if the delta needed to nullify the result was plausible, then from the clinical point of view there is reason to view the primary result with caution. Subject to clinical interpretation in the light of other study results, if a delta of less than 4 overturns the study result then there may be reason to view the primary result with caution.

Assessment of sensitivity analyses: The results from the sensitivity analyses will be collectively used to help interpret the overall study conclusions and in particular to judge the impact of the MAR assumption on differences in dropout rates between the treatment groups. With the exception of the tipping point analysis, absolute criteria have not been agreed as to when sensitivity analyses can be said to have confirmed the robustness of study results. Similarly, it is difficult to plan in advance how to decide whether the results of sensitivity analyses require that a study result be viewed with caution. Nevertheless, these sensitivity analyses will be discussed in the study report, and attempt will be made to use the analyses to justify the credibility of study results, or to qualify that credibility if the evidence warrants this.

Planned and exploratory presentations of missingness and missing values: Counts and percentages of subjects enrolled and in each study population will be presented by visit and treatment group. Counts and percentages will also be presented of discontinuations by treatment group and reason for discontinuation. The probability of remaining in the study over time will be presented in a Kaplan–Meier plot. Similar Kaplan–Meier plots will also be presented by treatment group separately for subjects who discontinued due to AE or lack of efficacy, and due to any other reason.

Plots of mean UPDRS subscore will be presented by visit, treatment group and time of discontinuation; a separate version of these plots will also be produced by reason for discontinuation. The plots will also include subjects who completed the study.

At the blind data review before database lock, the above plots will also be presented (without taking account of treatment group). The same plots will also be performed for the other subscores of UPDRS. Evidence from these plots of association between discontinuation and subscores of UPDRS will be used to finalize the full MI model used in sensitivity analyses. Logistic regression, with a missing/observed indicator as response, may be used to clarify associations between efficacy scores and missingness.

If warranted to help clarify aspects of missing data, spaghetti plots showing efficacy scores for selected individual subjects will be presented.

For the primary analysis and for each of the planned sensitivity analyses, the least squares mean estimate of treatment difference at Week 24 will be presented, together with its estimated standard error and the associated p-value. The models used in each analysis will be stated together with, as applicable, the covariance structure; the number of imputations and the MCMC tuning parameters and seed(s). Sample SAS code for each analysis will be included in an appendix to the SAP.

Post hoc analyses: If unexpected associations are seen between missingness and other study variables, or if any other aspects of the missing values suggest they might improve the understanding of the primary analysis, post-hoc sensitivity analyses will be performed (European Medicines Agency, 2010). These will not have the object of "rescuing" a failed study, but of clarifying the robustness of the primary analysis to missing data.

Responder analysis: If there is a noticeable imbalance between treatment groups in withdrawals due to AE, sensitivity to missing data may be assessed in addition by a responder analysis where "success" is defined as an improvement of 2.5 or more in the UPDRS subscore from baseline at Week 24, and subjects with missing data at Week 24 are counted as failures. The odds ratio for success for the experimental arm versus the control arm will be presented, together with its 95% confidence interval. If, as is expected, the experimental arm has a higher proportion of withdrawals than the control arm, this analysis will tend to favor the control arm, and thus be "conservative" in the sense of the EMA guidance.

Appendix 4.B: A formal definition of a sensitivity parameter

We adopt the notation of Daniels and Hogan (2008, p. 166) for this appendix which describes their argument as to what constitutes a sensitivity parameter. Daniels and Hogan write the factorization of the full data model as

$$p(\mathbf{y}, \mathbf{r} | \boldsymbol{\omega}) = p(\mathbf{y}_{mis} | \mathbf{y}_{obs}, \mathbf{r}, \boldsymbol{\omega}_E) p(\mathbf{y}_{obs}, \mathbf{r} | \boldsymbol{\omega}_0)$$

where the $\mathbf{r}$ indicate whether data are observed, and $\boldsymbol{\omega}_E$ and $\boldsymbol{\omega}_0 \in \boldsymbol{\omega}$ are parameters indexing the missing data model (Daniels and Hogan call it the "extrapolation model") and the observed data model, respectively.

They define ξ_S to be a sensitivity parameter if there exists a reparameterization $\xi(\omega) = (\xi_S, \xi_M)$ such that

1. ξ_S is a non-constant function of ω_E;
2. the observed data likelihood $L(\xi_S, \xi_M | Y_{obs}, r)$ is constant as a function of ξ_S; and
3. at a fixed value of ξ_S, the observed data likelihood is a non-constant function of ξ_M.

The above definition means that one or more of the parameters for the missing data should be completely non-identified by data. It may sound surprising at first that non-identification is a virtue, is indeed essential to, a sensitivity parameter, but they show how in fact a sensitivity parameter is not freely interpretable if it is tied to the observed data; furthermore, if a sensitivity parameter were tied to the observed data (i.e., if condition 2 above did not hold), then we would in effect be making the missing data dependent on the observed data, which is inconsistent with the largely MNAR approach of sensitivity analyses.

Daniels and Hogan give a helpful example to illustrate how for parametric selection models no sensitivity parameter as defined above is available. A selection model jointly models the full data and a binary missingness indicator. Daniels and Hogan posit observed data whose histogram suggests a normal distribution but truncated at the right. If it is assumed that the full data are normally distributed, any assumption about the missing data is forced to be compatible with that missing data "filling in" the truncated part of the full data distribution. But they point out that *any* assumption about the distribution of the full data will restrict our assumptions about the missing data in a similar way, for this or other similar selection models. (Non-parametric selection models are a way around this problem, if it is desired to use the selection model framework.)

References

Blumer J, Findling R, Welchung J, Soubrane C, Reed M (2009) Controlled clinical trial of zolpidem for the treatment of insomnia associated with attention-deficit/hyperactivity disorder in children 6 to 17 years of age. *Pediatrics* **123**(5): e770–e776, available at http://pediatrics.aappublications.org/content/123/5/e770.long, accessed 18 June 2013.

Bowden C, Mosolov S, Hranov L, Chen E, Habil H, Kongsakon R, Manfredi R, Lin H-N (2010) Efficacy of valproate versus lithium in mania or mixed mania: a randomized, open 12-week trial. *International Clinical Psychopharmacology* **25**: 60–67.

Bunouf P, Grouin J-M, Molenberghs G (2012) Analysis of an incomplete binary outcome derived from frequently recorded longitudinal continuous data: application to daily pain evaluation. *Statistics in Medicine* **31**: 1554–1571.

Burzykowski T, Carpenter J, Coens C, Evans D, France L, Kenward M, Lane P, Matcham J, Morgan D, Phillips A, Roger J, Sullivan B, White I, Yu L-M of the Statisticians in the Pharmaceutical Industry (PSI) Missing Data Expert Group (2009) Missing data; discussion points from PSI missing data expert group. *Pharmaceutical Statistics* **9**: 288–297.

Carpenter JR, Kenward MG (2007) *Missing Data in Randomised Controlled Trials – A Practical Guide*. National Health Service Co-ordinating Center for Research Methodology, Birmingham, available at www.hta.nhs.uk/nihrmethodology/reports/1589.pdf, accessed 18 June 2013.

Carpenter JR, Roger JH, Kenward MG (2013) Analysis of longitudinal trials with protocol deviation: a framework for relevant, accessible assumptions and inference via multiple imputation. *Journal of Biopharmaceutical Statistics* **23**:1352–1371.

Committee for Proprietary Medicinal Products (2001) Points to consider on missing data, available at http://www.ema.europa.eu/docs/en_GB/document_library/Scientific_guideline/2009/09/WC500003641.pdf, accessed 18 June 2013.

Cook R, Weisberg S (1982) *Applied Regression Including Computing and Graphics*. John Wiley & Sons, Ltd, New York.

Daniels M, Hogan J (2008) *Missing Data in Longitudinal Studies*. Chapman and Hall, Boca Raton, FL.

Draper N, Smith H (1981) *Applied Regression Analysis*. John Wiley and Sons, Ltd, New York.

Eli Lilly and Company (2008) *An Efficacy Study of Compound LY2624803 in the Treatment of Patients with Chronic Insomnia (SLUMBER)*, National Library of Medicine, Bethesda, MD, available at http://clinicaltrials.gov/ct2/results?term=NCT00784875&Search=Search, accessed 18 June 2013.

Emre M, Aarsland D, Albanese A, Byrne J, Deuschl G, De Deyn P, Durif F, Kulisevsky J, van Laar T, Lees A, Poewe W, Robillard A, Rosa M, Wolters E, Quarg P, Tekin P, Lane R (2004) Rivastagmine for dementia associated with Parkinson's disease. *New England Journal of Medicine* **351**: 2509–2518.

European Medicines Agency (2010) Guideline on missing data in confirmatory clinical trials, EMA/CPMP/EWP/1776/99 Rev.1, available http://www.ema.europa.eu/docs/en_GB/document_library/Scientific_guideline/2009/09/WC500003460.pdf, accessed 22 March 2013.

Guico-Pabia C, Fayyad R, Soares C (2012) Assessing the relationship between functional impairment/recovery and depression severity. *International Clinical Psychopharmacology* **27**: 1–7.

Hauser R, Auinger P, on behalf of the Parkinson Study Group (2011) Determination of minimal clinically important change in early and advanced Parkinson's disease. *Movement Disorders* **26**: 813–818.

Holm K, Goa K (2000) Zolpidem: an update of its pharmacology, therapeutic efficacy and tolerability in the treatment of insomnia. *Drugs* **59**: 865–889.

International Conference on Harmonisation of Technical Requirements for Registration of Pharmaceuticals for Human Use (1998) Statistical principles for clinical trials: E9, available at http://www.emea.europa.eu/docs/en_GB/document_library/Scientific_guideline/2009/09/WC500002928.pdf, accessed 23 June 2013.

Keene O (2010) Intent-to-treat analysis in the presence of off-treatment or missing data. *Pharmaceutical Statistics* **10**: 191–195.

Kelleher T, Thiry A, Wilber R, Cross A (2001) Missing data methods in HIV clinical trials: regulatory guidance and alternative approaches. *Drug Information Journal* **35**: 1363–1371.

Krystal A, Erman M, Zammit G, Soubrane C, Roth T; on behalf of the ZOLONG Study Group (2008) Long-term efficacy and safety of zolpidem extended-release 12.5 mg, administered 3 to 7 nights per week for 24 weeks, in patients with chronic primary insomnia: a 6-month, randomized, double-blind, placebo-controlled, parallel-group, multicenter study. *Sleep* **31**: 79 90.

Lipkovich I, Houston J, Ahl J (2008) Identifying patterns in treatment response profiles in acute bipolar mania: a cluster analysis approach. *BMC Psychiatry* **8**: 65, available at http://www.ncbi.nlm.nih.gov/pmc/articles/PMC2515837, accessed 18 June 2013.

Little RJA (1993) Pattern-mixture models for multivariate incomplete data. *Journal of the American Statistical Association* **88**: 125–134.

Little RJA, Rubin DB (2002) *Statistical Analysis with Missing Data*, 2nd edn. John Wiley & Sons, Ltd, New York.

Little RJA, Yau L (1996) Intent-to-treat analysis in longitudinal studies with dropouts. *Biometrics* **52**: 1324–1333.

Mallinckrodt CH (2013) *Preventing and Treating Missing Data in Longitudinal Clinical Trials*. Cambridge University Press, Cambridge.

Mallinckrodt CH, Lane PW, Schnell D, Peng Y, Mancuso J (2008) Recommendation for the primary analysis of continuous endpoints in longitudinal clinical trials. *Drug Information Journal* **42**: 303–319.

Mergl R, Henkel V, Allgaier A, Kramer D, Hautzinger M, Kohnen R, Coyne J, Hegerl U (2011) Are treatment preferences relevant in response to serotonergic antidepressants and cognitive-behavioral therapy in depressed primary care patients? Results from a randomized controlled trial including a patients' choice arm. *Psychotherapy and Psychosomatics* **80**: 39–47.

Molenberghs G, Kenward MG (2007) *Missing Data in Clinical Studies*. John Wiley & Sons Ltd, West Sussex.

Myers W (2000) Handling missing data in clinical trials: an overview. *Drug Information Journal* **34**: 525–533.

National Research Council. Panel on Handling Missing Data in Clinical Trials. Committee on National Statistics, Division of Behavioral and Social Sciences and Education (2010) *The Prevention and Treatment of Missing Data in Clinical Trials*. The National Academies Press, Washington, DC, available at http://www.nap.edu/catalog.php?record_id=12955, accessed 16 July 2013.

O'Neill RT (2011) The Prevention and Treatment of Missing Data in Clinical Trials, Some FDA Background, presentation at the *Prevention and Treatment of Missing Data in Clinical Trials* course sponsored by Johns Hopkins School of Public Health; Iselin, New Jersey.

Parkinson Study Group (2004a) A controlled, randomized delayed-start study of rasagiline in early Parkinson disease. *Archives of Neurology* **61**: 561–566.

Parkinson Study Group (2004b) Levodopa and the progression of Parkinson's disease. *New England Journal of Medicine* **351**: 2498–2508.

Permutt T (2011) Regulatory Considerations, presentation at the *Prevention and Treatment of Missing Data in Clinical Trials course* sponsored by Johns Hopkins School of Public Health; Iselin, New Jersey.

Post R, Altshuler L, Frye M, Suppes T, McElroy S, Keck P, Leverich G, Kupka R, Nolen W, Luckenbaugh D, Walden J, Grunze H (2005) Preliminary observations on the effectiveness of levetiracetam in the open adjunctive treatment of refractory bipolar disorder. *Journal of Clinical Psychiatry* **66**: 370–374.

Purdue Pharma LP (2007) *A Study of Zolpidem Tartrate Sublingual Tablet in Adult Patients With Insomnia*, National Library of Medicine, Bethesda, MD, available at http://clinicaltrials.gov/ct2/results?term=NCT00466193&Search=Search, accessed 18 June 2013.

Ratitch B, O'Kelly M (2011) Implementation of Pattern-mixture models using standard SAS/STAT procedures. In: Proceedings of Pharmaceutical Industry SAS User Group, Nashville, available at http://pharmasug.org/proceedings/2011/SP/PharmaSUG-2011-SP04.pdf, accessed 23 June 2013.

Ratitch B, O'Kelly M, Tosiello R (2013) Missing data in clinical trials: from clinical assumptions to statistical analysis using pattern mixture models. *Pharmaceutical Statistics* **12**:337–347. DOI:10.1002/pst.1549, available at http://onlinelibrary.wiley.com/doi/10.1002/pst.1549/pdf, accessed 20 June 2013.

Roger JH (2012) Fitting pattern-mixture models to longitudinal repeated-measures data, available at http://missingdata.lshtm.ac.uk/dia/Five_Macros20120827.zip, accessed 20 June 2013.

Roth T, Walsh J, Krystal A, Wessel T, Roehrs T (2005) An evaluation of the efficacy and safety of eszopiclone over 12 months in patients with chronic primary insomnia. *Sleep Medicine* **6**: 487–495.

Rubin DB (1976) Inference and missing data. *Biometrika* **63**: 581–592.

SAS Institute Inc. (2011) *SAS/STAT® 9.3 User's Guide*. SAS Institute Inc., Cary, NC.

Schenkman M, Ellis T, Christiansen C, Barón A, Tickle-Degnen L, Hall A, Wagenaar R (2011) Profile of functional limitations and task performance among people with early- and middle-stage Parkinson disease. *Physical Therapy* **91**: 1338–1354.

Shulman LM, Gruber-Baldini AL, Anderson KE, Fishman PS, Reich SG, Weiner WJ (2010) The clinically important difference on the unified Parkinson's disease rating scale. *Archives of Neurology* **67**(1): 64–70.

Siddiqui O, Hung HMJ, O'Neil R (2009) MRM vs. LOCF: a comprehensive comparison based on simulation study and 25 NDA datasets. *Journal of Biopharmaceutical Statistics* **19**: 227–246.

Tohen M, Greil W, Calabrese J, Sachs G, Yatham L, Oerlinghauser B, Koukopoulos A, Cassano G, Grunze H, Licht R, Dell'Osso L, Evans A, Risser R, Baker R, Crane H, Dossenbach M, Bowden C (2005) Olanzapine versus lithium in the maintenance treatment of bipolar disorder: a 12-month, randomized, double-blind, controlled clinical trial. *American Journal of Psychiatry* **162**: 1281–1290.

U.S. Food and Drug Administration (2010) FDA executive summary prepared for the 19 March 2010 meeting of the Circulatory System Devices Panel: P090013, REVO MRI SureScan Pacing System, Medtronic, Inc., available at http://www.fda.gov/downloads/advisorycommittees/committeesmeetinmaterials/medicaldevices/medicaldevicesadvisorcommittee/circulatorysystemdevicespanel/ucm204715.pdf, accessed 18 June 2013.

Yan X, Li H, Gao Y, Gray G (2008) Case study: sensitivity analysis in clinical trials. AdvaMed/FDA conference, available at http://www.amstat.org/sections/sigmedd/Advamed/advamed08/presentation/Yan_sherry.pdf, accessed 20 June 2013.

5

Mixed models for repeated measures using categorical time effects (MMRM)

Sonia Davis

Key points

- A mixed model for repeated measures using categorical time effects, often referred to as MMRM, is an extension of analysis of covariance (ANCOVA) for repeated assessments in a clinical trial. Treatment group differences are estimated at the primary time point, typically the final treatment phase visit, while incorporating available data for subjects who dropped out early under minimal modeling assumptions.

- Data is assumed to be missing at random (MAR).

- MMRM is a particular parameterization of the mixed linear model, often with no random effects, with the time of post-baseline visits modeled as a classification variable, and with a structure imposed on the variance–covariance pattern of the outcome across the visits. The variance–covariance structure is used by the model to estimate the outcome at each visit, assuming that missing data has the same correlation structure as observed data.

- An unstructured variance–covariance pattern has the least assumptions and is the best choice, although in some cases model convergence can be an issue.

Clinical Trials with Missing Data: A Guide for Practitioners, First Edition. Michael O'Kelly and Bohdana Ratitch.
© 2014 John Wiley & Sons, Ltd. Published 2014 by John Wiley & Sons, Ltd.

- The variance–covariance pattern must be pre-specified in an analysis plan, and an appropriate back-up pattern should be pre-specified in case the primary model does not converge.

- Before beginning an analysis, it is important to understand the amount and pattern of missing data through relevant descriptive displays.

- An extension of the MMRM for logistic regression can be applied to repeated binary data using a generalized linear mixed model (GLMM). This model assumes data are MCAR yet produces model-based estimates of fixed effects that can often be fairly robust in mild departures from MCAR.

- Detailed examples applying MMRM and logistic regression GLMM are provided.

- Sensitivity analysis should be pre-planned to explore the robustness of the results to the MAR assumption. See Chapter 7.

5.1   Introduction

Mixed linear models are a large family of likelihood-based models that estimate linear functions of correlated data by using a combination of fixed and random effects. This family of models is useful for evaluating repeated measurements over time, both by taking into account the relationship of the repeated measures within a person and by estimating parameters from the available data even when some observations are missing, such as due to patient discontinuation. A specific form of the mixed linear model for comparing treatment groups at the final time point of a clinical trial under minimal assumptions about trends in the outcome measure was coined "mixed model for repeated measures" by Mallinckrodt *et al.* and is widely referred to as MMRM (Mallinckrodt *et al.*, 2003; 2008).

A tempting approach to modeling repeated measurements is to fit a linear or quadratic regression slope to the responses over time. However, this approach assumes that the modeled slope is the *correct* trajectory of the symptoms over time. This major assumption is unacceptable for comparing treatment groups in a clinical trial, especially when the goal is to obtain regulatory approval of a treatment from a confirmatory trial. MMRM avoids making any assumption about the response profile over time by treating time as a classification variable. The method relies on the functionality of the mixed model to take into account the correlation of the repeated visits. MMRM uses the estimated correlation between the visits for the available data to estimate the result at the primary visit assuming that missing data from dropouts has the same correlation as the observed data.

Historically, analysis of covariance with the last observation carried forward (LOCF) imputation of missing values was used for efficacy analyses of primary continuous outcomes submitted to the FDA in new drug applications. LOCF's assumption of no change after discontinuation may not always be appropriate, and can often favor the experimental arm (see Sections 1.4 and 4.2.2.3). MMRM can often provide less biased estimates at the final time point than LOCF (Mallinckrodt *et al.*, 2001a; 2001b; 2004; Siddiqui *et al.*, 2009). It assumes that the missing data are missing at random (MAR), but otherwise, in its simplest form, imposes few assumptions about the data other than normally distributed errors. MMRM is frequently selected as the primary analysis method in Phase III pharmaceutical trials.

A benefit of MMRM is that the structure of the model is similar to ANCOVA. Therefore, it is easy to describe the model, and to present and interpret the results. The FDA-sponsored National Research Council report on prevention and treatment of missing data (National Research Council, 2010) stresses the importance of inter-pretability when deciding on a method for handling missing data (see Section 3.5.5). MMRM is readily implemented using standard statistical computing packages such as SAS.

An extension to the MMRM is available for binary outcomes such as responder status or relapse status. An odds ratio (OR) comparing treatments for categorical outcomes at the final time point is obtained by applying the MMRM modeling strategy to a generalized linear mixed model (GLMM).

This chapter provides a brief framework describing the MMRM model and the logistic GLMM for binary data, and shows detailed examples of each.

5.2   Specifying the mixed model for repeated measures

In this section, we will briefly introduce the mathematical mechanics of the mixed linear model and the MMRM as a special case. We then describe in detail several choices for the variance–covariance pattern, and when each is best used. We discuss strategies to help ensure convergence of the model, and steps to take when the model fails to converge.

Consider a dataset from a clinical trial, where each subject i has a number of repeated measurements across multiple post-baseline visits. All subjects are expected to follow the same visit structure for the repeated measurements, but some subjects might have one or more missing "skipped" visits, and some subjects might discontinue the trial early, therefore resulting in missing data from all visits after a certain point in time.

5.2.1   The mixed model

A linear model for a continuous outcome variable y for subject i at visit j receiving treatment t can be written as follows:

$$y_{ij} = \beta_{0jt} + \sum_{s} x_{ijs}\beta_s + e_{ij} \tag{5.1}$$

where β_{0jt} denotes a visit × treatment intercept term, β_1 to β_s are the regression coefficients for explanatory variables x_1 to x_s and e_{ij} is the residual. The explanatory variables can be at the subject level, so the value is the same for each visit of a subject, or can be at the subject-visit level. The middle term can be thought of as a subject's individual covariate offset from the general visit $\times$ treatment intercept β_{0jt}.

Formulas for linear models can be presented more conveniently and compactly using matrix rather than scalar algebra. Since this chapter focuses extensively on linear models, we will use matrix notation for the remainder of this chapter, in order to present methods clearly and succinctly. Using matrix notation, Equation 5.1 can be extended to encompass the linear model for all subject visits together as follows: define Y as a vector of outcomes for each visit for all N subjects $Y = [y_{11}, y_{12} \ldots, y_{1J}, \ldots y_{N1}, y_{N2}, \ldots, y_{NJ}]$, define X as the matrix of explanatory variables, including the indicators for visit, treatment, and the visit $\times$ treatment interaction, and define β as a vector of fixed regression coefficients including the visit $\times$ treatment intercept, and e as a vector of residuals. A longitudinal linear model for a continuous outcome variable Y can be written as follows:

$$Y = X\beta + e \tag{5.2}$$

Subjects are assumed to be independent. For one subject i, the vector of residuals e_i has a multivariate normal distribution with mean 0 and variance–covariance matrix Σ_i. The mean effect, or the expected value of Y, is

$$E[Y] = X\beta \tag{5.3}$$

For a standard linear model analysis of covariance, where each observation is assumed to be independent and identically distributed, the variance–covariance matrix V of the residual vector e simplifies to:

$$V = \text{Cov}[e] = \sigma^2 I_{NJ} \tag{5.4}$$

where σ^2 is the common variance term, and I_{NJ} is an identity matrix (with 1s on the diagonal) corresponding to the number of subject visits.

However, since repeated measurements for the same subject over time are correlated with each other, a standard linear model is not appropriate. Instead, we use a mixed effects linear model, which is a more general version of the linear model, where the correlation *between* independent subjects is zero, but *within* a subject i, the elements of the within-subject covariance matrix Σ_i are not assumed to be independent.

We specify the mixed linear model as

$$Y = X\beta + Z\gamma + e \tag{5.5}$$

The vector γ is an unknown vector of random parameters with design matrix Z, and e is the random error vector. Common choices for random factors in a clinical trial include a random subject intercept, or perhaps investigator site, if it can be argued that the sites in the trial are a random selection of all possible sites. Vectors γ and e are independent of each other and are both normally distributed with mean of 0. The variance–covariance matrices are Cov $[\gamma] = G$ and Cov $[e] = R$. For the vector of outcomes from all subject visits Y, the variance–covariance matrix V is specified as:

$$V = \text{Cov}[Y] = ZGZ^T + R \qquad (5.6)$$

Recall that the simple linear model has no random effects, and in this case Z and G are zero, and so Cov $[Y] = \text{Cov}[e] = \sigma^2 I$ as in Equation 5.4. In the most common form of the MMRM model, we do not specify any random effects, but we take into account the correlation of the observations within a subject, and so Z and G are zero, and Cov $[Y] = R$. Although referred to as the *mixed model* for repeated measures, the MMRM focuses on fitting a structure to the correlated errors R, and actually has no random effects. For the MMRM, within each subject i, a structured matrix R_i is imposed to describe the covariance pattern of the residuals for the observations from this subject, such that:

$$\Sigma_i = \text{Cov}[e_i] = R_i \quad \text{for all } i \text{ subjects.} \qquad (5.7)$$

Each subject has the same imposed structure. Extending the covariance structure to the vector of visits for all subjects in the trial $i = 1$ to N, subject is a "blocking" factor, where data from separate subjects are uncorrelated, and data within each subject is correlated. For the vector of outcomes from all subject visits Y, the variance–covariance matrix V is specified as:

$$V = \text{Cov}[e] = R \qquad (5.8)$$

where R is a block diagonal matrix with the form:

$$\begin{bmatrix} R_1 & 0 & 0 & \cdots & 0 \\ 0 & R_2 & 0 & \cdots & 0 \\ 0 & 0 & R_3 & \cdots & 0 \\ \vdots & \vdots & \vdots & \ddots & \vdots \\ 0 & 0 & 0 & 0 & R_N \end{bmatrix} \qquad (5.9)$$

For each subject i, R_i is a submatrix corresponding to the non-missing observations for subject i. For example, if subject 1 has complete data, then R_1 is a $J \times J$ matrix, if subject 2 missed the fifth visit then R_2 is a submatrix of R_1 obtained by deleting the fifth row and fifth column of R_1. A user-specified structure is imposed on the R matrix (see Section 5.2.2), and restricted maximum likelihood (REML) is used to estimate both the β coefficients and the R parameters.

In SAS PROC MIXED (SAS Institute Inc., 2011b), the random components are specified with the RANDOM statement, and the correlation components from repeated measurements for a subject are generally specified with the REPEATED statement. MMRM uses only the REPEATED statement, unless a random subject effect is specified. The fixed effects and variance–covariance parameters are estimated via REML using a ridge-stabilized Newton–Raphson algorithm. Since REML is an iterative estimation method, a complex model with many fixed effects and variance–covariance parameters may not converge.

5.2.2   Covariance structures

One can make a variety of choices for the covariance matrix R. It could be tempting to wait until the end of the study to identify the structure that best fits the data. However, such a strategy could be seen as data dredging in order to find the structure that would put the test treatment in the best light. To avoid this bias, one must specify the covariance structure a priori in the protocol or analysis plan. In the regulatory setting, pre-specifying the covariance structure is required.

There are two main issues to consider when selecting a covariance structure: (1) the capacity to represent correlations between measurements while imposing the least amount of assumptions, and (2) the ability of the MMRM model to converge. The following sections describe some of the most relevant covariance patterns: unstructured, Toeplitz and heterogeneous Toeplitz, spatial power and AR(1). The SAS documentation for PROC MIXED (SAS Institute Inc., 2011b) provides a description of many other available options that may sometimes be of interest, including compound symmetry and heterogeneous compound symmetry. Regardless of the covariance structure, it is important to note that, while the set of planned visits is assumed to be the same across all subjects, MMRM easily accommodates subjects with missed visits, either internally or due to early discontinuation, by using the available data.

5.2.2.1   Unstructured

Misspecifying the variance–covariance pattern can inflate the Type I error and negatively impact power (Mallinckrodt et al., 2008). If there are no concerns about converging, then the unstructured covariance pattern is the very best choice. The unstructured pattern lets the data drive the estimates, and has no assumptions about the underlying covariance pattern. The structure assumes that each visit has a different variance, and each pair of visits has a separate correlation. It is therefore reasonable to use in any longitudinal setting with a fixed visit structure for all subjects, typical for clinical trials. The drawback is that it requires the estimation of more parameters than any other structure. If there are small sample sizes and many visits in the study, then an unstructured pattern might lead to non-convergence. Due to the minimal assumptions, unstructured should always be the primary choice in regulatory settings. However, since at times it may not converge, the analysis plan for a clinical trial should *always* specify a second option to use in its place if the unstructured fails to converge.

The unstructured covariance pattern has the following form for a clinical trial with four visits:

$$
\begin{bmatrix}
\sigma_1^2 & \sigma_{12} & \sigma_{13} & \sigma_{14} \\
\sigma_{12} & \sigma_2^2 & \sigma_{23} & \sigma_{24} \\
\sigma_{13} & \sigma_{23} & \sigma_3^2 & \sigma_{34} \\
\sigma_{14} & \sigma_{24} & \sigma_{34} & \sigma_4^2
\end{bmatrix}
\tag{5.10}
$$

The subscripts correspond to the visit numbers; for example, σ_1^2 is the variance for Visit 1, and σ_{12} is the covariance of Visit 1 and Visit 2.

The unstructured covariance pattern has the following characteristics:

- Heterogeneous variances;

- Heterogeneous covariances;

- Fits $J(J + 1)/2$ parameters, where J is the number of visits. If there are $J = 4$ visits, the unstructured pattern estimates $(4 \times 5)/2 = 10$ parameters;

- In SAS modeling statements, specify TYPE=UN;

- Is appropriate for any fixed visit structure.

5.2.2.2   Toeplitz and heterogeneous Toeplitz patterns

To be prepared for cases when the unstructured pattern does not converge, a secondary pattern must be pre-specified in the analysis plan. The Toeplitz or, preferably, heterogeneous Toeplitz patterns are good choices.

The Toeplitz pattern requires estimation of substantially fewer parameters than unstructured, which aids in convergence. This pattern assumes that all visits have the same variance and that the correlations between any two visits that are the same number of visits apart from each other are the same. For example, the correlation between Visits 1 and 3 is assumed to be the same as the correlation between Visits 6 and 8. Since we might expect clinical trial data to be less correlated as visits get farther apart, this structure has a reasonable pattern, particularly if the time between visits is equally spaced across the study. However, if the correlations at the end of the study are believed to be very different from those at the beginning of the study, this structure would not be appropriate.

The Toeplitz covariance structure has the following form:

$$
\begin{bmatrix}
\sigma^2 & \sigma_1 & \sigma_2 & \sigma_3 \\
\sigma_1 & \sigma^2 & \sigma_1 & \sigma_2 \\
\sigma_2 & \sigma_1 & \sigma^2 & \sigma_1 \\
\sigma_3 & \sigma_2 & \sigma_1 & \sigma^2
\end{bmatrix}
\tag{5.11}
$$

The subscripts correspond to the difference between the visit numbers, so σ^2 is the variance for each visit, σ_1 is the covariance of all adjacent visits, and σ_2 is the covariance of all visits that have one visit between them, and so on.

The Toeplitz covariance pattern has the following characteristics:

- Homogeneous variances;

- Covariance structure is banded;

- Fits J parameters, where J is the number of visits;

- In SAS modeling statements, specify TYPE=TOEP;

- Is most appropriate for visit structures that are equally spaced in time.

In practice, variance of the outcome often increases with time on study. Therefore, the heterogeneous Toeplitz is preferable to the Toeplitz structure. The heterogeneous Toeplitz combines the banded correlation structure from the Toeplitz with heterogeneous variances as follows:

$$
\begin{bmatrix}
\sigma_1^2 & \sigma_1\sigma_2\rho_1 & \sigma_1\sigma_3\rho_2 & \sigma_1\sigma_4\rho_3 \\
\sigma_1\sigma_2\rho_1 & \sigma_2^2 & \sigma_2\sigma_3\rho_1 & \sigma_2\sigma_4\rho_2 \\
\sigma_1\sigma_3\rho_2 & \sigma_2\sigma_3\rho_1 & \sigma_3^2 & \sigma_3\sigma_4\rho_1 \\
\sigma_1\sigma_4\rho_3 & \sigma_2\sigma_4\rho_2 & \sigma_3\sigma_4\rho_1 & \sigma_4^2
\end{bmatrix}
\tag{5.12}
$$

The subscripts for σ correspond to visit number, and the subscripts for ρ correspond to the difference between the visit numbers, so σ_1^2 is the variance for Visit 1 and $\sigma_1\sigma_2\rho_1$ is the covariance between Visit 1 and Visit 2, which are one visit apart.

The heterogeneous Toeplitz covariance pattern has the following characteristics:

- Heterogeneous variances;

- Correlation structure is banded;

- Fits $2J - 1$ parameters, where J is the number of visits. If there are $J = 4$ visits, the heterogeneous Toeplitz pattern estimates $2 \times 4 - 1 = 7$ parameters;

- In SAS modeling statements, specify TYPE=TOEPH;

- Is most appropriate for visit structures that are equally spaced in time.

5.2.2.3 Spatial covariance patterns

In general, the correlation between visits is stronger when they are closer together and weaker when they are farther apart. Toeplitz and heterogeneous Toeplitz patterns assume that the visits are all equally spaced. Yet, in clinical trials, there are often unequally spaced intervals between visits: the visits at the beginning of a trial are more frequent (such as once a week) and the later visits may have more time between them (such as once a month). When there are unequally spaced visits, a patterned correlation matrix that takes into account the time between visits and has fewer covariance parameters than unstructured may be of interest. Such patterns are called spatial covariance patterns. For spatial patterns, the correlation between visits is assumed to be related to the duration of time between visits rather than the number of visits between them.

Since the spatial pattern is a function of the time between visits, there are fewer parameters required to fit the spatial functions compared to the Toeplitz. However, this structure may not always be a good fit to the data. Also, many spatial patterns assume that the variances are homogeneous over time. Before selecting a spatial structure, it would be good to evaluate if this structure is suitable from a similar previous study. One choice for a spatial covariance structure is the spatial power:

$$\sigma^2 \begin{bmatrix} 1 & \rho^{d_{12}} & \rho^{d_{13}} & \rho^{d_{14}} \\ \rho^{d_{12}} & 1 & \rho^{d_{23}} & \rho^{d_{24}} \\ \rho^{d_{13}} & \rho^{d_{23}} & 1 & \rho^{d_{34}} \\ \rho^{d_{14}} & \rho^{d_{24}} & \rho^{d_{34}} & 1 \end{bmatrix} \tag{5.13}$$

where $d_{jj'}$ corresponds to a standardized duration of time between Visits j and j', so d_{14} is, for example, the standardized duration of time between Visits 1 and 4.

The spatial power structure is a generalization of the AR(1) autoregressive structure. For AR(1), the visits are assumed to be equally spaced, and the correlation between adjacent visits is ρ, the correlation between visits separated by one visit is ρ^2, and separated by two visits is ρ^3, and so on. Under this structure, we can see that after several visits, even a moderate correlation falls to a small number. This is generally not a realistic pattern for clinical trial data. Adding a random subject intercept to the MMRM model allows for the estimation of an underlying within-subject covariance that is constant across visits. With this parameterization, the spatial structure imposes higher correlations at near-by visits and lower correlations at far-apart visits, and the overall within-subject covariance keeps the estimated correlation at visits that are far apart from each other from falling unreasonably low. In order to fit clinical trial data appropriately, spatial structures should always be fit with the addition of a random subject effect. The spatial power + random subject effect pattern for a trial with four visits is as follows:

$$\sigma_G^2 I_4 + \sigma^2 \begin{bmatrix} 1 & \rho^{d_{12}} & \rho^{d_{13}} & \rho^{d_{14}} \\ \rho^{d_{12}} & 1 & \rho^{d_{23}} & \rho^{d_{24}} \\ \rho^{d_{13}} & \rho^{d_{23}} & 1 & \rho^{d_{34}} \\ \rho^{d_{14}} & \rho^{d_{24}} & \rho^{d_{34}} & 1 \end{bmatrix} \tag{5.14}$$

where σ_G^2 corresponds to the underlying within-subject covariance, I_4 is a 4 × 4 identity matrix, and the other parameters are the same as in Equation 5.13. Note that the addition of a constant covariance term would have no impact on the unstructured and Toeplitz patterns (Equations 5.10 and 5.11) and would only add unnecessary complexity to those models.

Spatial power with a random subject effect is a particularly helpful option for a long-term trial with a large number of unequally spaced repeat visits per subject (such as 10 or more), and with a small number of subjects, such that estimation of many correlation parameters using an unstructured pattern could lead to convergence problems. However, it imposes a strong assumption that correlation from farther apart visits is multiplicatively less than near-by visits, which may not reflect the actual data for a particular trial.

The spatial power + random within-subject covariance pattern has the following characteristics:

- Homogeneous variances;

- Covariance structure that decreases multiplicatively as visits become more separated in time, towards an underlying covariance that is constant across visits;

- Fits three parameters (one for the random subject effect, two for the spatial power structure);

- In SAS modeling statements: (1) specify TYPE=SP(POW)(*varname*), where *varname* is a variable in the SAS dataset indicating the planned duration of time since the baseline visit. The duration must be provided in the same unit for all visits, but the unit itself has no impact on the estimation. Alternatively, the actual duration from baseline for each subject may be used; (2) specify RANDOM INTERCEPT / SUBJECT=subjid;

- Is applicable to visit structures that are unequally spaced in time, and is helpful when the trial consists of a small number of subjects followed for a long duration across many visits.

5.2.3   Mixed model for repeated measures versus generalized estimating equations

For MMRM, obtaining unbiased estimates requires that we have chosen the correct variance–covariance matrix. Using the unstructured pattern has the benefit of imposing minimal assumptions. However, any chosen pattern could be incorrect, leading to a biased estimate of the fixed effects. Because of this, when a pattern other than unstructured is specified, FDA regulatory authorities have at times requested modifying the primary analysis to include an empirical sandwich estimate of the variance–covariance matrix of the fixed-effects parameters.

The empirical sandwich estimator of the fixed effects variance–covariance terms is asymptotically consistent, and therefore the fixed effect estimates are asymptotically unbiased and robust against misspecification of the correlation pattern (Gardiner *et al.*, 2009; SAS Institute Inc., 2011b). On the other hand, the sandwich estimator requires data to be missing completely at random (MCAR), as opposed to the less rigorous assumption of MAR for the model-based estimator. When data are MAR but not MCAR, analyses using the empirical sandwich estimator may be biased (Liu and Zhan, 2011). Because of the MCAR assumption, we recommend using the sandwich estimator as a sensitivity analysis of the primary MMRM model when a structured correlation pattern is specified, but not *instead of* the model-based estimator.

A generalized estimating equations (GEE) model (Liang and Zeger, 1986) is somewhat similar to a mixed model with a sandwich estimator. GEE is more frequently applied to repeated binary data, but is also applicable for normally distributed data. In GEE, the asymptotic variance–covariance of the fixed effects is estimated with the empirical sandwich estimator (Gardiner *et al.*, 2009); however, the fixed effects are estimated by GEE, and the variance–covariance parameters are specified by a "working" correlation matrix which is estimated by the method of moments. Like MMRM with a sandwich estimator, GEE estimates are asymptotically unbiased no matter what covariance matrix is selected only when data is MCAR. GEE also requires a larger sample size for the asymptotic assumption than required for MMRM under MAR, and tends to produce wider confidence intervals. It has a loss in efficiency if the working correlation matrix is misspecified (Gardiner *et al.*, 2009).

Chapter 7 provides a description of other sensitivity analyses.

5.2.4   Mixed model for repeated measures versus last observation carried forward

Chapters 1 and 4 have provided a substantial description of assumptions and biases of MMRM and LOCF. A brief summary comparing these two methods is as follows:

- Like ANCOVA of LOCF data, MMRM requires the residual error to be normally distributed.

- MMRM requires that missing data is MAR, compared to LOCF, which assumes the data after a subject drops out is a constant. Simulations have shown that if data is missing not at random (MNAR), then both are biased. However, MMRM is generally less biased than LOCF (Mallinckrodt *et al.*, 2008; Siddiqui *et al.*, 2009).

- MMRM variance estimates are generally larger than LOCF, because LOCF often underestimates standard errors when there is missing data. We have also, though, found examples where the LOCF-estimated variance was higher than MMRM, when the LOCF values were very different from the observed values (and MMRM predicted values) at the final time point.

- LOCF can lead to estimates of treatment differences that are substantially different from those under the MCAR or the MAR assumption, either conservative or anti-conservative, depending on the situation. Under the MAR assumption, MMRM requires specifying the correct covariance structure to obtain an unbiased estimate, but simulations have shown that, even when the pattern is specified incorrectly, the MMRM Type I error is often better than LOCF (Mallinckrodt *et al.*, 2004).

- Because of its substantial use historically and relevance in some situations, the FDA might still want to see LOCF analyses in regulatory submissions, and so including the LOCF analysis as a supportive descriptive analysis is a reasonable strategy for indications that are not expected to worsen over time (see Sections 1.4 and 4.2.2.3).

5.3   Understanding the data

In the next section we will provide a detailed MMRM example. However, as described in Section 4.4, before doing an analysis designed to address missing data due to patient discontinuations, it is important to understand the amount and pattern of the missing data, including the number discontinued, the reasons for discontinuation, and the time the discontinuations happened. Therefore, in this section, we will describe the Parkinson's disease example introduced in Sections 1.2 and 1.10.1, so that the missing data is well understood before we complete an MMRM analysis in Section 5.4. A second example, from the NIMH CATIE study (Lieberman *et al.*, 2005) of antipsychotics for schizophrenia, is also presented here to highlight the strengths and importance of some of the displays for showing missing data patterns.

5.3.1   Parkinson's disease example

Our first example of the use of MMRM is the illustrative Parkinson's disease dataset. The multi-country multi-site parallel double-blind study of 114 subjects, 57 per treatment group, consisted of a baseline visit, followed by 8 visits 1 to 28 weeks after baseline. The primary outcome measure is the change from baseline in a sub-score of the United Parkinson's Disease Rating Scale (UPDRS), which measures the signs and symptoms of Parkinson's disease. Higher values indicate more severe symptoms (Fahn *et al.*, 1987). A change in this UPDRS sub-score of 2.5 corresponds to a minimal clinically important difference, a change of 5.2 is considered moderate, and 10.8 is a large clinically important difference (Shulman *et al.*, 2010). The average baseline score is 29. See Section 1.10.1 for a complete description of the Parkinson's disease dataset.

In total, 38% of subjects discontinued before 28 weeks: 32% on placebo, and substantially more (44%) on active treatment. Table 5.1 shows that 16% of placebo

Table 5.1   Discontinuation by reason in Parkinson's disease example.

Reason for discontinuation	Placebo (N = 57)	Active (N = 57)	Total (N = 114)
Completed	39 (68%)	32 (56%)	71 (62%)
Discontinued	18 (32%)	25 (44%)	43 (38%)
Adverse event	5 (9%)	22 (39%)	27 (24%)
Lack of efficacy	9 (16%)	0	9 (8%)
Withdrew consent/loss to follow-up	2 (4%)	3 (4%)	5 (4%)
Protocol violation	2 (4%)	0	2 (2%)

Table 5.2   Discontinuation by visit in Parkinson's disease example.

Visit	Placebo (N = 57)		Active (N = 57)	
	Completed	Discontinued	Completed	Discontinued
0 (Baseline)	57 (100%)	0	57 (100%)	0
1 (Week 2)	55 (96%)	2 (4%)	53 (93%)	4 (7%)
2 (Week 3)	52 (92%)	3 (5%)	48 (84%)	5 (9%)
3 (Week 4)	52 (88%)	0	45 (79%)	3 (5%)
4 (Week 6)	46 (88%)	6 (11%)	39 (68%)	6 (11%)
5 (Week 8)	42 (77%)	4 (7%)	35 (61%)	4 (7%)
6 (Week 12)	40 (72%)	2 (4%)	32 (56%)	3 (5%)
7 (Week 20)	39 (68%)	1 (2%)	32 (56%)	0
8 (Week 28)	39 (68%)	0	32 (56%)	0

subjects discontinued due to lack of efficacy, compared to no subjects on the active treatment. In contrast, 39% of subjects on active treatment and 9% on placebo discontinued due to adverse events. Table 5.2 shows the pattern of discontinuation over time. The active group had more subjects discontinued in the first 4 weeks, and after that, the discontinuation rates were similar. Figure 5.1 shows the Kaplan–Meier plot of time until discontinuation.

Figure 5.2 shows the observed data mean change from baseline by visit. In each treatment group, Parkinson's disease signs and symptoms decreased for the first 12 weeks, and then either flattened or worsened through Week 28. Since a large percentage of subjects discontinued, treatment group comparisons should not be made based on the observed data, except for descriptive purposes.

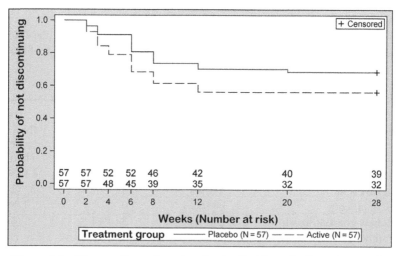

Figure 5.1   Time to discontinuation for the Parkinson's disease example.

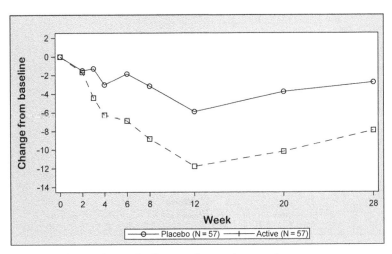

Figure 5.2   Parkinson's disease observed means by treatment group.

Response profile plots over time by visit of discontinuation and by reason for discontinuation can often show different patterns of response that might suggest a pattern-mixture analysis could be helpful. See Section 1.10 for further examples of response profile graphs, and Chapter 7 for pattern-mixture models. Figure 5.3 shows the mean UPDRS sub-score change from baseline over time for categories of reason for discontinuation (AE, other, completers) and treatment group. Regardless of reason for discontinuation, those who discontinued early had less improvement, or

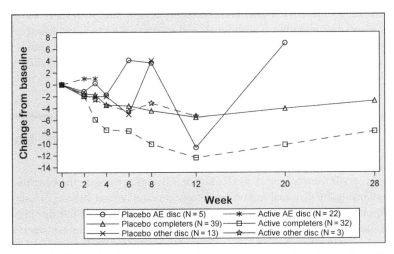

Figure 5.3   Parkinson's disease observed means by reason for discontinuation and treatment group.

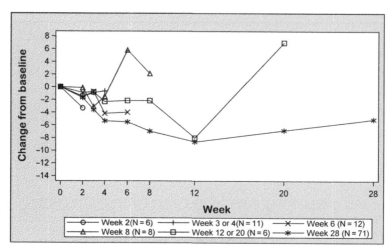

Figure 5.4   Parkinson's disease observed means by visit of discontinuation.

sometimes even a worsening in their PD signs and symptoms, compared to completers. Figure 5.4 combines subjects by their visit of discontinuation, regardless of the reason. Because of the small sample size, the treatment groups are combined, although it would be preferable to have them separate. We see that, except for the first visit at Week 2, the subjects who discontinued at a visit always had worse average scores than those who completed the trial.

Summarized together, the information from Figures 5.1, 5.2, 5.3 and 5.4 indicates that those who discontinue from the study after Week 2 have worsening symptoms at the time of discontinuation regardless of reason for discontinuation, and that the treatment groups have a differential discontinuation rate, with more subjects in the active arm discontinuing. The differential discontinuation rate, combined with the trend for worsening symptoms for all subjects in the later visits, would tend to make LOCF or completers analyses inaccurate estimates of the treatment group differences. A method that takes all information into account and addresses the missing data patterns is needed.

5.3.2   A second example showing the usefulness of plots: The CATIE study

Due to the small sample size in the Parkinson's disease example, the benefits of the graphs of means by visit and reason for discontinuation are not striking. To show the benefits of these graphing methods, we introduce here some similar displays from the National Institute of Mental Health Clinical Antipsychotic Trials of Intervention Effectiveness (CATIE) schizophrenia trial (Lieberman *et al.*, 2005; Davis *et al.*, 2011). The primary phase of the CATIE trial had 1432 subjects followed for up to 18 months, with a discontinuation rate of 74%. The primary outcome for CATIE was time until

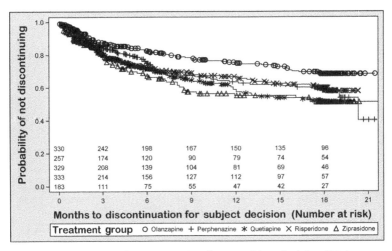

Figure 5.5   CATIE time to discontinuation due to subject decision (Lieberman et al.*, 2005).*

discontinuation. Time to discontinuation due to lack of efficacy, for intolerability, and for subject decision, including loss to follow-up were secondary outcomes. Figure 5.5 displays the time to discontinuation due to subject decision for the five treatment groups in the trial. One treatment group had less discontinuation for subject decision compared to the other treatment groups (24% vs. 30–35%). If discontinuation due to subject decision was unrelated to the treatment, then we would expect no difference between the groups.

Figure 5.6 provides a graph of the main efficacy assessment, the Positive and Negative Syndrome Scale (PANSS) total score change from baseline (Davis *et al.*, 2011), by both the visit of discontinuation and the reason for discontinuation, dichotomized into lack of efficacy and all other reasons combined. The five treatment groups are combined in this figure. Those who discontinued due to lack of efficacy clearly had a decline in their average PANSS scores at the visit in which they discontinued. However, subjects who discontinued for other reasons (intolerability or subject decision combined) also had a decline in their PANSS score at their final visit, compared to those who completed the trial.

These graphs from CATIE demonstrate the benefits of simple graphs of time to discontinuation and response means by time and reason of discontinuation to understand the relationship of the missing data with the outcome, and the potential impact of the missing data on treatment group comparisons.

5.4   Applying the mixed model for repeated measures

In this section, we will use the Parkinson's disease example to specify an MMRM analysis, show the SAS code to produce the results, review key SAS outputs from the

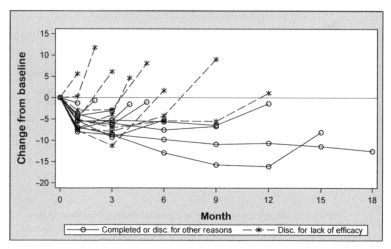

Figure 5.6   CATIE PANSS mean change from baseline by cohorts based on reason for discontinuation and duration of phase participation (Davis et al., 2011).

model and present and interpret the results. We also explore the MMRM results for this example using several different covariance patterns and modeling options, and compare them to LOCF.

5.4.1   Specifying the model

5.4.1.1   Analysis plan

An important step in preparing for the analysis is to provide a complete and clear description in a statistical analysis plan (SAP) prior to unblinding the trial. The following example is an adequate and appropriate description of MMRM for the Parkinson's disease trial. Complete SAP text for primary and sensitivity analyses for this example is provided in Appendix 4.A.

Treatment groups will be compared for the change from baseline in the Unified Parkinson's Disease Rating Scale (UPDRS) Total Score at Week 28 using a mixed effects ANCOVA model for repeated measures (MMRM). The observed change from baseline score at each scheduled post-baseline visit (Visits 1 to 8) is the dependent variable. The model will include the baseline UPDRS total score as a fixed effect covariate, with fixed effect categorical factors for geographic region (North America, South America, Western Europe, Eastern Europe and Asia), treatment group (Active and Placebo), visit and baseline × visit and treatment × visit interactions. The interactions will remain in the model regardless of significance. Treatment group comparisons at each visit will be estimated by differences between least squares (LS) means from the treatment × visit interaction, with accompanying *p*-values and 95% CIs. An unstructured covariance pattern will be used to estimate the variance–covariance of the within-subject repeated measures. Parameters will be estimated using REML with the Newton–Raphson algorithm and using the Kenward–Roger method for calculating the denominator degrees of freedom.

In case this model does not converge, a heterogeneous Toeplitz covariance pattern will be used in place of unstructured. In this case, to assess the robustness of the results, a supportive model using a sandwich estimator for the standard error of the fixed effects parameters will also be produced.

The objective of this analysis is to examine treatment differences at Week 28, the final time point, using LS means from the model. The treatment × visit interaction tests the hypothesis of parallel response profiles over time in the treatment groups. A significant treatment × visit interaction indicates that the magnitude of the difference between treatment groups varies over time. It remains in the model even if not significant so that we can test for differences at Week 28, which is our primary focus.

It is beneficial in a clinical trial to adjust for baseline, since baseline is often a strong predictor of the amount of change and can provide a substantial reduction in the residual variance, hence a gain in power. Adjustment for investigator site also has a similar impact. In some studies, there are many sites from different countries or regions, each with only a few subjects. Our illustrative Parkinson's disease trial had many small sites across many countries. Investigator site could not be included as a fixed effect in the model, since the model would likely not converge due to the small sample sizes within each site. Therefore, geographic region was used instead. Another option might be to fit site as a random effect. However, since investigator sites in clinical trials are a convenience sample and not a random sample representative of some larger population, we do not consider random sites appropriate for clinical trials.

The baseline × visit interaction allows the model to reflect potential differences in the relationship between baseline and the change from baseline at each post-baseline visit. Including this interaction can provide a better fit to the data. For example, those with more severe baseline symptoms often drop out sooner, and so the average baseline score for subjects present at later visits may be milder than the average baseline score for patients present at the initial post-baseline visits.

Kenward–Roger is a method for computing denominator degrees of freedom for the tests of fixed effects, proposed by Kenward and Roger (1997). It is preferred for models with small samples or missing data, and thus it is a standard option for MMRM. However, since there are other methods for computing degrees of freedom, an MMRM model is not fully specified without identifying the degrees of freedom estimation method.

5.4.1.2   Strategies to improve convergence

Site pooling   Often in a clinical trial, it is advantageous to adjust for investigator site. When there are small sample sizes within investigator sites, there may be concern that the model may not converge. Pre-planning to pool small sites can help with the MMRM model convergence. Yet it is preferable to minimize pooling to the extent possible in order to preserve randomization when subjects are randomized within site. Also, no pooled site should be too large relative to the size of other pooled or free-standing sites, so that no pooled site is overly dominant in the analysis. Sites should be pooled by similar characteristics such as geographical location, type of site and/or number of subjects randomized (e.g., very few versus several). The site pooling strategy should be specified in the analysis plan and implemented prior to unblinding. A reasonable strategy for a continuous primary outcome is to pool sites that have less than the equivalent of 5 subjects per treatment group (i.e., 10 total subjects per site for a 2-arm study). If the subject drop-out rate is expected to be very high, then the minimum number of subjects per stand-alone site might be increased, to ensure a reasonable number of completers per stand-alone site. Small sites are then combined into a number of pooled sites based on pre-specified site characteristics, such that pooled sites are at least the size of the smallest stand-alone site, but not larger than approximately three times the size of the smallest stand-alone site. Pooled sites should also not be larger than approximately twice the size of the *largest* stand-alone site. Sometimes it may be necessary to pool a small site with a stand-alone site if no other small sites are available with the same site characteristics. As an example, if a trial has three treatment groups with 1:1:1 allocation within site, then the sites with fewer than 15 subjects would be pooled with other small sites, such that the smallest pooled site is at least 15 subjects and the largest pooled site is not more than approximately 45 subjects. Sites with 15 subjects or more would not be pooled, unless a smaller site needs to be pooled with a larger one due to geographic proximity. Another example of site pooling strategy is described in Koch *et al.* (1993).

It is very common for a Phase III clinical trial to be multi-national, with a large number of sites and a very small number of subjects per site. In this case, a good pooling strategy is often to group by country or geographic region, as with the Parkinson's disease example. As discussed in Section 5.4.1.1, treating site as a random effect is not preferred for a trial with a convenience sample of sites. An alternate strategy to site adjustment is to substitute site with explanatory site-level variables, such as geographic region and site type, directly in the model (Koch *et al.*, 1998).

Baseline × visit interaction   If there are very many visits and a relatively small sample size, an additional option is to leave the baseline × visit interaction out of the primary model. However, it is always better to keep this term in the model if possible. Generally, due to sample sizes required for safety reporting, a Phase III clinical trial will have enough sample size for the unstructured model to converge with a reasonable set of pooled sites, and with the inclusion of the baseline × visit interaction.

5.4.1.3   SAS code

When producing the statistical analysis in a software package such as SAS, it can be good practice to provide sample SAS code of your primary efficacy analysis as

```
PROC MIXED DATA=updrs_v;
  CLASS subjid region trt visit ;
  MODEL change = base_upd region trt visit trt*visit
        base_upd*visit  / DDFM=KR ;
  REPEATED visit / TYPE=UN SUBJECT=subjid R RCORR;
  LSMEANS trt*visit / PDIFF CL;
  ESTIMATE "TRT 1 vn 2 at visit 8" TRT 1 -1
        TRT*VISIT 0 0 0 0 0 0 0 1  0 0 0 0 0 0 0 -1 /CL ;
RUN;
```

SAS Code Fragment 5.1 Standard MMRM SAS code for Parkinson's disease example.

an appendix to the SAP for additional documentation. SAS code for the Parkinson's disease trial is provided in SAS Code Fragment 5.1. It is good practice to first sort the dataset by the class variables, and to be sure the categorical variables listed in the CLASS and MODEL statements appear in the same order. The dataset UPDRS_V has a "vertical" structure, with one record per subject visit. The dependent variable is the UPDRS change from baseline.

In scalar notation, the model estimate for an observed value y_{ij} can be written as follows:

$$y_{ij} = \beta_0 + x_b\beta_b + \sum_{r=1}^{5} x_r\beta_r + \sum_{t=1}^{2} x_t\beta_t + \sum_{k=1}^{8} x_k\beta_k + \sum_{k=1}^{8} x_k x_b \beta_{bk} + \sum_{t=1}^{2}\sum_{k=1}^{8} x_{tk}\beta_{tk} \quad (5.15)$$

where β_0 is the intercept, x_b is the baseline value, x_r, x_t, x_k, x_{tk} are indicators for the 5 regions, 2 treatments, 8 visits and 16 treatment × visit combinations respectively, and $\beta_r, \beta_t, \beta_k$, and β_{tk} are the corresponding coefficients. The estimate for the treatment difference at Visit 8 can be obtained by calculating the estimate at Visit 8 for a given baseline value and region separately for each treatment group and then subtracting the coefficients for treatment group 2 from treatment group 1. In so doing, the intercept and coefficients for baseline, region, and baseline by Visit 8 interaction cancel out, leaving a difference of treatment 1 − treatment 2 for the estimates of both the overall treatment effect and the effect for Visit 8. The estimate statement is shown in SAS Code Fragment 5.1. Recall that terms in the model with all coefficients equal to zero are not required to be specified in the estimate statement.

The Kenward–Roger method is specified with the DDFM=KR option. REML is the default, but we could have added an option to the first line METHOD=REML. The REPEATED statement indicates that the variable *visit* uniquely identifies the repeated measurements for the subjects, and the variable *subjid* uniquely identifies each subject. TYPE=UN specifies the unstructured covariance pattern of the repeated visits per subject. R and RCORR do not affect the model, but request helpful SAS output for interpreting the model: the variance–covariance **R** matrix for an example subject and the same matrix converted to correlations. PDIFF and CL request pairwise differences and confidence intervals for each pairwise set of combinations of treatment and visit. We are only interested in some of these comparisons, and so we could specify our estimates of interest through the CONTROL= facility of the LSMEANS statement; or through ESTIMATE statements, as provided in the SAS code for the final time point.

5.4.2   Interpreting and presenting results

In this section we will review the SAS output and corresponding results from the model specified in the prior section, and then a series of comparisons if alternate analysis options or strategies were used.

5.4.2.1   Unstructured covariance pattern

Provided here are selected sections of SAS output obtained from the SAS code specified in SAS Code Fragment 5.1 for the Parkinson's disease trial. For comparison of methods, this same example dataset with monotone missingness is used in Chapters 6 and 7. SAS Output 5.1 provides general model fitting information, where we confirm that we have requested REML, Kenward–Roger degrees of freedom estimation, and an unstructured covariance pattern.

SAS Output 5.2 provides class level information, confirming that we have appropriately specified region, treatment, and visit as categorical factors, and confirming the number of subjects in the analysis.

Pay careful attention to confirm the expected model dimension information in SAS Output 5.3. There are 36 covariance parameters specified. The unstructured pattern estimates $J(J + 1)/2$ parameters (J is the number of visits, see Section 5.2.2.1), and with 8 visits, this corresponds to $(8 \times 9)/2 = 36$. The 41 columns in X correspond to each of the factors in the model: 1 for the intercept + 1 for baseline + 5 for region + 2

Model Information	
Dataset	Updrs_V
Dependent Variable	Change
Covariance Structure	Unstructured
Subject Effect	Subjid
Estimation Method	REML
Residual Variance Method	None
Fixed Effects SE Method	Kenward–Roger
Degrees of Freedom Method	Kenward–Roger

SAS Output 5.1   Parkinson's disease MMRM model information.

Class Level Information		
Class	**Levels**	**Values**
Region	5	1 2 3 4 5
Subjid	114	1 10 100 101 102 ... 114
Trt	2	1 2
Visit	8	1 2 3 4 5 6 7 8

SAS Output 5.2   Parkinson's disease MMRM class level information.

Dimensions	
Covariance Parameters	36
Columns in X	41
Columns in Z	0
Subjects	114
Max Obs Per Subject	8

SAS Output 5.3   Parkinson's disease MMRM dimension information.

for treatment + 8 for visit + 8 for the baseline × visit interaction + 16 for the treatment × visit interaction. There are no columns in Z reflecting that we have not specified any random effects in this model, which we would have specified with the RANDOM statement. All of the 114 subjects were included in the analysis, and the maximum number of visits per subject is 8.

SAS Output 5.4 shows the number of observations used and not used in the analysis. This can be helpful to identify missing values in covariates. In this case,

Number of Observations	
Number of Observations Read	912
Number of Observations Used	724
Number of Observations Not Used	188

SAS Output 5.4   Parkinson's disease MMRM observation information.

| \multicolumn{9}{c}{Estimated R Matrix for subjid 1} | | | | | | | | |
Row	Col1	Col2	Col3	Col4	Col5	Col6	Col7	Col8
1	25.3	17.8	21.3	21.1	16.4	12.8	16.7	21.1
2	17.8	33.6	28.5	28.5	20.7	15.5	18.4	22.6
3	21.3	28.5	52.5	45.3	36.2	22.7	36.5	41.7
4	21.1	28.5	45.3	84.1	41.8	30.8	36.6	55.0
5	16.4	20.7	36.2	41.8	59.5	33.2	53.8	56.1
6	12.8	15.5	22.7	30.8	33.2	39.1	38.9	41.1
7	16.7	18.4	36.5	36.6	53.8	38.9	77.5	72.5
8	21.1	22.6	41.7	55.0	56.1	41.1	72.5	103.7

SAS Output 5.5   Parkinson's disease MMRM R variance–covariance matrix – unstructured.

our dataset was designed to have a record for all eight visits, with missing values for the visits after a subject discontinued. Although this is not the usual way that we formulate our analysis datasets, it provides here a nice description of the number of total records used in the analysis (724), and the number of records that were missing due to early subject dropouts (188, 21% of all expected visits).

The variance–covariance matrix of the repeated visits per subject based on the unstructured pattern is provided in SAS Output 5.5 for an example subject (*subjid = 1*). The diagonal has been highlighted to point out the variances from each visit. We see that the variance tends to increase in the later visits, which is commonly the case. The off-diagonal elements are best evaluated in the R correlation matrix, displayed in SAS Output 5.6. Each entry of the correlation matrix are obtained from the covariance matrix by Corr(A, B) = Cov(A, B)/SQRT(Var(A) × Var(B)). We see that the correlations between visits are generally high and consistent, but decrease as the visits become farther apart from each other. This pattern may be appropriate for alternate structures that require fewer parameters to be estimated; however, for MMRM, we want to keep the model as unrestricted as possible. Therefore, we would not use a review of this matrix to consider alternate covariance patterns. It is important to evaluate the magnitude of the correlation between visits, since the MMRM depends on the correlation to predict the results at later visits for subjects who drop out early, based on the available data for that subject and the model-estimated correlation between later visits. In particular, if the estimated correlations between the later visits and earlier visits are *low*, the estimates for subjects who drop out early will depend less on the available data for those subjects than in a scenario where the estimated correlations are *high*.

| Estimated R Correlation Matrix for subjid 1 | | | | | | | |
Row	Col1	Col2	Col3	Col4	Col5	Col6	Col7	Col8
1	1.00	0.61	0.58	0.45	0.42	0.40	0.37	0.41
2	0.61	1.00	0.67	0.53	0.46	0.42	0.36	0.38
3	0.58	0.67	1.00	0.68	0.64	0.50	0.57	0.56
4	0.45	0.53	0.68	1.00	0.59	0.53	0.45	0.58
5	0.42	0.46	0.64	0.59	1.00	0.68	0.79	0.71
6	0.40	0.42	0.50	0.53	0.68	1.00	0.70	0.64
7	0.37	0.36	0.57	0.45	0.79	0.70	1.00	0.80
8	0.41	0.38	0.56	0.58	0.71	0.64	0.80	1.00

SAS Output 5.6   Parkinson's disease MMRM R correlation matrix – unstructured.

The degrees of freedom and p-values for the fixed effects are provided in SAS Output 5.7. We see that geographic region is a weak predictor, and both baseline and the baseline × visit interaction are highly significant in this trial. The treatment × visit interaction has $p < 0.05$, yet we are not particularly interested in the significance of treatment, visit and their interaction for MMRM. The primary interest is the one degree of freedom treatment comparison at Week 28, which is only one component of the interaction.

The LS estimated mean change from baseline for each treatment and visit from this interaction term are displayed in Table 5.3, and graphed in Figure 5.7. The active - placebo (trt 2 - trt 1) differences between the LS means, with corresponding 95% CIs

| Type III Tests of Fixed Effects | | | |
Effect	Num DF	Den DF	F Value	Pr > F
Region	4	110	2.19	0.0746
base_UPD	1	100	10.30	0.0018
Trt	1	102	11.87	0.0008
Visit	7	75	0.81	0.5807
base_UPD*visit	7	74.8	3.50	0.0027
trt*visit	7	74.7	2.71	0.0146

SAS Output 5.7   Parkinson's disease MMRM fixed effects – unstructured.

Table 5.3   MMRM estimates by treatment group and visit for Parkinson's disease example.

Visit	Placebo (N = 57)			Active (N = 57)		
	Est.	SE	95% CI	Est.	SE	95% CI
1 (Week 2)	−1.1	0.7	(−2.5, 0.4)	−1.5	0.7	(−2.9, −0.1)
2 (Week 3)	−0.9	0.8	(−2.6, 0.7)	−4.3	0.8	(−5.9, −2.7)
3 (Week 4)	−2.7	1.0	(−4.7, −0.7)	−6.0	1.0	(−8.0, −3.9)
4 (Week 6)	−1.6	1.3	(−4.1, 1.0)	−6.3	1.3	(−8.9, −3.6)
5 (Week 8)	−3.0	1.1	(−5.2, −0.7)	−8.0	1.2	(−10.4, −5.6)
6 (Week 12)	−4.9	1.0	(−6.8, −2.9)	−10.8	1.0	(−12.8, −8.7)
7 (Week 20)	−2.8	1.3	(−5.4, −0.0)	−8.4	1.4	(−11.3, −5.6)
8 (Week 28)	−1.2	1.6	(−4.3, 1.9)	−6.1	1.7	(−9.4, −2.7)

and p-values, are displayed in Table 5.4. The treatment groups are similar at Visit 1, and then diverge starting at Visit 2 (Week 3). The difference weakens at Visit 8 (Week 28), but is still within the level of a moderate clinically important difference according to Shulman et al. (2010) (LSmean difference $= -4.9$, SE $= 2.3$, $p = 0.033$). Figure 5.7 includes the observed means for the non-missing cases on the same plot, for comparison. We can see that the MMRM estimates have higher values, or, in other words, a smaller (worse) change from baseline than the observed cases. We would expect this, since we saw in Section 5.3.1 that, on average, when subjects dropped out early, their UPDRS scores were not as good as others who did not discontinue

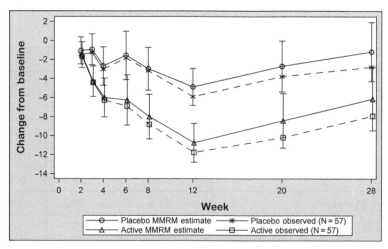

Figure 5.7   Parkinson's disease MMRM unstructured estimates and 95% CI and observed means.

Table 5.4   MMRM results of treatment group differences by visit for Parkinson's disease example.

Active vs. placebo at visit:	Est.	SE	95% CI	p-value
1 (Week 2)	−0.4	1.0	(−2.3, 1.4)	0.638
2 (Week 3)	−3.4	1.1	(−5.6, −1.1)	0.003
3 (Week 4)	−3.3	1.4	(−6.1, −0.5)	0.022
4 (Week 6)	−4.7	1.8	(−8.3, −1.1)	0.012
5 (Week 8)	−5.3	1.6	(−8.2, −1.8)	0.003
6 (Week 12)	−5.9	1.4	(−8.6, −3.1)	<0.0001
7 (Week 20)	−5.7	2.0	(−9.6, −1.8)	0.004
8 (Week 28)	−4.9	2.3	(−9.5, −0.4)	0.033

at that visit, or sometimes even worse than baseline. The MMRM model is using the observed data and the observed correlation of the non-missing data at later visits (based on the specified covariance structure) to make the LS mean estimate at each visit based on all available information, including information from partially observed subjects. Therefore, if later visits are fairly highly correlated with early ones, we would expect their scores would have continued to be poor had they stayed in the trial until Week 28.

SAS Output 5.7 shows us that the interaction between baseline score and visit is a strong predictor of the change score, indicating that the relationship between baseline and change in UPDRS during the study varies across visits. Table 5.5 presents results from an unstructured model without this term. In our example, removing the term reduced the number of fixed effects by seven and produced a somewhat larger estimate of the treatment group difference at Week 28 (LSmean = −5.1, Table 5.5), with the same standard error. We can compare the fit of these two models with the Corrected Akaike Information Criterion (AICC) (Hurvich and Tsai, 1989), the fit statistic provided by SAS PROC MIXED and presented in Table 5.5. The AICC for these models is numerically very similar, although the model without the interaction has a slightly better AICC because it estimates fewer parameters. The AICC is a function of the number of parameters in the model and the likelihood. It penalizes models with more parameters (Hurvich and Tsai, 1989). As noted earlier, when there is sufficient sample size to support convergence, we recommend always including the baseline × visit interaction.

Another option available for the MMRM model is, while still requiring the covariance *structure* to be the same for each subject, to allow the covariance *estimates* of this structure to vary across groups of subjects, for example, separate covariance estimates by treatment group. In this case, the *R* covariance matrix, as presented in Equation 5.9, is modified to estimate one set of R parameters per treatment group. This option provides more generality by not requiring the treatment groups to have the same covariance estimates, yet also adds complexity to the model by requiring estimation of more covariance parameters, for example, twice as many for two treatment groups.

Table 5.5   Parkinson's disease example active versus placebo at Visit 8 (Week 28) using different models.

Model	No. of covar parms	Est.	SE	95% CI	p-value	AICC
Unstructured	36	−4.9	2.3	(−9.5, −0.4)	0.033	4483.9
Unstructured without baseline × visit interaction	36	−5.1	2.3	(−9.6, −0.6)	0.028	4477.9
Unstructured with separate covariance parameters for each treatment group	72	−4.6	2.4	(−9.3, 0.2)	0.058	4487.6
Heterogeneous Toeplitz	15	−4.7	2.1	(−9.0, −0.5)	0.029	4475.7
Heterogeneous Toeplitz with sandwich estimator	15	−4.7	2.1	(−8.9, −0.6)	0.025	4475.7
Spatial power	2	−4.5	1.9	(−8.3, −0.8)	0.019	4651.8
Spatial power with random subject effect	3	−4.5	1.7	(−7.9, −1.1)	0.009	4565.3
Spatial power with random subject effect and sandwich estimator	3	−4.5	2.1	(−8.7, −0.3)	0.034	4565.3
LOCF	N/A	−3.8	1.7	(−7.2, −0.5)	0.025	N/A
Observed case (completers)	N/A	−4.3	2.3	(−9.0, 0.4)	0.072	N/A
GEE with exchangeable working correlation	1	−4.5	2.1	(−8.7, −0.3)	0.036	N/A

AICC = Akaike Information Criterion Corrected (smaller value indicates better model fit).

Operationally, separate parameters are obtained for the treatment groups by adding the option GROUP=*trt* to the REPEATED VISIT line in SAS Code Fragment 5.1. Compared to SAS Output 5.3, there are 72 instead of 36 covariance parameters. Table 5.5 shows that the estimated treatment group difference is somewhat similar to the original model with the same estimates across the treatment groups, although the standard error is larger. The AICC is higher (worse) for this model compared to the original model. In this example, the pre-specified model with the same parameters for the two treatment groups is a preferable fit to the data.

5.4.2.2   Heterogeneous Toeplitz covariance pattern

We have completed the MMRM analysis for the Parkinson's disease dataset according to the pre-specified SAP. In this section, results from other analysis options are provided as a comparison. An analysis of a confirmatory clinical trial would do such

			Estimated R Correlation Matrix for subjid 1					
Row	Col1	Col2	Col3	Col4	Col5	Col6	Col7	Col8
1	1.00	0.67	0.62	0.51	0.50	0.43	0.38	0.37
2	0.67	1.00	0.67	0.62	0.51	0.50	0.43	0.38
3	0.62	0.67	1.00	0.67	0.62	0.51	0.50	0.43
4	0.51	0.62	0.67	1.00	0.67	0.62	0.51	0.50
5	0.50	0.51	0.62	0.67	1.00	0.67	0.62	0.51
6	0.43	0.50	0.51	0.62	0.67	1.00	0.67	0.62
7	0.38	0.43	0.50	0.51	0.62	0.67	1.00	0.67
8	0.37	0.38	0.43	0.50	0.51	0.62	0.67	1.00

SAS Output 5.8   Parkinson's disease MMRM R correlation matrix – heterogeneous Toeplitz.

explorations only if pre-specified in the analysis plan. If the unstructured model had not converged, our plan specified the heterogeneous Toeplitz. The SAS code for this model is the same as in SAS Code Fragment 5.1, with TYPE=UN changed to TYPE=TOEPH. This model estimates $(2 \times 8) - 1 = 15$ variance–covariance parameters instead of 36, a substantial reduction in the number of parameters estimated. The estimated R correlation matrix for the heterogeneous Toeplitz structure is shown in SAS Output 5.8.

A visual comparison shows that the correlations are mostly similar to the unstructured matrix in SAS Output 5.6, except that the correlations are underestimated for Visit 8 with Visits 3, 5, 7 and for Visit 5 with Visit 7. The AICC is numerically very similar for these two models. The estimated treatment difference at Week 28 is -4.7, SE $= 2.1$, $p = 0.029$ (Table 5.5).

In summary, in this example, UN and TOEPH covariance patterns yielded similar fit and similar results, although TOEPH estimated 21 fewer covariance parameters. The comparison between these two variance patterns helps demonstrate the need to pre-specify the correlation pattern a priori. If the results are hovering around statistical significance, we do not want to open ourselves up to the possibility of selecting a pattern in a manner that could be viewed as biased because of having looked at the data.

Since, by using the heterogeneous Toeplitz, we have imposed a structure onto the covariance of the repeated measurements, there is the possibility that this structure may in fact not be the actual structure of the data. As we specified in our analysis plan, we will perform a sensitivity analysis of the MMRM results by requesting the empirical sandwich estimator.

To produce this variance estimator, we add the EMPIRICAL option to the PROC MIXED line in the SAS code. The Kenward–Roger method for degrees of freedom is not available with this option, so we allow SAS to use the default between-within degrees of freedom estimation method. For our Parkinson's disease example, the results comparing the treatment groups at Week 28 are practically identical to the model without the sandwich estimator (Table 5.5). The empirical variance estimator is less efficient, and so, in general, we would expect to see an increase in the standard error in most settings.

For our Parkinson's disease example, the visits are not equally spaced in time. It might be reasonable to expect that visits that are closer together, such as Visit 1 and Visit 2, which are 1 week apart, may have a different correlation than Visits 7 and 8, which are 8 weeks apart. For the heterogeneous Toeplitz, the correlations are banded. As we see in SAS Output 5.8, the estimated correlation between Visit 1 and Visit 2 is the same as between Visit 7 and Visit 8 (0.67). In our example data, the correlation between Visits 7 and 8 is actually stronger than between Visits 1 and 2, as we see from SAS Output 5.6 for the unstructured model. Although not seen in this case, we most often would expect the correlation to be smaller (and certainly not larger) the farther apart in time the two visits are from each other.

5.4.2.3 Spatial power covariance pattern

Since we have unequally spaced visits, we will explore how the model results would change if we had specified a spatial power covariance pattern in the analysis plan. Recall that spatial power structure decreases the correlation with increased time between visits, so this is likely not an optimal choice for this dataset. We will fit three models: one standard MMRM model (which is *not* recommended); one with the addition of the random subject effect; and one with both the random subject effect and the empirical sandwich estimator.

To fit the spatial power in SAS, we first create a continuous variable that corresponds to the planned number of weeks from baseline for each of the visits, which we will call *visweek*. In the MMRM model, we specify TYPE=SP(POW)(*visweek*). The complete PROC MIXED code for the sandwich estimator spatial power model with a random subject effect is provided in SAS Code Fragment 5.2.

```
PROC MIXED DATA=updrs_v EMPIRICAL;
  CLASS subjid region trt visit ;
  MODEL change = base_upd region trt visit trt*visit
        base_upd*visit ;
  REPEATED visit/TYPE=SP(POW)(visweek)SUBJECT=subjid R RCORR;
  RANDOM INTERCEPT / SUBJECT=subjid G V VCORR;
  LSMEANS trt*visit / PDIFF CL;
  ESTIMATE "TRT 1 vs 2 at visit 8" TRT 1 -1
        TRT*VISIT 0 0 0 0 0 0 0 1 0 0 0 0 0 0 0 -1 /CL;
RUN;
```

SAS Code Fragment 5.2 MMRM with spatial power, random subject effect and sandwich estimator.

Estimated R Correlation Matrix for subjid 1							
Row	Col1	Col2	Col3	Col4	Col5	Col6	Col7	Col8
1	1.00	0.81	0.67	0.44	0.30	0.13	0.03	0.01
2	0.81	1.00	0.81	0.54	0.36	0.16	0.03	0.01
3	0.67	0.81	1.00	0.67	0.44	0.20	0.04	0.01
4	0.44	0.54	0.67	1.00	0.67	0.30	0.06	0.01
5	0.30	0.36	0.44	0.67	1.00	0.44	0.09	0.02
6	0.13	0.16	0.20	0.30	0.44	1.00	0.20	0.04
7	0.03	0.03	0.04	0.06	0.09	0.20	1.00	0.20
8	0.01	0.01	0.01	0.01	0.02	0.04	0.20	1.00

SAS Output 5.9   Parkinson's disease MMRM R correlation matrix – spatial power.

The G, V and VCORR options do not affect the model, but request helpful SAS output for interpreting the model: the covariance parameter G for an example subject, the variance–covariance V matrix for an example subject (recall $V = ZGZ^T + R$) and the same matrix converted to correlations.

The spatial power model without the random effects parameter fits two covariance parameters. The estimated correlation matrix is shown in SAS Output 5.9.

Inspection of this matrix tells us right away that this was not a good fit to the data, since the imposed structure has a correlation of 0.81 between Visits 1 and 2 (1 week apart), only 0.2 for Visits 7 and 8 (8 weeks apart), and nearly zero correlation between visits that are 16 or more weeks apart. These estimates are very different from the unstructured estimates in SAS Output 5.6. The AICC for the model fit (Table 5.5) shows a substantially worse fit to the data than the unstructured model. The correlation misspecification has a substantial impact on both the LS mean treatment group difference at Week 28 and its standard error (LSmean = −4.5, SE = 1.9, $p = 0.019$, Table 5.5). In this example, both turned out smaller than other models.

The addition of the random subject covariance to the spatial power model adds an underlying within-subject covariance term, which allows for a decrease in correlations over time in the spatial power format, but not below the within-subject correlation. SAS Output 5.10 displays selected components of the SAS output for this model, showing that there are three covariance parameters, and that the Z matrix has one column per subject, corresponding to the intercept. SAS Output 5.11 displays the estimated V correlation matrix from the model. The addition of the random subject effect improved the model fit substantially according to the AICC (Table 5.5), yet still not as well as the unstructured or heterogeneous Toeplitz. With the better correlation fit than the simple MMRM spatial power structure, the LSmean estimate was the same, but the standard error was reduced (SE = 1.7, $p = 0.009$, Table 5.5). A supportive

Dimensions	
Covariance Parameters	3
Columns in X	41
Columns in Z Per Subject	1
Subjects	114
Max Obs Per Subject	8

Estimated G Matrix			
Row	Effect	Subjid	Col1
1	Intercept	1	29.3115

SAS Output 5.10   Parkinson's disease MMRM selected model information – spatial power + random subject.

analysis applying the sandwich estimator has a higher standard error, as expected (SE = 2.1, $p = 0.034$, Table 5.5).

5.4.2.4   Last observation carried forward

For comparison to the MMRM results, Table 5.5 includes estimates from a simple ANCOVA adjusting for baseline score and geographic region for the LOCF endpoint, and also for the observed Week 28 data for the subset of 71 subjects that completed

Estimated V Correlation Matrix for subjid 1								
Row	Col1	Col2	Col3	Col4	Col5	Col6	Col7	Col8
1	1.00	0.76	0.64	0.54	0.52	0.51	0.51	0.51
2	0.76	1.00	0.76	0.57	0.52	0.51	0.51	0.51
3	0.64	0.76	1.00	0.64	0.54	0.51	0.51	0.51
4	0.54	0.57	0.64	1.00	0.64	0.52	0.51	0.51
5	0.52	0.52	0.54	0.64	1.00	0.54	0.51	0.51
6	0.51	0.51	0.51	0.52	0.54	1.00	0.51	0.51
7	0.51	0.51	0.51	0.51	0.51	0.51	1.00	0.51
8	0.51	0.51	0.51	0.51	0.51	0.51	0.51	1.00

SAS Output 5.11   Parkinson's disease MMRM V correlation matrix – spatial power + random subject.

the trial. In our example, the LOCF analysis yielded an estimate of the treatment difference at Visit 8 (LSmean $= -3.8$) that is smaller than the MMRM estimate. This discrepancy is due to the larger percentage of subjects discontinuing the active treatment arm in the first three visits (Table 5.2 and Figure 5.1), combined with the fact that those who discontinued early generally had a worsening of symptoms (Figure 5.4). As often, the LOCF yields a relatively small estimate of the standard error (SE $= 1.7$). The completers analysis has a relatively high standard error (SE $= 2.3$) due to the smaller number of subjects, and in this particular example, like the LOCF analysis, yields an estimate of treatment difference at Week 28 that is smaller than the MMRM estimate. In situations where treatment group differences continue to diverge over time, the completers analysis would overestimate the actual treatment difference.

5.4.2.5 Generalized estimating equations

In practice, GEE is seldom used for analysis of normally distributed outcomes, in preference for the mixed model, due to the differences highlighted in Section 5.2.3. However, we present a GEE model in this section in order to provide a full comparison of methods for the Parkinson's disease example. In SAS, GEE is fit with PROC GENMOD (SAS Institute Inc., 2011c). The model is specified with the SAS Code Fragment 5.3. In SAS, GENMOD has fewer options for fitting the working correlation structure than MIXED, as less emphasis is placed on fitting the structure in GEE since GEE estimates are asymptotically unbiased regardless of the covariance matrix selected, under the MCAR assumption. Due to the relatively large sample size required for GEE estimation, and the small number of subjects in our example, the GEE algorithm would not converge with an unstructured pattern. Compound symmetry, also called exchangeable, was selected instead. The compound symmetry structure estimates one covariance term, and assumes homogeneous variances and covariances across all visits. Results for this example, presented in Table 5.5, are similar to the MMRM using the spatial power with random subject effect and sandwich estimator.

```
PROC GENMOD DATA=updrs_v ;
  CLASS subjid region trt visit ;
  MODEL change = base_upd region trt visit trt*visit
        base_upd*visit / DIST=NORMAL LINK=IDENTITY ;
  REPEATED SUBJECT=subjid / TYPE=CS CORRW;
  LSMEANS trt*visit / PDIFF CL;
  ESTIMATE "TRT 1 vs 2 at visit 8" TRT 1 -1
      TRT*VISIT 0 0 0 0 0 0 0 1 0 0 0 0 0 0 0 -1 ;
RUN;
```

SAS Code Fragment 5.3 GEE with compound symmetry working correlation matrix.

5.5   Additional mixed model for repeated measures topics

5.5.1   Treatment by subgroup and treatment by site interactions

Phase III clinical trials should have an assessment of the treatment by site interaction specified in the analysis plan. Treatment by subgroup interactions also must be assessed prior to submitting a new drug application to a regulatory authority.

Begin by evaluating the treatment by gender interaction for the Parkinson's disease example. Since the primary time point for this trial is at Week 28 (Visit 8), it is most appropriate to assess the interaction between treatment group and gender at Visit 8. Adding a one degree of freedom treatment × gender interaction to the MMRM model would assess if there is an interaction between treatment and genders averaged across all visits. Although this is of interest, it is not specifically targeted at our primary time point. In order to assess the interaction specifically at Visit 8, we will fit a seven degrees of freedom 3-way interaction of treatment × gender × visit, and assess the one degree of freedom interaction specifically at Visit 8 through a contrast. Appropriate parameterization and interpretation of the 3-way interaction requires fitting all three 2-way interactions. So, although it is of little interest in its own right, a gender × visit interaction is also added.

The SAS code for producing the test of the interaction at Visit 8 is shown in SAS Code Fragment 5.4. As noted earlier, it is best practice to sort the data by the items in the class statement, ensuring that the order of items listed in the class statement, the model statement, and the contrast statement are in a consistent order. The contrast

```
PROC MIXED DATA=updrs_v;
  CLASS subjid region trt gender visit ;
  MODEL change = base_upd region trt gender visit trt*visit
       base_upd*visit
       trt*gender gender*visit trt*gender*visit
       / DDFM=KR ;
  REPEATED visit / TYPE=UN SUBJECT=subjid R RCORR;
  CONTRAST "TRT BY GENDER INTERACTION AT VISIT 8"

  trt*gender 1 -1 -1 1 trt*gender*visit 0 0 0 0 0 0 0 1

                      0 0 0 0 0 0 0 -1

                      0 0 0 0 0 0 0 -1

                      0 0 0 0 0 0 1;
RUN;
```

SAS Code Fragment 5.4   MMRM SAS code for Parkinson's disease treatment × gender interaction at Visit 8.

Type III Tests of Fixed Effects				
Effect	**Num DF**	**Den DF**	**F Value**	**Pr > F**
Region	4	108	2.24	0.0696
base_UPD	1	99.6	8.99	0.0034
Trt	1	100	11.74	0.0009
SEX	1	99.7	0.23	0.6308
Visit	7	76.5	0.76	0.6216
base_UPD*visit	7	75.3	3.82	0.0013
trt*visit	7	74.7	2.37	0.0303
trt*gender	1	99.2	0.00	0.9782
gender*visit	7	74.7	1.04	0.4096
trt*gender*visit	7	74.8	0.99	0.4471
Contrasts				
Label	**Num DF**	**Den DF**	**F Value**	**Pr > F**
TRT by gender interaction at Visit 8	1	75.9	0.38	0.5381

SAS Output 5.12   Selected output produced by SAS Code Fragment 5.12.

for the treatment by gender interaction at Visit 8 can be derived by developing the contrast for the treatment difference at Visit 8 (see SAS Code Fragment 5.1) separately for each gender, and then subtracting the coefficients in one of the gender-specific contrasts from the other, forming a one degree of freedom test of a difference of differences. Recall that terms in the model that have coefficients of zero are not required to be specified in the contrast. SAS Output 5.12 shows the Type III tests of the fixed effects and the contrast. There is no evidence of treatment × gender interaction at Week 28.

Since we are adjusting for geographic region in our model because of the small sample size per site, we will evaluate the treatment × region interaction. Similar to the treatment × gender interaction, it is most relevant to assess the interaction at Visit 8, the primary time point. Adding a four degrees of freedom treatment × region interaction to the MMRM model would assess if there is an interaction between treatment and regions averaged across all visits. We will assess the interaction specifically at Visit 8 by fitting a 28 degrees of freedom 3-way interaction of treatment × region × visit, and assessing the 4 degrees of freedom interaction specifically at Visit 8 through a contrast. The 3-way interaction requires fitting all three 2-way interactions, so we also add a region × visit interaction term.

Table 5.6   Format for the four degrees of freedom treatment × region interaction at Visit 8 for Parkinson's disease.

TRT × region	Treatment × region × visit				
Placebo Active	Line 1: Placebo, Line 2: Active				
12345 12345	Region 1	Region 2	Region 3	Region 4	Region 5
	12345678	12345678	12345678	12345678	12345678
−10001 1000−1	0000000−1	00000000	00000000	00000000	00000001
	00000001	00000000	00000000	00000000	0000000−1
−10010 100−10	0000000−1	00000000	00000000	00000001	00000000
	00000001	00000000	00000000	0000000−1	00000000
−10100 10−100	0000000−1	00000000	00000001	00000000	00000000
	00000001	00000000	0000000−1	00000000	00000000
−11000 1−1000	0000000−1	00000001	00000000	00000000	00000000
	00000001	0000000−1	00000000	00000000	00000000

The SAS code to test the interaction is similar to the code for the treatment × gender interaction, except that, since there are five regions, the test of interaction between treatment and region at Visit 8 is four degrees of freedom, requiring a lengthy contrast statement. Table 5.6 shows the content of this contrast. As with the treatment by gender interaction, the contrasts can be derived by first developing the contrast for the active − placebo treatment difference at Visit 8 separately for each region; and secondly subtracting the coefficients in one of the region-specific contrasts from another one, forming one line of the four degrees of freedom contrast. The four lines of the contrast in Table 5.6 correspond to region 1 versus 5, 1 versus 4, 1 versus 3 and 1 versus 2. Terms in the model that have coefficients of zero are not required to be specified in the contrast.

SAS Output 5.13 shows the Type III tests of the fixed effects and the contrast. There is no strong evidence of treatment × region interaction at Week 28 ($p = 0.143$). Note that the power to detect a treatment × region × visit interaction is often low in most clinical trials. A forest plot of the mean difference between treatment groups ±95% CI by region would be a good tool to visually inspect the strength or pattern of a potential interaction in this case.

5.5.2   Calculating the effect size

It is often very useful to calculate the estimated treatment difference in terms of effect size, that is, the units of standard deviation. This is helpful for two reasons: to obtain

Type III Tests of Fixed Effects				
Effect	Num DF	Den DF	F Value	Pr > F
Trt	1	102	22.05	<.0001
Region	4	96.9	2.00	0.1011
base_UPD	1	92.3	11.09	0.0012
Visit	7	68.8	0.75	0.6331
base_UPD*visit	7	67.8	3.83	0.0015
trt*visit	7	70.1	4.86	0.0002
trt*region	4	96.4	2.71	0.0344
region*visit	28	158	2.14	0.0018
trt*region*visit	28	158	1.80	0.0133
Contrasts				
Label	Num DF	Den DF	F Value	Pr > F
TRT by Region Interaction at Visit 8	4	62.1	1.79	0.1427

SAS Output 5.13   Selected output for MMRM model with treatment × region × visit interaction.

a standardized value for the strength of the treatment effect, and to use for sample size calculations for future trials. The effect size, also called Cohen's d (Cohen, 1988), is calculated as the LS mean difference between the treatment groups divided by the standard deviation:

$$\text{Effect size} = \left| \frac{LSMean\ difference}{\sqrt{Variance}} \right| \qquad (5.16)$$

To calculate the standard deviation of change from baseline at a particular visit based on the MMRM model, we take the square root of the variance estimate for that visit, obtained from the SAS-estimated R matrix. For the unstructured MMRM model, the variance is obtained from the diagonal cells from SAS Output 5.5. Table 5.7 displays the effect size for each visit. Although the effect size is smaller at Week 28 compared to Weeks 8, 12 and 20, an effect size of approximately 0.5 is considered a medium strength (Cohen, 1988). Often an effect size as low as 0.2 is considered a small effect, yet still potentially approvable by regulatory agencies for some indications. An effect size of 0.8 or more is considered large.

Table 5.7   Effect size for Parkinson's disease from MMRM unstructured model.

Active – Placebo at Visit:	Estimate	Variance from the R matrix	Effect size
1 (Week 2)	−0.4	25.3	0.08
2 (Week 3)	−3.4	33.6	0.59
3 (Week 4)	−3.3	52.5	0.46
4 (Week 6)	−4.7	84.1	0.51
5 (Week 8)	−5.3	59.5	0.69
6 (Week 12)	−5.9	39.1	0.94
7 (Week 20)	−5.7	77.5	0.65
8 (Week 28)	−4.9	103.7	0.48

5.5.3   Another strategy to model baseline

An alternative to the MMRM model is one that fits a similar structure, but has the baseline score as another repeated measurement instead of as a covariate (Liang and Zeger, 2000). The dependent variable in this case is the observed total score rather than the difference from baseline. The model further constrains the mean of the baseline scores to be the same for the treatment groups, since mean baseline scores for treatment groups would be expected to be equal under randomization. Liu et al. (2009) refer to this as the constrained longitudinal data analysis (cLDA) method, and refer to our usual MMRM model as the ANCOVA method.

Disadvantages of this model include the loss of the ability to adjust for the baseline score and the baseline × visit interaction as covariates. We also have more covariance parameters to estimate, potentially impacting the power of the test of treatment group differences and increasing the chances for a convergence problem. For example, if there are eight post-baseline visits, an unstructured covariance pattern estimates $(8 \times 9)/2 = 36$ parameters. If we include the baseline visit as an additional repeated measure, there are $(9 \times 10)/2 = 45$ covariance parameters.

A potential benefit of this model is that the baseline records provide another repeated measurement from which to estimate the correlation structure, which could in turn aid the model in making a good estimate of treatment group differences when there is missing data. This also provides a framework for including subjects in the analysis who were randomized and have a baseline score but no post-baseline assessments.

Liang and Zeger (2000) and Liu et al. (2009) argue in preference to the cLDA model, while Kenward et al. (2010) argue that the two methods are similar. Operationally, the parameterization of this model in SAS is quite different from the ANCOVA method. It is more challenging to specify the model, program it in SAS and interpret the results. It requires using a set of indicator variables and interaction terms for the visit and treatment effects instead of two classification variables and

```
PROC MIXED DATA=updrs_v;
  CLASS subjid region trt visit ;
  MODEL updrs = region vis1 vis2 vis3 vis4 vis5 vis6 vis7 vis8
        trt*vis1 trt*vis2 trt*vis3 trt*vis4 trt*vis5
        trt*vis6 trt*vis7 trt*vis8 / DDFM=KR ;
  REPEATED visit / TYPE=UN SUBJECT=subjid R RCORR;
  ESTIMATE 'BL lsmean' INTERCEPT 1 region 0.2 0.2 0.2 0.2 0.2 ;

  ESTIMATE 'vis 8 chg from BL trt 1' vis8 1 trt*vis8 1 0 / cl;

  ESTIMATE 'vis 8 chg from BL trt 2' vis8 1 trt*vis8 0 1 / cl;

  ESTIMATE 'active - placebo at v8' trt*vis8 -1 1 / cl ;
RUN;
```

SAS Code Fragment 5.5   MMRM SAS code for Parkinson's disease cLDA model with baseline as a repeated measurement.

the CLASS statement, and requires a series of ESTIMATE statements instead of an LSMEANS statement. SAS Code Fragment 5.5 provides the SAS code to fit the cLDA model for the Parkinson's disease trial.

Selected results of the model are in SAS Output 5.14. We see that there are now 45 covariance parameters instead of 36, and 9 observations per subject. The model also has seven fewer fixed effect degrees of freedom from the removal of the baseline × visit interaction compared to the main MMRM model. Table 5.8 shows the cLDA treatment group comparisons at Week 28 as well as the original unstructured MMRM and the MMRM model without the baseline × visit interaction copied from Table 5.5 for reference. In our example, all three models had similar standard error estimates, but the cLDA estimate of the treatment group difference was somewhat lower than that of the other two models.

Dimensions	
Covariance Parameters	45
Columns in X	30
Columns in Z	0
Subjects	114
Max Obs Per Subject	9

SAS Output 5.14   SAS dimension information for the cLDA model.

Table 5.8   Parkinson's disease unstructured MMRM model compared to cLDA model.

Active vs. placebo at Visit 8 (Week 28) by various models	No. of covar parms	Est.	SE	95% CI	p-value
Unstructured cLDA with baseline as a repeated measurement	45	−4.7	2.3	(−9.2, −0.2)	0.042
Unstructured (see Table 5.5)	36	−4.9	2.3	(−9.5, −0.4)	0.033
Unstructured without baseline × visit interaction (see Table 5.5)	36	−5.1	2.3	(−9.6, −0.6)	0.028

5.6   Logistic regression mixed model for repeated measures using the generalized linear mixed model

The MMRM can be extended to binary data, such as repeated measurements of a response outcome when treatment group comparisons at the final time point are of primary interest and there is missing data due to early discontinuations.

As with continuous data, an extension of logistic regression for repeated measurements could be modeled by fitting a linear time effect. However, this implies a relationship over time that we would prefer not to assume while assessing treatment group comparisons. An alternate strategy that makes no assumption about the relationship of the response over time is a generalized version of the MMRM, which fits the fixed effects via a logistic model and takes into account the correlation between the visits for a subject through an estimated variance–covariance pattern.

5.6.1   The generalized linear mixed model

The GLMM is an extension of the linear mixed model, which assumes that the outcome is normally distributed, to a broader set of distributions. Broadening from the normal distribution adds substantial complexity to estimating the model parameters, which we briefly describe here. Fully specifying a GLMM requires specifying three components:

- A set of linear predictors $X\beta$;

- A monotonic mapping function (or link) between the mean of the dependent variable and the linear predictors;

- The distribution of the model error term for the dependent variable, which is specified from within the exponential family. For a generalized linear model, the observations are all considered to be independent, but a GLMM incorporates the correlation between related observations.

The mixed model used for MMRM is a simple form of GLMM with the identity mapping function and the multivariate normal error distribution. To model a binary random variable via a repeated measures version of logistic regression in the style of MMRM, the mapping function between the mean of Y and $X\beta$ is the logit, or log-odds, as in logistic regression, and the distribution of the error term is the binomial. If p is the probability of the event, then the logit is defined as:

$$\text{logit} = \ln\left(\frac{p}{1-p}\right) \tag{5.17}$$

Through the generalized linear model, we estimate the logit of the expected value of the response for a subject visit y_{ij} with the predictors:

$$\text{logit}(E[y_{ij}]) = x_{ij}\beta \tag{5.18}$$

We can back-transform from the logit to the estimated, or predicted, probability as follows:

$$\text{Predicted probability} = e^{x_{ij}\beta}/(1 + e^{x_{ij}\beta}) \tag{5.19}$$

The odds ratio, defined as $p/(1-p)$, is estimated by $e^{x_{ij}\beta}$. Using matrix notation for the vector of all subject-visit responses Y, the mean is estimated as:

$$\text{logit}(E[Y]) = X\beta \tag{5.20}$$

and the variance–covariance of Y is obtained by:

$$\text{Var}(Y) = A^{1/2} R A^{1/2} \tag{5.21}$$

where R is a variance–covariance matrix with a specified structure. For a logistic regression close to MMRM, the R matrix is defined the same as in Equation 5.9 for MMRM. The variance–covariance patterns in Section 5.2.2 are all applicable. A is a diagonal matrix containing the variance function of the specified error distribution. For the binomial distribution, the diagonal element for subject i at visit j is $p_{ij}(1 - p_{ij})$.

Unlike the linear mixed model, the GLMM cannot be estimated with maximum likelihood. Rather, it requires an iterative process called restricted pseudo-likelihood, which estimates a "pseudo-response" by maximizing the residual log pseudo-likelihood with a first-order Taylor series expansion around the solutions of the best linear unbiased predictors of the random effects (Wolfinger and O'Connell, 1993; SAS Institute Inc., 2011a).

Logistic regression MMRM is a special case of the GLMM with no random effects other than the correlation of the repeated measurements per subject. With the addition of random effects, the fully specified GLMM for the pseudo response variable P takes the following form:

$$P = X\beta + Z\gamma + e \tag{5.22}$$

where γ is an unknown vector of random parameters with design matrix Z, and e is a random error vector. The expected value is $g(E[Y|\gamma]) = X\beta + Z\gamma$, where $\text{Var}(\gamma) = G$ and $\text{Var}(Y|\gamma) = A^{1/2} R A^{1/2}$. Since logistic regression MMRM has no random effects other than the random subject effect from the correlated visits, Z is zero, and the formula simplifies to $P = X\beta + e$, and the variance is estimated as in Equation 5.21. The specification of random parameters in the GLMM are often called "G-side" random effects, whereas specification of correlated residuals are called "R-side" random effects.

For a continuous normally distributed response, estimates from MMRM have the attribute of being both subject-specific and marginal population-averaged estimates. A GLMM with R-side but no G-side random effects is a marginal population-average model. However, a GLMM with G-side random effects is a conditional or subject-specific model only (Liu and Zhan, 2011; SAS Institute Inc., 2011a). In clinical trials, we are interested in the population-average model, and so we will not address G-side random effects for the GLMM.

Restricted pseudo-likelihood allows for a variety of optimization methods for arriving at convergence. In our example, we use Newton–Raphson with ridging, which is similar to Newton–Raphson, used in mixed linear models and standard logistic regression. There is no single correct optimization method, and a handful of other methods are available. The methods may differ in the number of iterations or amount of computer time needed, and so selecting a different option may help if the chosen one does not converge (SAS Institute Inc., 2011a).

Due to the pseudo-likelihood estimation of the marginal population-average fixed effects, the logistic regression GLMM assumes data are MCAR. GEE, described in Section 5.2.3, is also a marginal population-average model and requires MCAR. GEE calculates parameter estimates with a working correlation matrix using the method of moments and an empirical sandwich estimator. Although GEE and the logistic regression GLMM both require MCAR, if data is MAR and the correlation structure of the repeated measurements are correctly specified, the logistic regression GLMM generally provides a more consistent estimate of the fixed effects than GEE (Liu and Zhan, 2011). Thus the pseudo-likelihood model-based parameters from logistic regression GLMM provide an advantage over GEE. As with the mixed model, the empirical sandwich estimator of the fixed effects variance-covariance terms can be applied to the GLMM, ensuring asymptotic unbiased estimates if the data are MCAR and an incorrect correlation structure is specified.

5.6.2   Specifying the model

In this section, we will use the mania example to specify a logistic regression MMRM analysis and show the SAS code to produce the results.

The mania trial is described in detail in Sections 1.10.3 and 7.4.7.1. Briefly, 1100 subjects, 550 per treatment arm, received either an experimental treatment or control treatment for the indication of mania in a double-blind fashion. Subject visits occurred at baseline, and 5 post-baseline visits at days 4, 7, 14, 21 and 28. Response to treatment at each visit was defined based on the subject's change from baseline

Table 5.9   Discontinuation by the reason in mania example.

Reason for discontinuation	Control (N = 550)	Experimental (N = 550)
Completed	385 (70%)	414 (75%)
Discontinued	165 (30%)	136 (25%)
Adverse event	7 (1%)	14 (3%)
Investigator decision	37 (7%)	38 (7%)
Withdrew consent/loss to follow-up	62 (11%)	52 (9%)
Other/sponsor decision	59 (11%)	32 (6%)

in the Young Mania Rating Scale (YMRS). Twenty seven percent of the subjects discontinued from the study (Table 5.9). The study was conducted in 30 investigator sites across 3 countries.

5.6.2.1   Analysis plan

The following example is an adequate and appropriate SAP description of a logistic regression MMRM for the mania example.

Treatment groups will be compared for odds of response at Day 28 using a logistic GLMM for repeated measures. Response or non-response at each scheduled post-baseline visit (Visits 1 to 5) is the dependent variable. Subjects who discontinued very early without providing a post-baseline YMRS score will be considered non-responders at Visit 1 (Day 4). The logistic GLMM is fit using the logit link and the binomial distribution. The model will include the baseline YMRS total score as a fixed effect covariate, with fixed effect categorical factors for pooled investigator site (defined elsewhere in the SAP), treatment group (Experimental and Control), visit and baseline × visit and treatment × visit interactions. The interactions will remain in the model regardless of significance. Treatment group comparisons at each visit will be estimated by differences between LS means from the treatment × visit interaction, and will be presented as odds ratios with accompanying p-values and 95% CIs. The predicted probability of response at each visit will also be presented. An unstructured covariance pattern will be used to estimate the variance–covariance of the within-subject repeated measures i.e., as R-side random effects. Parameters will be estimated using restricted pseudo-likelihood with Newton–Raphson ridging optimization and the Kenward–Roger method for calculating the denominator degrees of freedom.

In case this model does not converge, a heterogeneous Toeplitz covariance pattern will be used in place of unstructured. In this case, to assess the robustness of the results, a supportive model will also be produced using the bias-corrected sandwich estimator HC3 (MacKinnon and White, 1985) for the standard error of the fixed effects parameters.

5.6.2.2   Pooling investigator sites to improve convergence

In Section 5.4.1.2, we provided guidelines for the pooling of investigator sites for a linear model. For a binary response, it is the *number of subjects with events*, rather than the total number of subjects, that impacts convergence. Small event rates within site can cause a logistic model not to converge; yet, adjusting for sites can provide substantial variance reduction and power enhancement. Therefore, a site pooling strategy for logistic regression must often be more conservative (pooling more sites) than one based on a linear model. The method used to pool the sites, and preferably the pooled sites themselves, should be specified in the analysis plan prior to unblinding the study. In studies with both binary outcomes and continuous outcomes, the analysis plan might have two versions of site pooling: one that pools sites based on the criteria in Section 5.4.1.2, and a second strategy that pools sites further, based on the requirements for binary data.

For logistic regression, a guideline for the number of events needed per level of categorical predictor is 5–10 (Peduzzi *et al.*, 1996). There are more likely to be problems with model convergence when the number of events per category is less than 10, and especially when the number is below 5. Also keep in mind that if nearly all subjects have the event, then convergence may be impacted by the small number of subjects *without* the event. Logistic regression at a particular visit or at the LOCF endpoint therefore requires at least 5 and preferably 10 events per pooled site *at the specific visit*. Some modeling strategies for missing data including multiple imputation (MI, Chapter 6) and other sensitivity methods that are a modification of MI (described in Chapter 7) analyze binary data for all visits using a visit-by-visit process. Site adjustment for these techniques therefore requires a pooling strategy that meets the guidelines for the minimum number of events at *each* visit.

On the other hand, in a logistic GLMM repeated measures model, data from all visits are included in a single analysis, allowing for a more lenient pooling strategy compared to methods applied to each visit individually. One possible strategy for GLMM is to pool sites such that each pooled site has at least 15 subjects (from all treatment groups combined) who responded *for at least 1 visit*, and also at least 15 subjects who were non-responders *for at least 1 visit*. Additionally, it is preferable for pooled sites to be no more than approximately three times larger than the smallest stand-alone site.

Using this guideline for the mania study, 13 of the 30 sites had low event counts and were pooled with other sites within the same country. Twelve of the small sites were pooled to form three pooled sites, and one small site was pooled with an adjacent stand-alone site, producing twenty total sites after pooling. The largest pooled site had 66 subjects and the smallest stand-alone site had 23 subjects. To implement logistic regression at each visit, too many sites had small event counts at one or more visits in order to develop a reasonable site pooling strategy. However, there were enough events per visit within each country to support guidelines for logistic regression (the smallest number of events at any one visit within a country was

```
PROC GLIMMIX DATA=mania_v ;
  NLOPTIONS TECHNIQUE=NRRIDG;
  CLASS subjid poolinv trt visit ;
  MODEL RESPONSE = base_ymrs poolinv trt visit trt*visit
        base_ymrs*visit /
        DIST=BIN LINK=LOGIT DDFM=KR;
  RANDOM visit/TYPE=UN SUBJECT=subjid RSIDE ;
  LSMEANS trt*visit / ILINK CL; /*estimates event rates*/
  LSMEANS trt*visit / ODDSRATIO DIFF CL; /*estimates ORs*/
  ESTIMATE "Experimental vs Control at visit 5"
      TRT -1 1 TRT*VISIT 0 0 0 0 -1 0 0 0 0 1 /EXP CL;
  RUN;
```

SAS Code Fragment 5.6 Logistic GLMM SAS code for the mania study.

nine). Therefore, logistic models at the visit level could adjust for country but not pooled site.

5.6.2.3 SAS code

SAS Code Fragment 5.6 provides code for the mania study example, as specified in the analysis plan, with an unstructured covariance pattern. The optimization method in SAS GLIMMIX is specified with NLOPTIONS TECHNIQUE=NRRIDG. PROC GLIMMIX does not have a REPEATED statement; however, covariance structures are modeled with the RANDOM statement, using the RSIDE option. In the LSMEANS statement, we use the ILINK option to obtain estimates in terms of the event rate rather than the logit. Using the LSMEANS ODDSRATIO and DIFF options together provides ORs for pairwise comparisons. An appropriately specified ESTIMATE statement with the EXP option can be used to obtain the OR comparing the treatment groups at the final visit. As specified in the analysis plan, if this model does not converge, we will modify the code to specify TYPE=TOEPH, and run a supportive model by adding EMPIRICAL=HC3 on the first line to obtain the empirical sandwich estimator. For the generalized linear model, there are several options for calculating the empirical sandwich estimator. HC3 is recommended for small sample sizes (SAS Institute Inc., 2011a), and is a reasonable option for all cases, even though the mania example has a large sample size. The dataset MANIA_V has a "vertical" structure, with one record per subject visit.

5.6.3 Interpreting and presenting results

We will first present results from the planned analysis, and then present some supportive models, and compare and contrast the results to a logistic model at LOCF endpoint. Adjustment for pooled site and country are both explored.

5.6.3.1   Logistic generalized linear mixed model adjusting for pooled site

Selected results from the logistic GLMM are provided in SAS Output 5.15. Reviewing this output, we can confirm that we are using the binomial distribution with the logit link, residual pseudo-likelihood with Kenward–Roger degrees of freedom estimation, and Newton–Raphson with ridging optimization. There are 15 covariance parameters estimated, corresponding to $(5) \times (5 + 1)/2$ parameters for the unstructured pattern with 5 visits (see Section 5.2.2.1). There are 1100 subjects included in the analysis, with up to 5 visits per subject, no random effects, and 44 columns in the fixed effects X matrix, corresponding to intercept (1) + baseline YMRS (1) + pooled

Model Information	
Dataset	Mania_V
Response Variable	Response
Response Distribution	Binomial
Link Function	Logit
Variance Function	Default
Variance Matrix Blocked By	Subjid
Estimation Technique	Residual PL
Degrees of Freedom Method	Kenward–Roger
Fixed Effects SE Adjustment	Kenward–Roger
Optimization Information	
Optimization Technique	Newton–Raphson with Ridging
Parameters in Optimization	15
Dimensions	
R-side Cov Parameters	15
Columns in X	44
Columns in Z per Subject	0
Subjects (Blocks in V)	1100
Max Obs per Subject	5

SAS Output 5.15 Mania study selected model fitting information for logistic GLMM – unstructured.

Type III Tests of Fixed Effects				
Effect	Num DF	Den DF	F Value	Pr > F
base_YMRS	1	1216	33.21	<.0001
Poolinv	19	1101	14.65	<.0001
Trt	1	1205	27.95	<.0001
Visit	4	1051	17.92	<0.0001
trt*visit	4	1048	2.83	0.0235
base_YMRS*visit	4	1043	9.33	<0.0001

SAS Output 5.16 Fixed effects for the logistic GLMM for the mania study – unstructured with adjustment for pooled site.

investigator (20) + treatment (2) + visit (5) + treatment × visit (10) + baseline YMRS × visit (5). The Type III tests of the fixed effects in SAS Output 5.16 show strong effects from each covariate, as well as each interaction. Recall that we are not specifically interested in the statistical significance of treatment or the treatment × visit interaction, and the primary analysis is the comparison of the treatment groups at Visit 5.

Results from the model are provided in Table 5.10 and Figure 5.8. For the control group, the estimated response rate is similar to the observed rate. For the experimental treatment, the estimated response rate is higher than the observed rate, starting at Day 14. This could be caused by a combination of two effects: the estimation of missing data due to the observed correlation between visits; and/or the adjustment for the fixed effects of pooled site, baseline, or baseline × visit. At Day 28, the estimated OR for experimental versus control is 1.57, $p = 0.006$.

Table 5.10   Logistic GLMM results for the mania study – unstructured with adjustment for pooled site.

Visit	Observed response rate		Estimated response rate		Experimental vs. control odds ratio	95% CI	p-value
	Control	Exp.	Control	Exp.			
1 (Day 4)	0.03	0.09	0.02	0.07	3.45	(2.01, 5.92)	<0.001
2 (Day 7)	0.21	0.22	0.19	0.22	1.20	(0.83, 1.73)	0.335
3 (Day 14)	0.46	0.53	0.48	0.60	1.59	(1.21, 2.08)	0.001
4 (Day 21)	0.55	0.63	0.58	0.69	1.62	(1.20, 2.18)	0.002
5 (Day 28)	0.64	0.68	0.65	0.74	1.57	(1.14, 2.16)	0.006

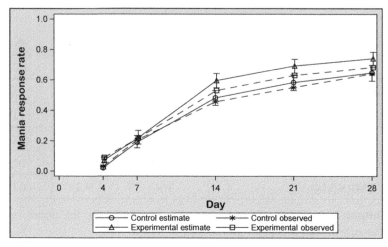

*Figure 5.8   Mania response observed data and GLMM estimates and 95% CIs –
pooled site adjustment.*

5.6.3.2   Alternate repeated measures models

The planned analysis identified in the SAP is complete. Several additional models
are presented in Table 5.11 in order to provide a more in-depth evaluation of this
example. Table 5.11 shows us that excluding the baseline × visit interaction yields
essentially similar results. Heterogeneous Toeplitz, which estimated 9 rather than
15 covariance parameters, also yielded similar results, with a slightly lower OR
of 1.49, either with or without the empirical sandwich estimator. A GEE model
with an unstructured working covariance matrix also had similar results, yielding an
OR of 1.54 (Table 5.11). The SAS code to produce the GEE model (SAS Institute
Inc., 2011c) is presented in SAS Code Fragment 5.7. In our example with large

```
PROC GENMOD DATA=mania_v DESCENDING;
  CLASS subjid poolinv trt visit ;
  MODEL RESPONSE = base_ymrs poolinv trt visit trt*visit
        base_ymrs*visit /
          DIST=BIN LINK=LOGIT TYPE3 ;
  REPEATED SUBJECT=subjid / TYPE=UN CORRW ;
  LSMEANS trt*visit / DIFF CL;
  ESTIMATE "Experimental vs Control at visit 5"
     TRT -1 1 TRT*VISIT 0 0 0 0 -1 0 0 0 0 1 /EXP;
  RUN;
```

SAS Code Fragment 5.7   Logistic GEE SAS code for the mania study.

Table 5.11 Mania example experimental treatment versus control at Visit 5 (Day 28) using different models.

Model	Site adjustment	No. of covar parms	Logit	SE (logit)	Odds ratio	95% CI	p-value
Unstructured GLMM	Pooled site	15	0.45	0.163	1.57	(1.14, 2.16)	0.006
Unstructured GLMM excluding baseline × visit interaction	Pooled site	15	0.44	0.163	1.54	(1.12, 2.13)	0.008
Heterogeneous Toeplitz	Pooled site	9	0.40	0.161	1.49	(1.09, 2.05)	0.013
Heterogeneous Toeplitz with sandwich estimator	Pooled site	9	0.40	0.169	1.49	(1.07, 2.08)	0.018
GEE with unstructured working correlation	Pooled site	15	0.43	0.164	1.54	(1.12, 2.12)	0.009
LOCF (logistic regression)[a]	Pooled site	—	0.47	0.141	1.60	(1.21, 2.10)	0.001
Unstructured GLMM	Country	15	0.28	0.143	1.32	(1.00, 1.75)	0.050
LOCF (logistic regression)	Country	—	0.29	0.122	1.33	(1.05, 1.69)	0.018
Observed case (completers logistic regression)	Country	—	0.18	0.153	1.20	(0.89, 1.61)	0.244
Logistic regression with all dropouts counted as non-responders	Country	—	0.27	0.122	1.31	(1.03, 1.67)	0.025

[a]Note: quasi-complete separation.

Type III Tests of Fixed Effects				
Effect	Num DF	Den DF	F Value	Pr > F
base_YMRS	1	1178	17.47	<0.0001
Country	2	1085	6.74	0.0012
Trt	1	1156	14.99	0.0001
Visit	4	1027	14.90	<0.0001
trt*visit	4	1028	3.30	0.0107
base_YMRS*visit	4	1023	10.71	<0.0001

SAS Output 5.17 Fixed effects for the logistic GLMM for the mania study – unstructured with adjustment for country.

sample size, it is not surprising that the GEE and GLMM models have similar results.

Since some analysis strategies based on a by-visit analysis such as MI (Chapter 6), tipping point analysis (Chapter 7), and logistic regression at LOCF endpoint require adjusting for country rather than pooled site due to the required number of events per visit and site/country, Table 5.11 and SAS Output 5.17 also present results from the logistic regression GLMM model with adjustment for country instead of pooled site. Replacing the 19 degrees of freedom factor for pooled site with the 2 degrees of freedom factor for country changes the results substantially, yielding an estimated OR of 1.32, $p = 0.050$ (Table 5.11, SAS Output 5.17).

Figure 5.9 shows that the expected values for the experimental group from the logistic GLMM model adjusting for country are similar to the observed rates, in contrast to Figure 5.8, where there was an adjustment for pooled site.

5.6.3.3 Univariate logistic models

For comparison purposes, Table 5.11 also presents a logistic regression of the LOCF endpoint, once adjusting for pooled site and once adjusting for country. The model adjusting for pooled site yielded quasi-complete separation. Two of the pooled sites had zero non-responders at the final visit, and therefore the estimated response rate at these two sites was not estimable. Treatment comparison results were still available from the model in spite of this problem, showing a fairly similar estimated treatment effect (OR = 1.60, $p = 0.001$) compared to the GLMM model. Note that the standard error at LOCF is substantially less than the repeated measures model. As described in Section 5.2.4, LOCF estimates tend to be more biased than MMRM and can underestimate the variance. The results should be interpreted with caution because of the quasi-complete separation. Note that SAS GENMOD and GLIMMIX might not provide warnings of quasi-complete separation, and so SAS output should be

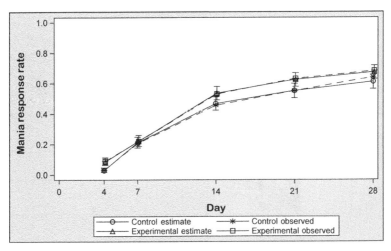

Figure 5.9   Mania response observed data and GLMM estimates and 95% CIs – country adjustment.

inspected for very large estimates and standard errors at each level of the classification variables, indicative of quasi-complete separation.

The logistic regression model at LOCF using country instead of pooled site had no convergence or estimation problems, and resulted in an OR of 1.33 comparing the experimental and control treatments, similar to the GLMM estimate with adjustment for country, yet apparently underestimating the standard error (Table 5.11). For completers, a logistic regression of Visit 5 response adjusting for country found an OR of 1.20. A noteworthy univariate logistic regression sensitivity analysis defines all dropouts as non-responders and otherwise uses the observed response at Visit 5 for all completers. This model resulted in an OR of 1.31, similar to the GLMM estimate, yet still underestimating the standard error. See Chapter 7 for an in-depth description of sensitivity analyses. In the face of missing data, the logistic GLMM will tend to produce less biased results and take better account of the trajectory of symptoms in the observed data than LOCF or completers analysis. In this example, ORs from the logistic GLMM were similar to logistic regression at LOCF, although LOCF models underestimated the standard error.

5.6.3.4   Adjustment for pooled site versus country

In our example, adjusting for pooled investigator site instead of country had a substantial impact on the treatment effect of all analyses. This example displays the benefit of adjusting for investigator site whenever possible, and also the need to pre-plan the site pooling strategy for binary outcomes based on observed event rates to avoid non-convergence or quasi-complete separation. We are also reminded of the importance of pre-specifying how sites will be pooled prior to unblinding, so

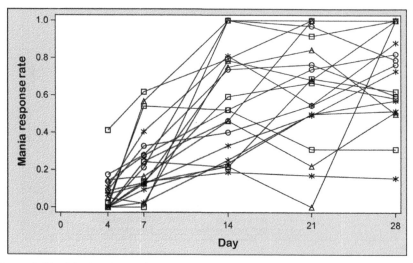

Figure 5.10   Mania observed response rates over time by pooled investigator site.

that bias is not introduced by selecting from a variety of site pooling strategies after unblinding.

Figure 5.10 shows the observed response over time for the 20 pooled investigator sites, for the 2 treatment groups combined. The event rate per site is quite variable. Some sites have very high overall response rates; others have moderate or low rates. This graph explains why pooled site is a strong predictor of response: adjusting for site takes into account the between-site variation, providing a site-adjusted treatment group comparison. In contrast, when sites are combined according to country, Figure 5.11 shows that there is less variability in response rates between the countries than there is for the individual pooled sites. Examining Table 5.11 shows that the OR estimates adjusting for pooled site are higher than when adjusting for country, yet the standard errors are also larger. The p-value comparing treatment groups is smaller when adjusting for pooled site because compared to country, the OR estimate had a larger relative increase than the increase in standard error. This phenomenon of logistic regression is described by Tangen and Koch (1999). Because of the nonlinear nature of logistic regression, covariate adjustment often results in an increase in the estimated treatment effect and a corresponding smaller increase in the standard error. In Section 5.6.1, we described that logistic GLMM with no random effects is a population-average (rather than conditional subject-specific) model, yet more precisely any logistic model with covariate adjustment produces conditional treatment group comparisons that are subpopulation-average ORs applicable to the subpopulation of people with the same covariates (Tangen and Koch, 1999).

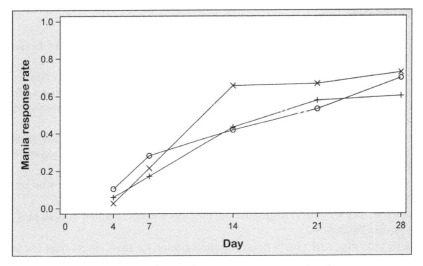

Figure 5.11   Mania observed response rates over time by country.

In summary, we found a stronger treatment effect for GLMM models that adjust for pooled site, compared to country. Methods that analyze binary repeated measurements on a visit-by-visit basis are more limited in their ability to adjust for investigator sites than a GLMM that models data from all visits together in one model. In all cases, treatment by site interaction can be very difficult to test within a model, and so graphical evaluations such as forest plots can provide an alternative method to evaluate interactions.

Site adjustment issues should be carefully considered in the analysis planning stages when specifying a binary outcome as the primary parameter. When specifying a series of sensitivity analyses in an analysis plan, it would be important to ensure that all models adjusted for the same covariates, so the comparison of results is limited to a comparison of methods without also including a comparison of covariates.

5.6.4   Other modeling options

A strategy to avoid convergence and site adjustment limitations of the GLMM is to define the primary outcome in a different way, such as change from baseline in the total YMRS score on a continuous scale instead of response based on percentage improvement in YMRS. When a continuous parameter is available, this is always preferable to defining a binary response, although there are some outcomes that are defined only on the basis of a binary classification with no underlying continuous parameter. In such cases, other analysis strategies to consider include time until the first response, or duration of sustained response.

References

Cohen J (1988) *Statistical Power Analysis for the Behavioral Sciences,* 2nd edn. Lawrence Erlbaum Associates.

Davis SM, Stroup TS, Koch GG, Davis CE, Rosenheck RA, Lieberman JA (2011) Time to all-cause treatment discontinuation as the primary outcome in the Clinical Antipsychotic Trials of Intervention Effectiveness (CATIE) schizophrenia study. *Statistics in Biopharmaceutical Research* 3(2): 253–265.

Fahn S, Elton RL, UPDRS Development Committee (1987) Unified Parkinson's disease rating scale. In: S Fahn, CD Marsden, DB Calne, M Goldstein (eds), *Recent Developments in Parkinson's Disease.* Macmillan, Florham Park, NJ, pp. 153–163.

Gardiner JC, Luo ZH, Roman LA (2009) Fixed effects, random effects and GEE: what are the differences? *Statistics in Medicine* **28**: 221–239.

Hurvich CM, Tsai CL (1989) Regression and time series model selection in small samples. *Biometrika* **76**: 297–307.

Kenward MG, Roger JH (1997) Small sample inference for fixed effects from restricted maximum likelihood. *Biometrics* **53**: 983–997.

Kenward MG, White IR, Carpenter JR (2010) Should baseline be a covariate or dependent variable in analyses of change from baseline in clinical trials? by Liu GF, Lu K, Mogg R, Mallick M, Mehrotra DV in *Statistics in Medicine* **28**: 2509–2530. *Statistics in Medicine* **29**: 1455–1456.

Koch GG, Amara IA, Forster J, McSorley D, Peace KE (1993) Statistical issues in the design and analysis of ulcer healing and recurrence studies. *Drug Information Journal* **27**: 805–824.

Koch GG, Davis SM, Anderson RL (1998) Methodological advances and plans for improving regulatory success for confirmatory studies. *Statistics in Medicine* **17**(15–16): 1675–1690.

Liang K-Y, Zeger S (1986) Longitudinal data analysis using generalized linear models. *Biometrika* **73**(1): 13–22.

Liang K-Y, Zeger S (2000) Longitudinal data analysis of continuous and discrete responses for pre-post designs. *Sankhya Indian Journal of Statistics* **62B**: 134–148.

Lieberman JA, Stroup TS, McEvoy JP, Swartz MS, Rosenheck RA, Perkins DO, Keefe RSE, Davis SM, Davis CE, Lebowitz BD, Severe J, and Hsiao JK (2005) Effectiveness of antipsychotic drugs in patients with chronic schizophrenia. *The New England Journal of Medicine* **353**(12): 1209–1223.

Liu GF, Lu K, Mogg R, Mallick M, Mehrotra DV (2009) Should baseline be a covariate or dependent variable in analyses of change from baseline in clinical trials? *Statistics in Medicine* **28**: 2509–2530.

Liu GF, Zhan X (2011) Comparisons of methods for analysis of repeated binary responses with missing data. *Journal of Biopharmaceutical Statistics* **21**: 371–392.

MacKinnon JG, White H (1985) Some heteroskedasticity-consistent covariance matrix estimators with improved finite sample properties. *Journal of Econometrics* **29**: 305–325.

Mallinckrodt CH, Clark WS, David SR (2001a) Accounting for dropout bias using mixed-effects models. *Journal of Biopharmaceutical Statistics* **11**(1–2): 9–21.

Mallinckrodt CH, Clark WS, David SR (2001b) Type I error rates from mixed effects model repeated measures versus fixed effects ANOVA with missing values imputed via last observation carried forward. *Drug Information Journal* **35**: 1215–1225.

Mallinckrodt CH, Kaiser CJ, Watkin JG, Molenberghs G, Carroll RJ (2004) The effect of correlation structure on treatment contrasts estimated from incomplete clinical trial data with likelihood- based repeated measures compared with last observation carried forward ANOVA. *Clinical Trials* **1**: 477–489.

Mallinckrodt CH, Lane PW, Schnell D, Peng Y, Mancuso J (2008) Recommendation for the primary analysis of continuous endpoints in longitudinal clinical trials. *Drug Information Journal* **42**: 303–319.

Mallinckrodt CH, Sanger TM, Dubé S, DeBrota DJ, Molenberghs G, Carroll RJ, Potter WZ, Tollefson GD (2003) Assessing and interpreting treatment effects in longitudinal clinical trials with missing data. *Biological Psychiatry* **53**: 754–760.

National Research Council. Panel on Handling Missing Data in Clinical Trials. Committee on National Statistics, Division of Behavioral and Social Sciences and Education (2010) *The Prevention and Treatment of Missing Data in Clinical Trials*. The National Academies Press, Washington, DC, available at http://www.nap.edu/catalog.php?record_id=12955, accessed 16 July 2013.

Peduzzi P, Concato J, Kemper E, Holford TR, Feinstein AR (1996) A simulation study of the number of events per variable in logistic regression analysis. *Journal of Clinical Epidemiology* **49**(12): 1373–1379.

SAS Institute Inc. (2011a) *SAS/STAT® 9.3 User's Guide: The GLIMMIX Procedure (Chapter)*. SAS Institute Inc., Cary, NC.

SAS Institute Inc. (2011b) *SAS/STAT® 9.3 User's Guide: The MIXED Procedure (Chapter)*. SAS Institute Inc., Cary, NC.

SAS Institute Inc. (2011c) *SAS/STAT® 9.3 User's Guide: The GENMOD Procedure (Chapter)*. SAS Institute Inc., Cary, NC.

Shulman LM, Gruber-Baldini AL, Anderson KE, Fishman PS, Reich SG, Weiner WJ (2010) The clinically important difference on the unified Parkinson's disease rating scale. *Archives of Neurology* **67**(1): 64–70.

Siddiqui O, Hung HMJ, O'Neil R (2009) MMRM vs. LOCF: a comprehensive comparison based on simulation study and 25 NDA datasets. *Journal of Biopharmaceutical Statistics* **19**: 227–246.

Tangen CT, Koch GG (1999) Complementary nonparametric analysis of covariance for logistic regression in a randomized clinical trial setting. *Journal of Biopharmaceutical Statistics* **9**(1): 45–66.

Wolfinger R, O'Connell M (1993) Generalized linear mixed models: a pseudo-likelihood approach. *Journal of Statistical Computation and Simulation* **48**: 233–243.

Table of SAS Code Fragments

5.1 Standard MMRM SAS code for Parkinson's disease example.

5.2 MMRM with spatial power, random subject effect and sandwich estimator.

5.3 GEE with compound symmetry working correlation matrix.

6

Multiple imputation

Bohdana Ratitch

Key points

- Multiple imputation (MI) is a useful tool for conducting analyses under both missing at random (MAR) and missing not at random (MNAR) assumptions.

- There are several methods for performing imputations. Those methods that can be used with monotone missing datasets are notably useful, and will serve as the basis for the implementation of various sensitivity analyses in Chapter 7.

- There are methodologies for analysis and overall inference with multiply-imputed data for both continuous and categorical outcomes.

- All details of MI-based analyses should be pre-specified.

6.1 Introduction

Multiple imputation (MI) is a methodology for dealing with missing data by explicitly imputing missing items with values that are estimated under assumptions made by the analyst regarding the missingness mechanism. A distinguishing feature of MI is that it uses several slightly different values for each missing data item thus creating multiple imputed datasets – complete versions of the original data. In each of the

---

Clinical Trials with Missing Data: A Guide for Practitioners, First Edition. Michael O'Kelly and Bohdana Ratitch.
© 2014 John Wiley & Sons, Ltd. Published 2014 by John Wiley & Sons, Ltd.

imputed datasets, observed values remain unchanged but missing items differ from one dataset to another. We will often refer to this collection of imputed datasets using a singular noun, a multiply-imputed dataset, with an understanding that this dataset contains multiple copies of the data, differing in terms of imputed values.

MI was formally introduced by Rubin (1978) with a comprehensive treatment of the underlying theory provided in Rubin (1987). This methodology was initially developed in the domain of sample surveys, but since then, its use has spread to other areas including observational and randomized clinical trials. Although it was considered complex and computationally demanding at first, many software packages, such as SAS, R, Stata and so on, now contain modules for the application of MI, which greatly facilitated the adoption of this methodology by analysts in different areas. An interesting overview of some successes and challenges in using MI observed during an 18-year period after its introduction is presented in Rubin (1996). A recent book by van Buuren (2012) covers many aspects of MI application with illustrative programming examples in R. A book by Carpenter and Kenward (2013) also provides an extensive treatment of MI theory and its applications in both medical and social sciences for dealing with missingness in continuous, categorical, cross-sectional and survival data. The use of MI in randomized clinical trials has been increasing in recent years as analysts and regulators become more familiar with this methodology, as the computational resources become more powerful and, especially, as it is being recognized as a very useful and flexible tool for implementing a variety of analyses with missing data under both MAR and MNAR assumptions.

6.1.1   How is multiple imputation different from single imputation?

The use of *multiple* plausible values to impute each missing item is in contrast with single imputation methods, for example, last observation carried forward (LOCF) and baseline observation carried forward (BOCF), which use a single value to fill in missing data. Single imputation methods establish a rule, most often a deterministic one, for deriving an imputed value (e.g., by directly using a previously observed value from the same subject or a mean from a group of subjects) and then use this imputed value in the analysis on an equal footing with the truly observed values. There is no distinction between the observed data and imputed data at the analysis stage, and thus the fact that imputed values are mere uncertain guesses is not taken into account during statistical inference. This inability to account for the uncertainty of imputed data in a statistically principled manner has been a target for criticism directed at single imputation methods, even though the underlying clinical assumptions for deriving imputed values in a certain way (e.g., BOCF) may be reasonable for some trials. For example, in symptomatic treatment trials for some chronic conditions, it may be clinically plausible to assume that, after treatment discontinuation, subjects would revert to their baseline severity of symptoms (an assumption reflected in the BOCF method). However, using each subject's baseline value for imputing their post-baseline missing data and treating this value as a real observed post-baseline assessment at the analysis stage can result in an artificially reduced standard error of the estimate of mean treatment difference and inflate the Type I error rate. MI addresses this concern by creating multiple plausible versions of the imputation, explicitly modeling the uncertainty about the imputed values and incorporating this uncertainty into the subsequent statistical analysis and inference. For the above example, MI can be used to model assumptions that are clinically similar to BOCF, while also handling uncertainty about imputed values in a more statistically rigorous way. An example of such analysis is provided in Chapter 7.

6.1.2   How is multiple imputation different from maximum likelihood methods?

Methods based on maximum likelihood estimation (Hartley and Hocking, 1971; Dempster *et al.*, 1977) use a log-likelihood function in order to estimate parameters of a statistical model (probability distribution) likely to have generated the observed data. Statistical inference, for example, hypothesis tests and estimation of mean effects, is then carried out based on this single statistical model corresponding to the maximum likelihood parameter estimates.

Analysis using a mixed model with repeated measures (MMRM), discussed in Chapter 5, is an example of a maximum likelihood-based approach for longitudinal data. Recall that in the MMRM analysis no imputation was performed. The method made use of all available data, including subjects with partial data (i.e., with missing values at some time points) in order to arrive at an estimate of the mean treatment effect without filling in missing items. This was made possible by modeling longitudinal relationships (covariances) between data across all the time points based on observed data, and then using these longitudinal relationships for inference about the mean treatment effect at the final time point over all subjects regardless of whether they had observed data at that time point or not. An MMRM estimate of the treatment effect at the final time point is based on the maximum likelihood parameters of the longitudinal model and is implicitly adjusted for the values observed at the previous time points and their correlation with the final time point.

MI, on the other hand, differs from maximum likelihood methodology in two ways: explicit imputation; and use of multiple draws from the distribution of model parameters, instead of a single set of maximum likelihood estimates of parameters. In order to produce imputed values, MI uses available data to estimate a statistical model (referred to as imputation model) that includes a primary outcome measure along with appropriate covariates. This model is then used to produce predicted values for the cases where outcome is missing based on observed predictors, and these predicted values serve as explicit imputations to fill in missing items. However, instead of using a single instance of an imputation model (as might be done using the maximum likelihood parameter estimates), MI uses multiple draws from the posterior distribution of the parameters of the imputation model, reflecting the fact that this model itself is not certain, and that its parameters have a variance. Analyzing data that has imputations based on the distribution of model parameters (rather than just the point estimates of those parameters), and "averaging" the results from such imputations allow us to account for uncertainty associated with modeling (predicting) missing data.

6.1.3   Multiple imputation's assumptions about missingness mechanism

Theoretical bases for MI have been rigorously developed for analyses under the MAR assumptions (Rubin, 1978; 1987). We sometimes refer to such use of MI in a MAR setting as *standard* MI. Standard MI and MMRM approaches belong to the same class of analysis methods in terms of their basic assumptions regarding the missingness mechanism, both assuming that unobserved outcomes of subjects who discontinued do not systematically differ from observed outcomes of subjects who remained in the study, provided that we account for relevant observed factors prior to discontinuation in our statistical model.

Despite the similarity in terms of a basic underlying MAR framework, standard MI can be used to explore sensitivity to some details of the modeling assumptions and can be compared to MMRM. As discussed in Chapter 1, MAR assumptions are formulated in the specific context of each clinical study. MAR assumes that missingness is independent of the unobserved responses, given the observed responses and the model. Therefore, MAR assumptions could be adopted given one model while not being appropriate given another model. In other words, an MAR-based approach could be used if the observed variables that are included in the statistical model sufficiently account for missingness in a sense that, given those variables, missingness is independent of the unobserved outcome. As will be discussed in greater detail in Section 6.1.5, MI allows us to make use of *ancillary variables* in the imputation model. Ancillary (otherwise known as auxiliary) are those variables that may be correlated with missingness but would not be of relevance to the overall inference had the data been complete. MI permits the use of such variables during the imputation process, whereas they can be subsequently excluded from the analysis of the imputed data. MMRM approach, on the other hand, uses a single model, so that if a variable is required to model MAR assumptions, it must be included in the overall inference model, which is not always desirable. For example, if a variable that is related to the missingness mechanism but not to the outcome itself is included in the analysis model, it might dilute the estimate of the treatment effect. By including different ancillary variables in the imputation model with standard MI, we can test sensitivity to a variety of assumptions, all of which may aspire to achieve an MAR approach. Section 6.3 provides a discussion on how to choose ancillary variables in either a prospective or a retrospective (exploratory) manner.

MI can also be used under various MNAR assumptions, for example, as discussed in Little and Yau (1996), Thijs *et al.* (2002), Molenberghs and Kenward (2007) and the National Research Council report (2010). MI is a valuable tool for implementation of pattern-mixture models typically used in the MNAR framework. The remainder of this chapter focuses on the standard use of MI (in the MAR framework), whereas Chapter 7 makes an extensive use of MI methodology to implement various analyses under various MNAR assumptions.

6.1.4   A general three-step process for multiple imputation and inference

Analysis based on MI is carried out by performing the following three steps:

1. *Imputation:* missing data are filled in using M different sets of values which results in M imputed datasets.

2. *Analysis:* each of the M imputed datasets is analyzed separately using the method that would have been chosen had the data been complete, for example, analysis of covariance (ANCOVA).

3. *Pooling:* analysis results from M imputed datasets are combined into one overall set of results.

The first step, imputation, can be performed in a variety of different ways depending primarily on whether the variables with missing values are continuous or categorical, on the type of predictors (covariates) that are included in the imputation model and on the type of a missing data pattern (monotone vs. non-monotone). In Section 6.2, we will discuss some general principles about how multiple imputations are obtained and review several widely used imputation methods, focusing particularly on those available in SAS. In Section 6.6.1, we will address the question of how to choose variables to be included in the imputation model.

The choice of the analysis method (step two) is guided by the objectives of the study and does not depend in any way on a specific method used for imputation. Any analysis method that would have been deemed appropriate had the data been complete can be used. The same analysis method should be applied to analyze each of the M imputed datasets.

Similarly, pooling the results of analysis obtained in step two does not depend on the imputation method used in step one. The methodology is very general and is essentially the same no matter what kind of statistic is estimated at the analysis stage (e.g., an estimate of the mean or of a regression parameter), but does assume that the statistic is approximately normally distributed (see Section 6.4.3 for examples of how to deal with analyses where this assumption is not satisfied). Both univariate and multivariate inferences can be performed by pooling the analysis results from multiple imputed datasets (Rubin, 1987; Schafer, 1997).

The fact that the methodology for analysis of the multiply-imputed data and pooling the results does not depend on the imputation method used in step one has an advantage in that it is possible to assess sensitivity to the method of handling missing data while keeping other aspects of analysis constant. When sensitivity analyses are performed under different assumptions regarding the missingness mechanism (e.g., MAR vs. different MNAR scenarios), the imputation phase is the only one that would be affected.

In SAS, the three basic steps outlined above can be performed using the MI procedure for the imputation step, any statistical analysis procedures (e.g., PROC GLM, PROC MIXED, PROC GENMOD, PROC LOGISTIC, etc.) for the analysis step and PROC MIANALYZE for the pooling step.

In the remainder of this chapter, we will further discuss all three stages of MI mentioned above. We will use several example datasets described in Section 1.10 (insomnia, Parkinson's disease and mania) in order to illustrate how each of these steps can be implemented in SAS.

6.1.5   Imputation versus analysis model

When modeling data and using predictions from a statistical model where the objective is to use the result to make important decisions, it is only natural to strive for a model that is as complete and accurate as possible. In this respect, one would wish to construct an imputation model that predicts missing values accurately with respect to the assumptions about the missingness mechanism. One important measure for ensuring this accuracy is to include into the imputation model all the variables that explain missingness or are highly correlated with a variable containing missing values. This is very intuitive, but may raise a concern: in practice, some of these variables may have little relevance for the purposes of main analysis and would not be considered for inclusion in the analysis model if the data were complete. If we include such variables in the imputation model to ensure quality of imputations, will we be bound to account for these variables in the analysis model used to analyze the imputed data, given that doing so may dilute the estimate of the effect of treatment?

Fortunately, the answer to this question is no. In MI, the process of imputation is completely separate from the analysis and pooling of results from multiple imputed datasets. A model that is used for analysis (often referred to as a *substantive model*) can be different from the imputation model, and the difference can, among other things, be in terms of the variables that are included in these respective models. For example, a variable that represents a secondary endpoint in a clinical trial might represent an important symptom that affects a subject's decision to continue with the treatment or not and might be highly correlated with a future trajectory of the primary endpoint. This variable would not normally be included in the analysis model for the primary outcome if all data were available. Nevertheless, with MI, it is possible (and recommended) to include such a variable into the imputation model in order to obtain more accurate predictions for the missing primary outcome. But once imputations are generated, there is no requirement to retain this variable in the analysis model.

However, the imputation method has to satisfy certain conditions for the so-called "proper imputations" as per Rubin's terminology. A formal theoretical framework for these conditions was presented in Rubin (1987) and summarized in Schafer (1997). The underlying theory is quite complex and, in most realistic applications, it is difficult to construct formal checks of validity. However, as the decade-long practical experience of using MI indicates, it can be successfully used if the following general principles are respected (Rubin, 1987, pp. 126–127).

(a) Draw imputations following the Bayesian paradigm as repetitions from a Bayesian posterior distribution of the missing values under the chosen models for non-response and data, or an approximation to this posterior distribution that incorporates appropriate between-imputation variability.

(b) Choose models for non-response appropriate for the posited response mechanism.

(c) Choose models for the data that are appropriate for the complete-data statistics likely to be used – if the model for the data is correct, then the model is appropriate for all complete-data statistics.

We will elaborate on these points shortly, but first, we will briefly explain the term *Bayesian posterior distribution* which will be referred to on several more occasions in this chapter. Bayesian statistics relies on three key elements. Prior distribution represents a probability distribution of one or more statistical variables, related to some data generation process, postulated prior to observing any (additional) evidence. Likelihood function represents a probability of some observed outcomes (data) given specific settings of these statistical variables. Finally, a posterior distribution represents the prior distribution updated based on the observed data (additional evidence). It is obtained by weighting the relative probabilities of different settings, as defined by the prior distribution, by the likelihood of observed data under these settings. In other words, in the posterior distribution, the probability of settings that have a greater likelihood of producing the observed evidence would be reinforced. Often, a so-called uninformative prior is used which gives an equal prior probability to all settings. In this case, the posterior distribution is driven entirely by observed data.

With these concepts in mind, the first principle of proper imputations (a) can be satisfied by first recognizing that both the missing data and imputation model parameters are governed by some underlying probability distributions. Starting from some prior distribution (which may be uninformative), we can estimate a conditional posterior distribution over the imputation model parameters given clinical trial data. Then imputed values should be obtained by first drawing a sample of the model parameters from this Bayesian posterior distribution, and then generating predictions for the missing values from the imputation model corresponding to the drawn parameter settings. This process is referred to as drawing imputed values from a Bayesian posterior predictive distribution.

The last two points (b) and (c) refer to the aspect of proper imputation which requires the imputation and analysis models to be compatible (Meng, 1994; Rubin, 1996; Collins *et al.*, 2001; Schafer, 2003) in the sense that the variables involved in the definition of estimands (complete-data statistics estimated from the analysis model) should be appropriately predicted by the imputation model. The variables involved in the response mechanism (related to its likely value or related to the probability of it being missing) should be included as covariates in the imputation model in order to reflect relevant correlations in the imputed portion of the data. For example, if a covariate X_1 is correlated with an outcome Y_1 but is excluded from the imputation model, then the multiply-imputed data will lead to estimates of the correlation between X_1 and Y_1 biased towards zero in the analysis model because this correlation was not modeled and thus would be diluted in the multiply-imputed dataset.

When MI is used under MAR assumptions, the requirement is that the imputation model should be at least as complex as the subsequent analysis model. In other words, the imputation model may contain factors not included in the analysis model, but it should not omit terms included in the latter. However, when used under MNAR assumptions, we may, in fact, want to dilute or change some relationships present in the observed data in order to reflect specific assumptions about the differences between subjects with missing data and those with observed data. Thus, the requirement for the imputation model to be at least as complex as the substantive model will not be always adhered to in the case of MNAR analyses. We will see some examples of this approach in Chapter 7.

6.1.6   Note on notation use

As previously mentioned, the imputation model may be based on a variety of variables considered related to missingness. They may include demographic characteristics or baseline disease assessments as well as post-baseline evaluations, such as the primary outcome measure and relevant secondary endpoints collected at multiple visits. We will use the following algebraic notation when presenting general descriptions of imputation methods in Section 6.2. We will denote by $X = (X_1, \dots, X_S)$ a set of variables whose values are observed for all subjects (typically baseline or demographic characteristics). We will assume that the imputation process is focused on a set of variables $Y = (Y_1, \dots, Y_J)$ representing the primary outcome measure collected at post-baseline visits 1 through J, and assume that any of them can have missing values for some subjects. In other words, the imputation process is generally applied to multiple variables with missing values in a unified manner so that at the end of the imputation phase, missing values of all these variables ($Y_1, \dots, Y_J$ in our case) get imputed. For the sake of succinctness and without loss of generality, we will limit our discussions to the primary outcome variables Y, but this set can be augmented by other post-baseline ancillary variables, which would be handled by the imputation method in the same manner as Y and within the same unified imputation model. This will be illustrated with some practical examples using the insomnia dataset described in Section 1.10.2.

6.2   Imputation phase

6.2.1   Missing patterns: Monotone and non-monotone

Methods that can be used for the imputation depend, among other things, on the pattern of missingness: monotone versus non-monotone. It is useful to picture this in terms of the location of missing values within subject records, where a dataset contains one record per subject and a record contains all variables of a subject that are used in the imputation, including the outcome and covariates at all assessment time points (a horizontal dataset structure). In the case of a monotone pattern, it is possible to arrange variables so that for all subjects, missing values are always located only in a block at the end of data records, whereas in the case of a non-monotone pattern, missing values may occur in the middle of a subject record. In the context of clinical trials, monotone missingness corresponds to data missing because a subject discontinues from the study. Non-monotone missingness happens

```
PROC MI DATA=sleeph NIMPUTE=0;
   VAR tst_0 - tst_5;
   ODS OUTPUT MISSPATTERN=mp_tst;
RUN;
```

SAS Code Fragment 6.1 Using PROC MI to examine patterns of missingness of TST in the insomnia example.

when a subject simply misses an intermediate visit, but then returns and provides data for subsequent assessments. The attribute of monotone versus non-monotone missingness is determined for the entire dataset. If all subjects in the dataset have a monotone pattern, then a dataset is said to have the monotone pattern. However, if at least one subject has a non-monotone pattern, the entire dataset is considered to be non-monotone.

In SAS, a summary of missing patterns can be easily obtained using PROC MI functionality. SAS Code Fragment 6.1 provides an example, using the insomnia dataset described in Section 1.10.2, where PROC MI is invoked with an option NIMPUTE=0, instructing the procedure not to perform any imputation (requested number of imputations is 0), which nevertheless results in the production of some summaries about the missing patterns. The input dataset *sleeph* has a horizontal structure with one record per subject, with variables *tst_0* through *tst_5* corresponding to total sleep time (TST) values at baseline and post-baseline Visits 1 through 5, as well as variables *mss_0* through *mss_5* corresponding to morning sleepiness scores (MSS) at the same visits. In this code fragment, statement VAR specifies a list of variables *tst_0, tst_1, ..., tst_5*, representing the TST per night at Visits 0 through 5.

This invocation of PROC MI produces a summary of the missing patterns, part of which is shown in SAS Output 6.1. It is directed to the SAS output window and can also be captured in an ODS OUTPUT dataset MISSPATTERN as shown in the SAS Code Fragment 6.1. In this summary, each unique pattern (configuration of observed and missing values) is represented by one row. Positions marked by "X" represent cases where the corresponding variables (named in the top row) are observed, whereas positions marked by dots (".") represent cases where the variables have missing values. For example, row 2 represents a group of subjects that have all

	tst_0	tst_1	tst_2	tst_3	tst_4	tst_5	%
1	X	X	X	X	X	X	81.25
2	X	X	X	X	X	.	3.75
3	X	X	X	X	.	.	5.31
4	X	X	X	.	.	.	3.59
5	X	X	.	.	.	.	6.09

SAS Output 6.1 Summary of patterns of missingness of TST in the insomnia example produced by PROC MI.

	tst_0	tst_1	tst_2	tst_3	tst_4	tst_5	mss_0	mss_1	mss_2	mss_3	mss_4	mss_5	%
1	X	X	X	X	X	X	X	X	X	X	X	X	81.25
2	X	X	X	X	X	.	X	X	X	X	X	.	3.75
3	X	X	X	X	.	.	X	X	X	X	.	.	5.16
4	X	X	X	X	.	.	X	X	X	.	.	.	0.16
5	X	X	X	.	.	.	X	X	X	.	.	.	3.59
6	X	X	.	.	.	.	X	X	.	.	.	.	5.31
7	X	X	.	.	.	.	X	.	.	.	.	.	0.78

SAS Output 6.2 Summary of patterns of missingness of TST and MSS in the insomnia example when the list of variables does not follow a chronological order across two endpoints.

TST values from baseline to Visit 4 observed (variables *tst_0* through *tst_4*) but have missing values at Visit 5 (variable *tst_5*). The last column provides a percentage of subjects in each such group. From this summary, we can see that all groups have a monotone pattern of missingness for the TST endpoint, because missing values (dots) appear only at the end of each row.

It is important to note that ordering of the variables specified in the VAR statement of PROC MI is used directly to determine the monotone versus non-monotone patterns. This is especially important to bear in mind when we include more than one endpoint assessed at multiple post-baseline visits, for example, a primary outcome (a primary object of the imputation process) and a secondary endpoint (as an ancillary variable), both collected at all study visits. In the case of the insomnia dataset, all subjects have a monotone missing pattern with respect to TST and morning sleepiness score. However, if variables are specified in the order of *tst_0, tst_1, ..., tst_5, mss_0, mss_1,..., mss_5* (i.e., TST assessments at all visits followed by MSS assessments at all visits), the pattern of missingness would appear as being non-monotone, as shown in SAS Output 6.2, because missing values appear in the middle of each row 2 through 7.

On the other hand, if we reorder variables in such a way as to group all assessment chronologically by visit with TST at a given visit followed by MSS at the same visit (*tst_0, mss_0, tst_1, mss_1,..., tst_5, mss_5*), the dataset will represent monotone missingness, as shown in the SAS Output 6.3.

	tst_0	mss_0	tst_1	mss_1	tst_2	mss_2	tst_3	mss_3	tst_4	mss_4	tst_5	mss_5	%
1	X	X	X	X	X	X	X	X	X	X	X	X	81.25
2	X	X	X	X	X	X	X	X	X	X	.	X	3.75
3	X	X	X	X	X	X	X	X	.	.	.	.	5.16
4	X	X	X	X	X	X	X	.	.	.	.	.	0.16
5	X	X	X	X	X	X	.	.	.	.	.	.	3.59
6	X	X	X	X	.	.	.	.	.	.	.	.	5.31
7	X	X	X	.	.	.	.	.	.	.	.	.	0.78

SAS Output 6.3 Summary of patterns of missingness of TST and MSS in the insomnia example when the list of variables follows a chronological order across two endpoints.

	mss_0	tst_0	mss_1	tst_1	mss_2	tst_2	mss_3	tst_3	mss_4	tst_4	mss_5	tst_5	%
1	X	X	X	X	X	X	X	X	X	X	X	X	81.25
2	X	X	X	X	X	X	X	X	X	X	.	.	3.75
3	X	X	X	X	X	X	X	X	.	.	.	.	5.16
4	X	X	X	X	X	X	.	X	.	.	.	.	0.16
5	X	X	X	X	X	X	.	.	.	.	.	.	3.59
6	X	X	X	X	.	.	.	.	.	.	.	.	5.31
7	X	X	.	X	.	.	.	.	.	.	.	.	0.78

SAS Output 6.4 Summary of patterns of missingness of TST and MSS in the insomnia example when using an alternative chronological order across two endpoints.

It should be noted, that even when using a chronological ordering, it may not always be possible to obtain monotone missingness. For example, if in the above example we simply switched the order of the TST and MSS parameters at each visit (*mss_0, tst_0, mss_1, tst_1,..., mss_5, tst_5*), the pattern would appear to be non-monotone because of the group of subjects represented by row 7 in the SAS Output 6.4 – subjects who had TST data but no MSS data for Visit 1.

The analyst should attempt to find an ordering of variables that could produce an overall monotone pattern, because, as we will see in the following sections, there are imputation methods that we may want to take advantage of which are available exclusively for monotone missingness. This being said, a chronological order should still be preserved.

If we examine in a similar way the patterns of missingness in the Parkinson's disease dataset (see Section 1.10.1), we can see from SAS Output 6.5 that there are several groups of subjects with intermittent missing values (rows 7, 9, 10, 12 and 14) for the primary endpoint (UPDRS score), thus presenting a non-monotone missingness for this dataset overall.

In Section 6.2.3, we will discuss some general principles underlying different methods for monotone and non-monotone missingness.

6.2.2   How do we get multiple imputations?

In order to fill in missing values, we would like to use an imputation model $P_{imp}(Y|X,\theta)$, characterized by a vector of parameters θ, to draw predictions for missing values of Y given observed covariates X. This imputation model is estimated based on a finite set of available trial data, and therefore its parameters have a nonzero variance. We can obtain point estimates for the parameters θ but only within a certain precision, that is, model parameter estimates are uncertain quantities. Recall from Section 6.1.5 that one of the basic principles of MI is that we should draw imputed values as samples from a Bayesian posterior predictive distribution, that is, first drawing a sample θ^* from its Bayesian posterior, and then draw predictions for missing Y from a predictive distribution $P_{imp}(Y|X,\theta^*)$. Moreover, we should not pick just

	upd_0	upd_1	upd_2	upd_3	upd_4	upd_5	%
1	X	X	X	X	X	X	61.70
2	X	X	X	X	X	X	2.13
3	X	X	X	X	X	X	1.06
4	X	X	X	X	X	X	3.19
5	X	X	X	X	X	X	3.19
6	X	X	X	X	X	.	4.26
7	X	X	X	X	.	X	8.51
8	X	X	X	X	.	.	4.26
9	X	X	X	.	X	X	1.06
10	X	X	X	.	.	X	1.06
11	X	X	X	.	.	.	1.06
12	X	X	.	X	X	X	1.06
13	X	X	.	.	.	.	6.38
14	X	.	X	X	X	X	1.06

SAS Output 6.5 Summary of patterns of missingness of the UPDRS score in the Parkinson's disease example.

a single sample of parameters θ and generate one imputed dataset using predictions from the corresponding model as if from the ultimate true model. Instead, MI uses M different samples of the parameters $\widehat{\theta^m}, m = 1, \ldots, M$. Once a sample $\widehat{\theta^m}$ is drawn, an instance of the imputation model $P_{imp}\left(Y|X, \widehat{\theta^m}\right)$ is used to produce the mth imputed dataset by generating predictions for missing values of Y given observed values of X from this model.

Different imputation methods can be devised depending on the assumed form of $P_{imp}(Y|X, \theta)$, Bayesian methodology for deriving posterior distribution of θ, and a method for sampling $\widehat{\theta^m}$ from this posterior. The same general principles also apply when using semi- or non-parametric approaches to perform imputation. For example, an approximate Bayesian bootstrap algorithm can be used in a non-parametric setting to draw samples for M imputed datasets (Rubin 1987). We will review several specific imputation methods in Section 6.2.4.

A Bayesian posterior distribution for model parameters is generally estimated based on available data, that is, cases where values of Y are observed (subjects with non-missing data). This effectively means that when using predictions from the imputation model $P_{imp}\left(Y|X, \widehat{\theta^m}\right)$ to impute cases with missing values of Y, we assume that the probability distribution for subjects with missing data is the same as the probability distribution in subjects with observed data used for model estimation, conditional on X. In this chapter, we discuss a setting where this process corresponds to MAR assumptions, whereas Chapter 7 discusses how the imputation procedure can be tailored to reflect different, MNAR assumptions instead.

6.2.3   Imputation strategies: Sequential univariate versus joint multivariate

In general, an imputation model would represent a joint probability distribution over all included variables (such as X and Y). However, depending on the missingness pattern, estimation of and draws from a Bayesian posterior for such a model can be performed in two ways. For monotone missingness, conditional independence between variables can be assumed, and the joint distribution can be approximated using a factorization based on univariate models, each representing a probability distribution of one variable conditional on some other variables. More specifically, univariate models are constructed for one variable at a time starting from left to right in an ordered list and using preceding variables in that list as predictors. The ordering in that list is the one under which a monotone missing pattern was established. By univariate we mean a model that has one variable on the left-hand side and may have multiple predictor variables on the right-hand side, such as a regression model. Drawing samples of parameters from Bayesian posterior distributions for univariate models tends to be much simpler compared to doing so for multivariate models.

Imputation can be performed in a sequential manner as follows. Assume that variables $X_1, \ldots, X_S, Y_1, \ldots, Y_J$ are included in the imputation model, where variables $Y_1, \ldots, Y_J$ have some missing values. Then Y_1 is imputed first using a univariate model of Y_1 based on variables $X_1, \ldots, X_S$ as predictors. This step imputes only missing values of Y_1 and does not fill missing values of other variables $Y_2, \ldots, Y_J$. Then the next variable, Y_2, would be imputed using $X_1, \ldots, X_S$ and Y_1 as predictors, and so on for each variable Y_j using variables $X_1, \ldots, X_S, Y_1, \ldots, Y_{j-1}$ as predictors. This process can be summarized as follows (SAS Institute Inc., 2011, pp. 4586–4587):

1. Obtain an imputation model for the variable Y_j:

$$\theta_j^{(m)} \sim P(\theta_j | x_1, \ldots, x_S, y_{1(obs)}, \ldots, y_{j-1(obs)}, y_{j(obs)})$$

2. Impute missing values of the variable Y_j:

$$y_{j(imp)}^{(m)} \sim P(Y_j | \theta_j^{(m)}, x_1, \ldots, x_S, y_{1(obs+imp)}^{(m)}, \ldots, y_{j-1(obs+imp)}^{(m)})$$

where

- $y_{j(obs)}$ represent observed values of the variable Y_j;

- $y_{j(obs+imp)}^{(m)}$ represent values of the variable Y_j that are observed and those that were imputed on the previous step;

- $\theta_j^{(m)}$ represent parameters of the imputation model drawn from the Bayesian posterior of θ_j given the available data; and

- $y_{j(imp)}^{(m)}$ represent imputed values for the variable Y_j drawn from a predictive distribution of Y_j given model parameters $\theta_j^{(m)}$ and predictor variables.

Steps (1) and (2) are performed for each variable $Y_j, j = 1, \ldots, J$ and for multiple imputations $m = 1, \ldots, M$.

In order to estimate Bayesian posterior distribution of parameters θ_j, subjects with observed values of Y_j are used. With monotone missingness, these subjects also have observed values for $Y_1, \ldots, Y_{j-1}$. So the model is estimated entirely from observed data. On the other hand, subjects with missing values of Y_j may also have missing values of preceding variables, and imputations generated for any of the $Y_1, \ldots, Y_{j-1}$ on the previous steps are used as predictors when imputing missing values of Y_j.

With this sequential procedure, it is possible to use a different model or method of imputation for each variable (Raghunathan et al., 2001). This is useful if some endpoints are continuous and some categorical. This can happen, for example, when ancillary variables are of a different type than the primary response variables. In this case, for example, a regression model can be used for continuous variables and a logistic regression model for categorical variables.

The sequential imputation procedure is valid primarily for monotone missing data, although even in this case, theoretical validity can be shown only under conditions of multivariate normal distribution over all variables included in the imputation model. Nevertheless, the method has been successfully used in practice when multivariate normality assumptions were violated, and has been reported to perform well even when binary variables are included in the model (Carpenter and Kenward, 2007; Demirtas et al., 2008). This strategy is used as the basis for several methods available in SAS PROC MI for the monotone missing patterns. Section 6.2.4 and Appendix 6.A provide a brief overview of such methods.

Analogs of the above sequential imputation procedure, often referred to as fully conditional specification (FCS) methods (Oudshoorn et al., 1999; van Buuren et al., 2006) have also been applied with non-monotone missing patterns. However, they do not have the same theoretical properties and there is less evidence regarding the performance of these approaches in practice. SAS version 9.3 introduced an experimental version of the FCS approach for non-monotone missingness, which includes methods for cases where all variables are continuous and where some or all variables are categorical (SAS Institute Inc., 2011).

A method that has been typically applied for patterns with non-monotone missingness when all variables are continuous works directly with a multivariate probability distribution. The implementation available in SAS is based on a multivariate normal distribution over all variables. In order to draw samples from a Bayesian posterior for a multivariate normal distribution, a Markov Chain Monte Carlo (MCMC) simulation methodology is used, which will be summarized in Section 6.2.4.

For data with non-monotone missingness, imputation in SAS can also be done in two steps. First the MCMC method can be used to impute data partially, filling in only those missing values that create a non-monotone pattern. Once this is done, other methods, designed for monotone missingness, can be used to fill in the rest of the missing data if deemed more appropriate. This method is most suitable when all variables included in the imputation model are continuous because the MCMC method is based on the multivariate normal distribution. However, this approach has also been applied even when some variables are categorical. Nominal categorical values can be dummy-coded using a set of binary variables (see Section 6.2.4), while ordinal variables can sometimes be treated as continuous in this partial imputation step. Although it is not an ideal method for categorical variables, it may be acceptable if the number of non-monotone missing values is not large and/or if the ordinal or dummy-coded variables are approximately normally distributed.

6.2.4   Overview of the imputation methods

Depending on the pattern of missing data (monotone vs. non-monotone), type of the variables included in the imputation model (continuous vs. categorical) and assumptions regarding the distribution of these variables, different imputation methods may be employed. Table 6.1 summarizes different methods that are available in SAS PROC MI.

We will briefly review the functionality of these methods in the remainder of this section and in Appendix 6.A.

6.2.4.1   Regression method

We will start with an overview of a regression method that can be used for monotone missing patterns or with an FCS approach for non-monotone patterns as part of the sequential imputation procedure, where variables are imputed one at a time. This overview is intended to illustrate in more detail the process where, for each of the imputed datasets, first a new instance of the imputation model is obtained from a Bayesian posterior distribution, and then the imputed values are generated as predictions from this model instance.

As discussed in Section 6.2.3, the idea is to use a univariate linear regression model for a continuous variable on the left-hand side and a set of effects on the right-hand side which can include both continuous and categorical variables and their interactions, just as in a regular linear regression methodology. We will focus on one step where imputations are obtained for a variable Y_j using the following linear regression model:

$$Y_j = \beta_0 + \beta_1 W_1 + \beta_2 W_2 + \cdots + \beta_{K_j} W_{K_j} \tag{6.1}$$

where $W_k, k = 1, \ldots, K_j$ represent model effects constructed from variables $X_1, \ldots, X_S, Y_1, \ldots, Y_{j-1}$. In other words, W_k may represent either main effects corresponding to some or all of these variables or their interactions. Note that each variable Y_j may have a different number of predictors included in the model, thus the use of notation K_j dependent on j.

Model parameters are represented by a vector $\boldsymbol{\beta} = (\beta_0, \beta_1, \beta_2, \ldots, \beta_{K_j})$. This model is first estimated based on available values of Y_j and $W_1, \ldots, W_{K_j}$ (the latter are based on available values of $X_1, \ldots, X_S, Y_1, \ldots, Y_{j-1}$). Fitting this model results in parameter estimates $\hat{\boldsymbol{\beta}} = (\hat{\beta}_0, \hat{\beta}_1, \hat{\beta}_2, \ldots, \hat{\beta}_{K_j})$ and the associated covariance matrix $\hat{\sigma}_j^2 Var_j$, where Var_j is the $\boldsymbol{w}'\boldsymbol{w}$ inverse matrix derived from the intercept and model

Table 6.1   Imputation methods available in SAS PROC MI.

Pattern of missingness	Type of imputed variable	Type of covariates	Available methods
Monotone	Continuous	Arbitrary	Parametric: • Regression method • Predictive mean matching Non-parametric: • Propensity score
Monotone	Categorical (ordinal)	Arbitrary	Logistic regression
Monotone	Categorical (nominal)	Continuous	Discriminant function method
Arbitrary	Continuous	Continuous	Markov Chain Monte Carlo • Full imputation • Partial imputation to obtain monotone pattern
Arbitrary	Continuous	Arbitrary	• FCS regression • FCS predictive mean matching • MCMC partial imputation + a monotone method
Arbitrary	Categorical (ordinal)	Arbitrary	• FCS logistic regression • MCMC partial imputation + a monotone method
Arbitrary	Categorical (nominal)	Arbitrary	• FCS discriminant function method • MCMC partial imputation + a monotone method

effects w_k, $k = 1, \ldots, K_j$. After these initial estimates are obtained, the following steps are repeated M times in order to generate M imputed datasets (Rubin, 1987).

(a) New parameters $\beta^{(m)} = (\beta_0^{(m)}, \beta_1^{(m)}, \beta_2^{(m)}, \ldots, \beta_{K_j}^{(m)})$ and $\sigma_j^{(m)}$ are sampled from the Bayesian posterior distribution for each imputed dataset $m = 1, \ldots, M$. The variance sample is obtained as follows:

$$\sigma_j^{2\,(m)} = \hat{\sigma}_j^2 (n_j - K_j - 1)/g \tag{6.2}$$

where g is a $\chi^2_{n_j - K_j - 1}$ random variate and n_j is the number of non-missing values of Y_j.

The regression coefficients are drawn as follows:

$$\beta^{(m)} = \hat{\beta} + \sigma_j^{(m)} Var_{hj}' z \qquad (6.3)$$

where Var_{hj}' is the upper triangular matrix in the Cholesky decomposition of Var_j and z is a vector of $K_j + 1$ independent standard normal variates.

(b) Using a model instance corresponding to the newly drawn regression parameters $\beta^{(m)} = (\beta_0^{(m)}, \beta_1^{(m)}, \beta_2^{(m)}, \ldots, \beta_{K_j}^{(m)})$ and $\sigma_j^{(m)}$, missing values of Y_j are replaced by predictions from this model:

$$y_{j,i}^{(m)} = \beta_0^{(m)} + \beta_1^{(m)} w_{1,i} + \beta_2^{(m)} w_{2,i} + \cdots + \beta_{K_j}^{(m)} w_{K_j,i} + z_i \sigma_j^{(m)} \qquad (6.4)$$

where $w_{k,i}$ are the values of the model effects W_k based on non-missing values of variables $X_1, \ldots, X_S, Y_1, \ldots, Y_{j-1}$ from subject i, and z_i is a normal deviate simulated for each subject i with a missing value of Y_j.

Steps (a) and (b) above are repeated M times, which results in a generation of M imputed datasets.

SAS Code Fragment 6.2 provides an illustration of how the regression imputation can be performed with PROC MI. For this purpose, the MONOTONE statement is used with the keyword REGRESSION. This code fragment illustrates a syntax where there is one MONOTONE statement per variable that needs to be imputed (*tst_2* through *tst_5*), and each variable is specified in parentheses. With this syntax, if a variable, say *tst_2*, were not specified in a MONOTONE REGRESSION statement, it would not be imputed in the output dataset, even though it has missing values. Another, shorter syntax will be shown in later examples.

This particular syntax allows specifying the option DETAILS, which produces the details of the imputation models used for each variable, captured in the ODS dataset MONOREG. The dataset MONOREG contains some information that is very

```
PROC MI DATA=sleeph NIMPUTE=1000 SEED=883960001 OUT=tst_reg1;
   VAR trt tst_0 - tst_5;
   CLASS trt;
   MONOTONE REGRESSION (tst_2 / DETAILS);
   MONOTONE REGRESSION (tst_3 / DETAILS);
   MONOTONE REGRESSION (tst_4 / DETAILS);
   MONOTONE REGRESSION (tst_5 / DETAILS);
   ODS OUTPUT MONOREG=tst_regmod1;
RUN;
```

SAS Code Fragment 6.2 Imputation using monotone regression with a default model for each imputed variable corresponding to TST assessments in the insomnia example.

	ImpVar	Effect	trt	ObsVal	_1	_2	...
1	tst_2	Intercept	.	−0.02070	0.015503	−0.024413	
2	tst_2	TRT	1	0.01646	0.039139	0.000485	
3	tst_2	tst_0	.	0.20648	0.225214	0.248183	
4	tst_2	tst_1	.	0.65002	0.672662	0.624879	
5	tst_3	Intercept	.	−0.0004529	−0.043600	−0.036245	
6	tst_3	TRT	1	−0.02721	−0.048728	−0.026133	
7	tst_3	tst_0	.	−0.03009	0.004039	−0.060933	
8	tst_3	tst_1	.	0.28547	0.265238	0.301038	
9	tst_3	tst_2	.	0.66304	0.663934	0.685014	
10	tst_4	Intercept	.	−0.02649	−0.015529	−0.035053	

...

SAS Output 6.6 ODS dataset MONOREG from the imputation of TST in the insomnia example using monotone regression method from SAS Code Fragment 6.2.

instructive for understanding how the sequential imputation process works. In this dataset, a fragment from which is shown in SAS Output 6.6, contains a variable *ImpVar*, which represents variables on the left-hand side of the regression models. Records 1–4 represent the model for the variable *tst_2*, records 5–9 represent the model for the variable *tst_3* and so on. The variable *Effect* represents the effects (predictor variables) included in each model. Examining the values of this variable, we can see that when imputing the variable *tst_2*, the model includes an intercept and all other variables listed in the VAR statement of PROC MI before *tst_2*, that is, *trt, tst_0* and *tst_1*. Similarly, the model for the variable *tst_3* uses all preceding variables as effects, which now also includes the variable *tst_2*. This is a default manner in which PROC MI builds each of the regression models. We will see in the next example how this can be changed, if desired. The dataset MONOREG includes variables for effects specified in the CLASS statement (*trt* in our case) with their corresponding levels. Variable *ObsVal* contains estimates of model parameters $\hat{\beta} = (\hat{\beta}_0, \hat{\beta}_1, \hat{\beta}_2, \ldots, \hat{\beta}_{K_j})$ (see Equation 6.1) obtained from observed data, while the variables $\_1, \_2, \ldots, \_M$, contain model parameters $\beta^{(m)}$ sampled from the Bayesian posterior distribution (see Equation 6.3) that are used for each of the MIs, respectively.

Multiply-imputed data are stored in the output dataset named as specified in the OUT option of the PROC MI statement (*tst_reg1* in this case). This dataset has all the variables contained in the input dataset *sleeph* (specified in the DATA option), plus one new variable, *_Imputation_*, added by SAS to distinguish between multiple copies of the dataset, each corresponding to one of the M imputations. We used the option NIMPUTE = 1000 which results in the production of $M = 1000$ imputations. Finally, the option SEED is used to specify a seed for the random number generator. If no seed is provided by the user, SAS will generate a different seed every time the procedure is invoked. Therefore, in order to be able to reproduce the exact numeric results, the seed should always be specified.

```
PROC MI DATA=sleeph NIMPUTE=1000 SEED=883960001 OUT=tst_reg2;
   VAR trt tst_0 - tst_5;
   CLASS trt;
   MONOTONE REGRESSION (tst_2 = trt tst_0 tst_1 / DETAILS);
   MONOTONE REGRESSION (tst_3 = trt tst_0 tst_2 / DETAILS);
   MONOTONE REGRESSION (tst_4 = trt tst_0 tst_3 / DETAILS);
   MONOTONE REGRESSION (tst_5 = trt tst_0 tst_4 / DETAILS);
   ODS OUTPUT MONOREG=tst_regmod2;
RUN;
```

SAS Code Fragment 6.3 Imputation using monotone regression with a user-specified model for each imputed variable corresponding to a TST assessment in the insomnia example.

SAS Code Fragment 6.3 shows an example of a different syntax for the MONO-TONE REGRESSION statement which can be used in order to specify a particular, non-default model for each imputed variable. In this case, the model for each variable includes only treatment arm (*trt*), baseline value (*tst_0*) and value from the time point immediately preceding the one being imputed.

For example, examining records 5–8 in the MONOREG dataset shown in SAS Output 6.7, we can see that the imputation model for *tst_3* now does not include an effect for *tst_1*, as was the case in the previous example.

Figure 6.1 illustrates the imputations resulting from the two regression methods discussed above. The left panel of the figure (Imputation Method 1) represents the regression implemented in SAS Code Fragment 6.2, where a default model is used for each imputed variable (including all variables preceding the one being imputed in the list specified in the VAR statement). The right panel (Imputation Method 2) represents

	ImpVar	Effect	trt	ObsVal	_1	_2	...
1	tst_2	Intercept	.	−0.02070	0.015503	−0.055733	
2	tst_2	TRT	1	0.01646	0.039139	0.032984	
3	tst_2	tst_0	.	0.20648	0.225214	0.197447	
4	tst_2	tst_1	.	0.65002	0.672662	0.596868	
5	tst_3	Intercept	.	0.00816	−0.037139	−0.007274	
6	tst_3	TRT	1	−0.05719	−0.079870	−0.062399	
7	tst_3	tst_0	.	0.04442	0.077930	0.030399	
8	tst_3	tst_2	.	0.82824	0.802903	0.811223	
9	tst_4	Intercept	.	−0.02643	−0.008937	−0.063563	
				...			

SAS Output 6.7 ODS dataset MONOREG from the imputation using monotone regression method for TST in the insomnia example as shown in SAS Code Fragment 6.3.

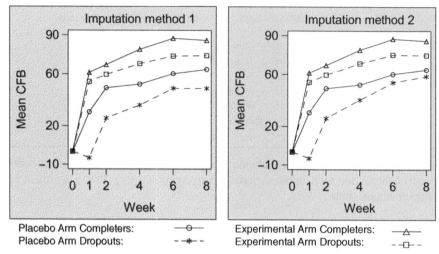

Figure 6.1   Plot of mean change from baseline (CFB) in TST over time based on observed and imputed data using regression method in the insomnia example. Imputation Methods 1 and 2 represent the methods shown in SAS Code Fragments 6.2 and 6.3, respectively.

the regression from the SAS Code Fragment 6.3, where each model includes only those effects that were specified in the MONOTONE REGRESSION statement for each variable. Both plots represent mean change from baseline in TST over time, with solid lines representing study completers and dashed lines representing subjects that discontinued early. Means for discontinued subjects are based on observed data prior to discontinuation and imputed data afterwards. We can see that there is some difference in the imputations depending on the models used (mostly in the imputations for the placebo arm, where the second method predicts a more optimistic outcome).

SAS Code Fragment 6.4 shows another, shorter syntax that would implement the default imputation models. It uses only one MONOTONE REGRESSION statement with no further details, which will result in imputation of all variables with missing data using the regression method and using all variables preceding the one being imputed in the VAR statement as effects. Note that in this case, we added ancillary

```
PROC MI DATA=sleeph NIMPUTE=1000 SEED=883960001 OUT=tst_mss_reg;
   VAR trt tst_0 mss_0 tst_1 mss_1 tst_2 mss_2
           tst_3 mss_3 tst_4 mss_4 tst_5 mss_5;
   CLASS trt;
   MONOTONE REGRESSION;
RUN;
```

SAS Code Fragment 6.4   Imputation of TST using MSS assessments as ancillary variables in the insomnia example using monotone regression with a default model.

Table 6.2 LSM estimates of the difference between experimental and placebo arms for the change from baseline to Week 8 in TST in the insomnia example. Imputation Methods 1, 2 and 3 represent the methods shown in SAS Code Fragments 6.2, 6.3 and 6.4, respectively.

Imputation Method	Estimate	SE	95% CI	p-value
Imputation Method 1	18.7399	6.4161	6.1644, 31.3154	0.0035
Imputation Method 2	17.3039	6.3873	4.7846, 29.8231	0.0067
Imputation Method 3	19.2888	6.3908	6.7630, 31.8146	0.0025

variables – mss_0 through mss_5 – MSS collected at baseline and post-baseline visits. They are listed in the VAR statement using an order of variables that would represent a chronological order of assessments across both measures and would result in a monotone pattern, as discussed in Section 6.2.1. Based on this ordering, a variable tst_2, for example, would be imputed using a model with trt, tst_0, mss_0, tst_1 and mss_1 as predictors, that is, all preceding variables. Note that this procedure will result in the imputation of both TST and MSS variables.

We will see in Sections 6.3 and 6.4 how to obtain overall results with multiply-imputed data, but for now, Table 6.2 provides a quick snapshot of how the differences in the imputation methods used above affect the final analysis results at the last time point (Week 8). This table presents least squares mean (LSM) estimates of the difference between experimental and placebo arms for the change from baseline to Week 8 in TST in the insomnia example obtained from an analysis model applied to the imputed data. As would be expected after the examination of the imputation plots in Figure 6.1, the second imputation method produces a slightly smaller estimate for the difference between the experimental and placebo arms for the change from baseline to Week 8 in TST compared to the first method (17.3 vs. 18.7 min). The third method (including MSS assessments as ancillary variables), results in a slightly larger estimate (19.3 min) compared to the other two methods. The differences between the methods in this case are rather insignificant, especially given the fact that the p-values are quite small and are unambiguously below the significance threshold of 0.05 for all three methods. But it illustrates the point that the imputation model affects the results, and thus should be fully pre-specified in advance in order to avoid speculation in case of results that are border-line significant.

As a final note, we would like to emphasize again that with the monotone regression (as with other monotone methods that we will review next), PROC MI imputes one variable at a time following the order of variables specified in the VAR statement. One could obtain equivalent results by invoking the MI procedure multiple times, once per variable (time point) that needs to be imputed, that is, tst_2,..., tst_5. In this case, we would specify just one variable for the imputation in the MONOTONE statement each time, and use the output dataset from one invocation of PROC MI as input to the next one. There is no reason to go into such trouble when performing the MAR-based analyses, but this feature will be very useful for carrying out some variants of MAR and some MNAR-based analyses, as will be shown in Chapter 7.

For example, in order to reflect some MNAR assumptions (deviations from MAR), we may need to modify the imputed values at a given time point before using them as predictors for the next time point. In order to do that, we can invoke PROC MI to impute values at one time point, appropriately modify the imputed values in the output dataset and then pass this post-processed dataset as input to the next invocation of PROC MI.

6.2.4.2   Logistic regression for categorical variables

Logistic regression method can be used to impute binary and ordinal categorical variables. The method for generating imputed values is in essence very similar to that of the linear regression, but is based on fitting a logistic regression model instead. For example, for a binary variable Y_j, the following model would be used:

$$logit(p_j) = \beta_0 + \beta_1 W_1 + \beta_2 W_2 + \cdots + \beta_{K_j} W_{K_j}$$

$$\text{where } p_j = Pr(Y_j = 1 | W_1, \ldots, W_{K_j}), \text{ and } logit(p) = log\left(\frac{p}{1-p}\right) \quad (6.5)$$

Detailed formulas for how to draw new model parameters from a Bayesian posterior distribution for each imputed dataset $m = 1, \ldots, M$ similar to Equation 6.3 above, and how to generate categorical values to fill in missing items similar to Equation 6.4 can be found in Rubin (1987).

Logistic regression can be invoked with the use of the LOGISTIC keyword in the MONOTONE statement. The same principles about the inclusion of model effects based on the order of variables in the VAR statement applies in this case, similar to what was discussed for the regression method. We will see an example of its use in Section 6.4.

6.2.4.3   Markov chain Monte Carlo

The MCMC method is often used to generate pseudorandom draws from complex multidimensional distributions when analytical methods for drawing random samples are intractable. In MCMC, the sampling process is based on a Markov chain which is a sequence of elements (random variables) $E_1, E_2, \ldots, E_\eta$, and so on, each having a distribution that depends on the value of the preceding element (see Equation 6.6).

$$Pr\left(E_{\eta+1}|E_\eta, E_{\eta-1}, \ldots, E_1\right) = Pr\left(E_{\eta+1}|E_\eta\right) \xrightarrow[\eta\to\infty]{} \pi(E) \quad (6.6)$$

Stationary Markov chains have a characteristic that, as their elements are generated for a sufficiently long time based on the conditional distribution $Pr\left(E_{\eta+1}|E_\eta\right)$, the elements stabilize to some stationary distribution $\pi(E)$. This property can be very useful for the generation of pseudorandom samples: while the stationary distribution $\pi(E)$ could be quite complex, the conditional distribution $Pr\left(E_{\eta+1}|E_\eta\right)$ of each element in the chain may be relatively simple. This may provide practical means to obtain samples from a complex stationary distribution while performing repeated draws from a simpler distribution. The MCMC method is often used for the simulation of joint Bayesian posterior distributions, for example, for drawing samples of model parameter estimates from their joint posterior distribution when analytical methods are intractable.

In the context of missing data, the observed-data posterior distribution $P\left(\theta|x,y_{obs}\right)$ of multivariate normal model parameters is intractable, while the complete data posterior $P\left(\theta|x,y_{obs},y_{mis}\right)$ would be much easier to simulate. In this case, a data augmentation algorithm (Tanner and Wong, 1987) can be applied with a Markov chain generation process, where the set of observed data y_{obs} is augmented by the estimated or simulated values of missing data y_{mis}, so that the easier, complete-data posterior could be utilized. A data augmentation step is used as a building block for the generation of each element of a Markov chain, which is intended to ultimately produce pseudorandom samples of missing data y_{mis} from a joint Bayesian posterior predictive distribution $P\left(Y_{mis},\theta|x,y_{obs}\right)$. The whole process can be summarized as follows, assuming that the data follow a multivariate normal distribution.

(a) Start with some initial estimates for the multivariate normal distribution parameters $\theta(0)$, that is, a mean vector and covariance matrix $\theta(0) = (\mu(0), \Sigma(0))$.

(b) Generate an element of the Markov chain, $\{y_{mis}(\eta), \theta(\eta)\}$, $\eta = 0, 1, 2, 3, \ldots$ and so on, as well as prepare for the generation of the next element using a two-step data augmentation algorithm as follows.

   (b.1) The imputation step (I-step): using the current estimate $\theta(\eta)$ for the mean vector and covariance matrix, draw a sample for missing values from a conditional distribution $P(Y_{mis}|x,y_{obs},\theta(\eta))$. This step produces a sample for the missing part of the data matrix, $y_{mis}(\eta)$, which provides us with a complete (augmented) data matrix $(y_{obs},y_{mis}(\eta))$.

   (b.2) The posterior step (P-step): simulate a new draw of parameter estimates $\theta(\eta + 1)$ from the posterior of the population mean and covariance matrix given the current complete-data matrix, $P\left(\theta|x,y_{obs},y_{mis}(\eta)\right)$. This step prepares a new estimate of the parameters θ to be used for the creation of the next element of the Markov chain.

(c) Repeat step (b) for a sufficiently large number of iterations so that the Markov chain $\{y_{mis}(0), \theta(0)\}$, $\{y_{mis}(1), \theta(1)\}$, $\{y_{mis}(2), \theta(2)\}$ and so on converges to a stationary distribution. This stationary distribution is what we are interested in, that is, $P(Y_{mis}, \theta|x, y_{obs})$. Samples for missing values $y_{mis}(\eta)$, generated sufficiently far from the start of this chain, can be considered as approximately independent draws of the missing values from this stationary distribution.

An interested reader is referred to Schafer (1997) for more technical details involved in the I- and P-steps. We will only briefly touch on the following aspects concerning practical use of the MCMC method.

First of all, it is important to note that imputations produced on individual iterations of I-step (b.1) are not all used for multiply-imputed data. The I-step is a component of an iterative Markov chain generation process, and many I-step imputations are produced simply to generate sufficient number of elements of the Markov chain so that it converges. It is only after the convergence is considered to have been achieved that the samples $y_{mis}(\eta)$ from the I-step can be used for the actual MIs.

Contrary to the maximum likelihood estimation, where convergence represents a situation where parameter estimates do not change significantly in successive iterations (converge to a point in the parameter space), the data augmentation algorithm is expected to converge to a stationary distribution instead of a specific point estimate. A stationary distribution would appear as a stable distribution without any systematic changes in a span of many iterations. If the process converges, parameter values are expected to move randomly around some mode of the distribution but not to exhibit any systematic trends.

At the same time, while the parameter estimates would appear to behave randomly from one iteration to the next after convergence, it is important to remember that each element of the Markov chain depends on the previous one, so there is a correlation between successive parameter samples $\theta(\eta)$ and thus the corresponding I-step imputations $y_{mis}(\eta)$. For MI, it is necessary to ensure that samples used for M different imputations are independent, and therefore, we cannot use I-step imputations $y_{mis}(\eta)$ from successive I-step iterations for that purpose even after convergence.

There are two approaches for ensuring independence of imputations in multiply-imputed datasets. One option is to use M draws, $y_{mis}(\eta_1)$, $y_{mis}(\eta_2)$, ..., $y_{mis}(\eta_M)$, from the same Markov chain based on iterations $\eta_1, \eta_2, ..., \eta_M$ that are sufficiently far apart from each other so that they can be considered approximately independent samples. This process is sometimes referred to as "thinning out" of the Markov chain. Software packages typically allow the user to specify the number of iterations (Markov chain elements) between their for MI to ensure independence. In SAS PROC MI, the option NITER in the MCMC statement serves this purpose with a default value being 100. Also, a user may wish to specify a number of "burn-in" iterations to be performed before the first draw $y_{mis}(\eta_1)$ is used to allow for convergence to the stationary distribution and to remove the effects of the starting point of the parameter values. In the MCMC statement, a user can specify this parameter using the NBITER option, which otherwise has a default value 200.

Another option would be to generate M different chains altogether, one for each of the MIs, and to use only one draw $y_{mis}(\eta_m)$ from each chain for the mth imputed dataset. Using multiple chains may result in less correlation between MIs. On the other hand, if a very long burn-in period is required to reach a stationary distribution, then a single long chain may be better than multiple shorter chains if they do not reach the desired distribution. Using multiple chains requires somewhat more computational time, but this is not a limiting factor with today's technology. Option CHAIN in the MCMC statement of PROC MI can be used to request either one chain or multiple chains (option values SINGLE or MULTIPLE, respectively). When multiple chains are used, option NBITER for the number of burn-in iterations is applied to each chain.

In order to kick off the generation of a Markov chain, it is necessary to have some initial estimates for the parameters θ as mentioned in step (a) above. Most often, it is done by applying an Expectation-Maximization (EM) algorithm (Dempster *et al.*, 1977) which produces maximum likelihood estimates of the parameters given observed data y_{obs}. In general, it is considered to be a good choice because these estimates tend to be located close to the center of the posterior distribution. Alternatively, if the analyst has estimates of the parameters θ from other sources, these estimates can be used directly. In the MCMC statement, the choice between these two methods can be specified using the INITIAL option with values EM (default) or INPUT, respectively.

The P-step described in (b.2) above involves the estimation of a posterior distribution $P\left(\theta|x, y_{obs}, y_{mis}(\eta)\right)$ based on the current I-step imputation $y_{mis}(\eta)$ in order to draw a new sample $\theta(\eta + 1)$ from this posterior. The form of the posterior depends on the form of the prior distribution over θ. The most commonly used prior distribution is a Jeffrey's or uninformative prior. As the name suggests, this prior does not introduce any assumptions about the parameter values, and so the posterior distribution is completely driven by the data. In the MCMC statement of PROC MI, this is the default choice for the option PRIOR. Other alternatives include providing a specific distribution directly in a user dataset (informative prior), or a ridge prior. The latter may be recommended when there is a high degree of missingness, very strong correlations among the variables or when the number of observations is only slightly greater than the number of parameters. Ridge prior effectively biases the estimate of the covariances among the variables toward zero.

SAS Code Fragment 6.6 illustrates the use of the MCMC method for imputation of the UPDRS score in the Parkinson's disease dataset introduced in Section 1.10.1. It uses the MCMC statement with the options CHAIN=SINGLE for the use of a single Markov chain across all M imputed datasets, NBITER=200 to perform 200 burn-in iterations before starting sampling for the first imputed dataset, and NITER=100 to perform 100 iterations between sampling from the same chain for different imputed datasets. Option IMPUTE=FULL instructs PROC MI to impute all missing values in the dataset for the variables specified in the VAR statement.

When the MCMC statement is used, PROC MI models all variables specified in the VAR statement as continuous and the use of the CLASS statement is not allowed. Because of this, the user has to take extra measures for categorical covariates. First of all they have to be represented by numerical variables, with numeric codes representing different categories. For binary variables, numeric levels of 0 and 1, or 1 and 2 can be used, and this is what is done for the treatment arm variable *trt*. In the case of the Parkinson's disease dataset, we would also like to include geographic region as an effect in the model, which takes five different values representing five regions in which the trial was conducted. It is not appropriate to use a numeric variable with values 1 through 5 and to treat it as a continuous one in this model. In this case, the region should be encoded by several binary variables, the process is often referred to as dummy coding. Dummy coding for a variable with C categories refers to a procedure where this variable is replaced by a set of $C - 1$ dummy binary variables $D_1, D_2, \ldots, D_{C-1}$. One category, say the last one C, is designated as reference and all

```
PROC MI DATA= updrsh NIMPUTE=1000 SEED=883960001 OUT=upd_mcmc;
   VAR trt region1 region2 region3 region4 upd_0 - upd_8;
   MCMC CHAIN=SINGLE NBITER=200 NITER=100 IMPUTE=FULL;
RUN;
```

SAS Code Fragment 6.5   Full imputation with the MCMC method for the UPDRS score in the Parkinson's disease example.

records with the original values corresponding to this reference category would have values of 0 assigned to all $C-1$ dummy variables ($D_1 = 0, D_2 = 0, \ldots, D_{C-1} = 0$). Then each of the $C-1$ dummy variables would represent the remaining categories, so that a record with the original value equal to category c would have a value of 1 assigned to the dummy variable $D_c = 1$, and the values of 0 to the remaining ones. (Note that a similar coding can be obtained using PROC GLMMOD functionality which produces a dataset containing binary coding of classification effects based on the conventional MODEL and CLASS statements). We encoded the region in this manner using four binary variables, *region1* through *region4*, which are included in the VAR statement in SAS Code Fragment 6.5. Variables *upd_0* through *upd_8* represent UPDRS scores collected at baseline and eight post-baseline visits.

The next example in the SAS Code Fragment 6.6 demonstrates how the MCMC method can be used instead for partial imputation of the data with a non-monotone pattern in order to obtain a dataset with a monotone pattern. This is achieved with the use of option IMPUTE=MONOTONE in the MCMC statement. Then, the rest of the missing data can be imputed using monotone regression, as is done with the second invocation of PROC MI in SAS Code Fragment 6.6. Note that the output dataset *upd_mcmc_part* produced by the first PROC MI with the MCMC method in SAS Code Fragment 6.6 (which contains imputations for records with non-monotone

```
*** Use MCMC for partial imputation ***;
PROC MI DATA=updrsh NIMPUTE=1000 SEED=883960001 OUT=upd_mcmc_part;
   VAR trt region1 region2 region3 region4 upd_0 - upd_8;
   MCMC CHAIN=SINGLE NBITER=200 NITER=100 IMPUTE=MONOTONE;
RUN;

*** Complete imputation with monotone regression method ***;
PROC MI DATA=upd_mcmc_part NIMPUTE=1 SEED=883960001 OUT=upd_reg;
   VAR trt region upd_0 - upd_8;
   CLASS trt region;
   MONOTONE REGRESSION;
   BY _Imputation_;
RUN;
```

SAS Code Fragment 6.6   Partial imputation using the MCMC method with the remaining imputations done by monotone regression for the UPDRS score in the Parkinson's disease example.

missingness) is used as the input dataset for the next PROC MI with the MONOTONE statement so that other missing values can be filled in. The partially imputed output dataset *upd_mcmc_part* already contains 1000 copies of the original dataset since option NIMPUTE=1000 was used in the first PROC MI. With the next invocation of MI procedure, we do not need to further multiply the number of imputations, but rather we fill in missing data in the existing copies. This is why, in the second PROC MI in SAS Code Fragment 6.6, we specify NIMPUTE=1 and use a BY *_Imputation_* statement.

Note that in this example, we used dummy-coded binary variables representing geographic region in the first PROC MI, but then we used the original multi-level categorical variable *region* in the second PROC MI, where the use of CLASS statement is permitted in conjunction with the MONOTONE statement. Often, in clinical trials, the analysis models include the effect for the investigator site. When the number of sites is large, it may be planned not to include this effect in the multivariate normal model for the partial MCMC imputation, but then to include it in the monotone regression imputation for the rest of the missing data, where it would be modeled appropriately.

Figure 6.2 depicts the mean change from baseline in the UPDRS scores over time based on observed and imputed data from a full MCMC imputation (left panel) and from a partial MCMC imputation followed by monotone regression (right panel). There are no differences between the two methods perceivable from the plots for this example.

Examining the numerical results from the analysis of data imputed by the two methods in Table 6.3, we can see that the estimated LSMs for the difference between treatment arms are extremely close. The full MCMC method has a slightly smaller

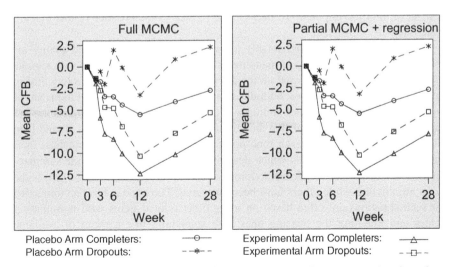

Figure 6.2   Plot of mean change from baseline in UPDRS score over time based on observed and imputed data from a full MCMC imputation, and from a partial MCMC imputation followed by monotone regression for the Parkinson's disease example.

Table 6.3   LSM estimates of the difference between experimental and placebo arms for the change from baseline to Week 28 in UPDRS scores for the Parkinson's disease example.

Imputation method	Estimate	SE	95% CI		p-value
Full MCM	−5.1813	2.2299	−9.5521	−0.8104	0.0202
Partial MCMC + regression	−5.1709	2.3348	−9.7474,	−0.5943	0.0268

standard error, but the difference is so small that it might very well be attributed to randomness involved in the imputation process.

While the results from the two methods (full and partial MCMC imputation) appear to be very similar in this example, it may not always be the case (see some additional discussions in Section 6.6.2). Moreover, as we will see in Chapter 7, proceeding with monotone methods after a partial MCMC imputation provides us with a flexibility of implementing different kinds of analyses based on MNAR assumptions.

6.2.5   Reusing the multiply-imputed dataset for different analyses or summary scales

One feature of MI is that once the imputation is performed, the same set of M imputed datasets can be reused for multiple analyses, just like it would have been done with complete data. For example, if subgroup analyses were planned based on the trial data, imputation can be produced for the entire group of study subjects, and then the same multiply-imputed dataset can be used both for the overall analysis and for the subgroup analyses. In fact, this strategy is preferred to an alternative of generating a new set of multiple imputations, because the former would produce results that are more internally consistent.

In many therapeutic areas, notably in psychiatry, health-related and quality-of-life questionnaires consisting of many items (questions) are often used with various summary scales computed based on the answers to individual questions (e.g., using sums or averages). Sometimes, both the summary scales and individual items are of interest for analysis. With such multiple-item data, it happens that subjects answer some but not all questions, or that the questionnaire is not answered at all and then all items are missing at a given time point. For many health questionnaires, their authors offer scoring manuals which describe the algorithms to compute summary scales and which often include methodologies for dealing with cases where only some items are missing while others have been answered. The approaches recommended for such situations are often based on using other related items with non-missing values and imputing the missing ones with something like a mean of available items. These guidelines should, in general, be applied first to fill in the items as per recommendations of the questionnaire authors. However, some cases will not be handled by the prescribed scoring algorithms, for example, when all items are missing for a given time point as a result of a missed visit, or if more than half of the items are missing while the scoring algorithm provides imputation rules only for the situations where at least half of the items are answered.

For such remaining cases, MI can be performed at the level of individual items. Once the individual items are imputed, the summary scales can be computed based on observed and imputed data, and finally all the planned analyses, both on summary scales and individual items, can be carried out. Even in the cases where only the summary scales are of interest for the analysis, there may be good reasons to impute data at the item level and to compute the summary scales afterwards. For example, Gottschall *et al.* (2012) conducted a simulation study which led to a conclusion that performing the item-level imputation provides meaningful power advantages over the scale-level imputation.

In order to perform an item-level imputation, one option could be to use one imputation model that encompasses all items in order to maximize the available information and model all relevant correlations. This approach, however, may not be optimal or even feasible for the questionnaires that involve dozens of items. First of all, the number of variables/parameters in a model cannot exceed the number of observations in a dataset. The problem would be most severe for non-monotone missing patterns, where a method such as MCMC must use a multivariate normal model including all items across multiple time points, which would have a large number of parameters. For the monotone or FCS methods, the problem is somewhat less severe because a univariate model would be used for each item and time point, and the predictor variables can be restricted to, for example, a subset of item values at baseline and a previous time point. Nevertheless, for large questionnaires, even this can result in models that are too large compared to the available sample size. Moreover, questionnaires often contain questions that are partially redundant which would create colinearities among predictor variables and could be problematic for such methods as, for example, regression. In such cases, the statistician should carefully consider a model for each item trying to balance the parsimony of the model and attempt to model as much correlation between the items as possible. Unfortunately, general methodologies for efficient item-level imputation in large questionnaires are not abundant in the current literature. Some strategies can be found in Enders (2010) and Little *et al.* (2011).

6.3   Analysis phase: Analyzing multiple imputed datasets

After the imputation phase has produced a multiply-imputed dataset, the analysis can begin. Each of the M imputed datasets needs to be analyzed using the same complete-data method. For example, if the primary objective of the study was to estimate a difference in the change from baseline in the primary endpoint between treatment arms, then an ANCOVA analysis can be performed on each of the imputed datasets using the observed and imputed values at the time point of interest in order to estimate this difference. Once the estimates for the difference and their standard errors are obtained from the analysis of each imputed dataset, these estimates must

```
*** Dataset tst_reg1v contains imputed data in vertical structure;
DATA tst_reg1vc; SET tst_reg1v;
   tstc=tst-tst_0; /* Compute change from baseline */
RUN;


PROC SORT DATA=tst_reg1vc; BY visit _Imputation_ trt subjid; RUN;

PROC MIXED DATA=tst_reg1vc;
   CLASS trt;
   MODEL tstc = trt tst_0 / solution;
   LSMEANS trt / DIFF=CONTROL("1") CL;
   ODS OUTPUT DIFFS=lsmdiffs LSMEANS=lsm SOLUTIONF=parms;
   BY visit _Imputation_ ;
RUN; QUIT;
```

SAS Code Fragment 6.7   An ANCOVA analysis by time point on multiply-imputed data for the insomnia example.

be combined to compute an overall estimate, as well as its p-value according to the methodology that will be described in Section 6.4.

As discussed in Section 6.1.5, the analysis model does not have to be the same as the imputation model, so ancillary variables may be omitted from the analysis model. Any appropriate complete-data analyses can be applied at this stage.

SAS Code Fragment 6.7 represents an ANCOVA analysis for each time point on multiply-imputed data for the insomnia dataset. We used the imputed output dataset *tst_reg1* from the SAS Code Fragment 6.2 for this analysis. Recall that this dataset has a horizontal structure with one record per subject and with values of TST at different time points represented by variables *tst_0* through *tst_5*. We transformed this dataset into one with a vertical structure, so that the resulting dataset *tst_reg1v* has one record per subject and time point (represented by variable *visit*), with a variable *tst* containing the TST values. Baseline value is stored as the *tst_0* variable in this dataset. Using this vertically structured dataset, we first calculated the change from baseline in TST at each time point and stored it in the new variable *tstc* (see DATA step in the SAS Code Fragment 6.7). Then the resulting dataset is analyzed using PROC MIXED. In this case, an ANCOVA model is specified for each time point (using a BY *visit* statement), where the model includes treatment effect and baseline value as covariate. The BY statement also contains the *_Imputation_* variable, which ensures that the analysis is done separately for each imputed dataset.

The results of this analysis are captured in the ODS output datasets: DIFFS (containing LSM estimates of differences between treatment arms), LSMEANS (containing LSM estimates for each treatment arm), and SOLUTIONF (containing ANCOVA model parameter estimates). Each of these output datasets contains the *visit* and *_Imputation_* variables to distinguish the results for each time point and imputation. SAS Output 6.8 contains a fragment of the ODS output dataset DIFF, where the variable *Estimate* contains the LSM estimates for the difference between

visit	_Imputation_	Effect	TRT	_TRT	Estimate	Std Err	DF	Probt	Lower	Upper
1	1	TRT	2	1	32.2	5.62	637	0.0000	21.14	43.20
1	2	TRT	2	1	32.2	5.62	637	0.0000	21.14	43.20
	...									
2	1	TRT	2	1	17.3	5.45	637	0.0016	6.57	27.95
2	2	TRT	2	1	17.7	5.49	637	0.0013	6.95	28.51
	...									
3	1	TRT	2	1	24.7	5.50	637	0.0000	13.90	35.49
3	2	TRT	2	1	24.4	5.55	637	0.0000	13.45	35.25
	...									
4	1	TRT	2	1	21.5	5.81	637	0.0002	10.13	32.96
4	2	TRT	2	1	22.9	5.81	637	0.0001	11.51	34.33
	...									
5	1	TRT	2	1	19.7	6.02	637	0.0011	7.90	31.54
5	2	TRT	2	1	17.2	6.04	637	0.0045	5.37	29.08
	...									

SAS Output 6.8 ODS output dataset DIFF from an ANCOVA analysis of the multiply-imputed data for the insomnia example.

treatment arms in the change from baseline for the TST, the variable *StdErr* contains the corresponding standard error for the LSM, the variable *DF* represents complete-data degrees of freedom in each of the imputed datasets, the variable *Probt* contains the p-value for the test of no difference between the treatment arms, and the variables *Lower* and *Upper* contain lower and upper limits of the confidence interval around the LSM estimate. We can see that there is one record per visit and imputation number. This dataset (as well as ODS datasets LSMEANS and SOLUTIONF) will be used to combine the results from individual imputations into one overall result. We will discuss how it is done in Section 6.4.

In some cases, MI is used for sensitivity analyses while the primary analysis is performed using an MMRM. Even under MAR assumptions ("standard MI"), this may be of interest if ancillary variables are included in the imputation model to enhance MAR-based modeling. In this case, some statisticians prefer to perform an MMRM-based analysis on the multiply-imputed dataset even if the estimation of time trends is not of importance and only the contrasts of treatment differences at specific time points are obtained at the end. This may be justified by a desire to apply exactly the same model at the analysis phase with imputed data as for the primary analysis using an MMRM where data have not been imputed. It should be noted that estimates obtained with time-point-specific contrasts from an MMRM analysis of imputed data would be equivalent to the estimates obtained from an ANCOVA model if the MMRM includes interactions of all variables with time point (e.g., baseline by time point).

SAS code Fragment 6.8 shows how PROC MIXED is used to perform an MMRM analysis using data imputed with a method shown in SAS Code Fragment 6.4, where the imputation model included the MSS scores as ancillary variables. The MMRM includes the effects for treatment arm, visit, treatment arm by visit interaction and

---

```
*** Dataset tst_mss_regvc contains imputed data in vertical structure
and a variable tstc representing change from baseline;

PROC SORT DATA=tst_mss_regvc; BY _Imputation_ trt visit subjid; RUN;

PROC MIXED DATA= tst_mss_regvc;
    CLASS trt visit subjid;
    MODEL tstc = tst_0 trt visit trt*visit/  DDFM=KR SOLUTION;
    REPEATED visit / TYPE=UN SUBJECT=subjid;
    LSMEANS trt*visit /CL DIFF=CONTROL("1" "5");
    ODS OUTPUT DIFFS=lsmdiffs LSMEANS=lsm SOLUTIONF=parms;
    BY _Imputation_ ;
RUN; QUIT;
```

SAS Code Fragment 6.8   MMRM analysis on multiply-imputed data for the insomnia example.

baseline value as covariate. Note that the ancillary MSS variables are no longer used during this analysis phase. Unstructured correlation matrix is used (TYPE=UN option). As in the previous example with ANCOVA, a BY _Imputation_ statement is used in PROC MIXED to analyze each imputed dataset separately, and the results are retrieved from the same ODS output datasets DIFFS, LSMEANS and SOLUTIONF.

In summary, the analysis on a multiply-imputed dataset is carried out in exactly the same way as it would be on complete data, with the only difference being the inclusion of the _Imputation_ variable in the BY statement of any SAS analysis procedure. We will see some additional examples for the analysis of categorical outcomes in Section 6.4.

6.4   Pooling phase: Combining results from multiple datasets

6.4.1   Combination rules

After missing data have been multiply imputed and each of the imputed datasets analyzed using a method suitable for the complete-data analysis, the results from multiple datasets need to be combined for an overall inference. The good news is that no matter what method has been used to impute missing data or to analyze them, the general principles for combining the results are the same and are based on the methodology developed by Rubin (1978, 1987). We provide a high-level overview of these principles in this section.

Assume that the objective of the complete-data analysis is to obtain the point and variance estimates for some parameter Q. Each of the M imputed datasets provided the corresponding estimates $\hat{Q}^m$ and $\widehat{Var(Q)}^m$, $m = 1, \ldots, M$. The combined point estimate for Q is then obtained as the average of the complete-data estimates:

$$\hat{Q} = \frac{1}{m} \sum_{m=1}^{M} \hat{Q}^m \tag{6.7}$$

The overall variance estimate consists of two components. Within-imputation variance is defined as the average of the M complete-data variance estimates:

$$\widehat{Var_{within}}(Q) = \frac{1}{m} \sum_{m=1}^{M} \widehat{Var(Q)}^m \tag{6.8}$$

The second component, between-imputation variance, is defined as follows:

$$\widehat{Var_{between}}(Q) = \frac{1}{m-1} \sum_{m=1}^{M} (\hat{Q}^m - \hat{Q})^2 \tag{6.9}$$

Finally, the total overall variance associated with $\hat{Q}$ is defined as:

$$\widehat{Var(Q)} = \widehat{Var_{Within}}(Q) + (1 + \frac{1}{M-1})\widehat{Var_{Between}}(Q) \tag{6.10}$$

A hypothesis test about the estimated parameter can be performed using the t-statistic:

$$\frac{(\hat{Q} - Q_{null})}{\sqrt{\widehat{Var(Q)}}} \tag{6.11}$$

where Q_{null} is the parameter value corresponding to the assumed null hypothesis. For example, if $\hat{Q}$ represents an estimate of a mean, then $Q_{null} = 0$ corresponds to a null hypothesis that the mean is equal to 0. The t-statistic is used in many complete-data analyses where it is known to follow the Student's t-distribution with appropriate degrees of freedom. When used with MI, the degrees of freedom, v_M, are computed according to the formula developed by Rubin (1987) which takes into account the number of imputations as well as the within- and between-imputation variance:

$$v_M = (M-1)\left[1 + \frac{\widehat{Var_{Within}}(Q)}{\left(1 + \frac{1}{M}\right)\widehat{Var_{Between}}(Q)}\right]^2 \tag{6.12}$$

The following ratio, which is a component of the formula defining the degrees of freedom in Equation 6.12, is referred to as the relative increase in variance due to non-response:

$$r = \frac{\left(1 + \frac{1}{M}\right) \widehat{Var}_{between}(Q)}{\widehat{Var}_{within}(Q)} \qquad (6.13)$$

When there is no missing data, the values of $\widehat{Var}_{between}(Q)$ and r in (6.13) are zero. With a large number of imputations M or a small value of r, the degrees of freedom v_M will be large and the distribution of the t-statistic in Equation 6.11 will be approximately normal.

This formula may, however, be inappropriate when the complete-data degrees of freedom are small and there is a small proportion of missing data. In this case, the above formula may provide inappropriately large number of degrees of freedom compared to what would have been used in complete-data analysis. The following adjusted degrees of freedom are recommended for such situations (Barnard and Rubin, 1999):

$$v_M^* = \left[\frac{1}{v_M} + \frac{1}{\hat{v}_{obs}}\right]^{-1} \qquad (6.14)$$

where $\hat{v}_{obs} = \frac{(1-r)v_0(v_0+1)}{(v_0+3)}$, v_0 are the complete-data degrees of freedom and r is defined as in (6.13)

While the degrees of freedom v_M do not depend on the sample size at all, the adjusted degrees of freedom defined in Equation 6.14 increase as the sample size increases but never exceed those of the complete-data analysis.

Confidence intervals around the combined point estimates can be obtained using the critical values from the t-distribution, $t_{v,\,1-\frac{\alpha}{2}}$, with the appropriate degrees of freedom v:

$$\hat{Q} \pm (t_{v,1-\frac{\alpha}{2}})\sqrt{\widehat{Var(Q)}} \qquad (6.15)$$

Multivariate inferences based on Wald tests and testing hypotheses about linear combinations of parameters can also be done based on a generalization of the approach described above (Rubin, 1987; Schafer, 1997).

In SAS, the procedure MIANALYZE implements combining results from the analysis of multiple imputed datasets based on the above methodology. It is designed to accept output datasets containing the results produced by other SAS procedures, for example, PROC REG, PROC MIXED, PROC LOGISTIC and so on, to apply the appropriate combination rules, and to perform hypothesis tests. Options DATA, PARMS, PARMINFO and COVB in the PROC MIANALYZE statement serve the purpose of conveying the analysis results and the information about the structure of the datasets containing them.

6.4.2   Pooling analyses of continuous outcomes

SAS Code Fragment 6.9 provides an example of how to combine the results of an ANCOVA analysis. First, it shows the analysis performed using PROC MIXED (as was described in SAS Code Fragment 6.8).

Recall that the ODS output datasets produced by PROC MIXED contain the results for each imputation, identified by the variable _Imputation_. These datasets

```
*** Analyze imputed data using an ANCOVA model;
PROC MIXED DATA=tst_reg1vc;
    CLASS trt;
    MODEL tstc = trt tst_0 / solution;
    LSMEANS trt / DIFF=CONTROL("1") CL;
    ODS OUTPUT DIFFS=lsmdiffs LSMEANS=lsm SOLUTIONF=parms;
    BY visit _Imputation_ ;
RUN; QUIT;


*** Combine LMS estimates for difference between treatments;
PROC MIANALYZE PARMS(CLASSVAR=FULL)=lsmdiffs;
    CLASS trt;
    MODELEFFECTS trt;
    ODS OUTPUT PARAMETERESTIMATES=mian_lsmdiffs;
    BY visit;
RUN;


*** Combine estimates of LMSs in each treatment arm;
PROC MIANALYZE PARMS(CLASSVAR=FULL)=lsm;
    CLASS trt;
    MODELEFFECTS trt;
    ODS OUTPUT PARAMETERESTIMATES=mian_lsm;
    BY visit;
RUN;


*** Combine ANCOVA model parameter estimates;
PROC MIANALYZE PARMS(CLASSVAR=FULL)=parms;
    CLASS trt;
    MODELEFFECTS Intercept trt tst_0;
    ODS OUTPUT PARAMETERESTIMATES=mian_parms;
    BY visit;
RUN;
```

SAS Code Fragment 6.9   Combining results from ANCOVA analysis of multiply-imputed data for the insomnia example.

are passed as input datasets to PROC MIANALYZE in separate invocations of this procedure. The PARMS option in the PROC MIANALYZE statement is used to pass a dataset which contains parameter estimates and the associated standard errors computed based on the imputed datasets. This type of output dataset is created in procedures such as PROC MIXED and PROC REG. With the PARMS option, the MIANALYZE procedure expects to find effect names stored in a variable *Parameter*, *Effect*, *Variable* or *Parm*. It then reads parameter estimates for the corresponding effect from the values of the variable *Estimate*, and the standard error of the estimate from the values of the variable *StdErr*. In our example, the dataset *lsmdiffs*, passed as input to the first invocation of PROC MIANALYZE, has a structure similar to the one shown in SAS Output 6.8.

When the effects contain classification variables, the CLASS statement can be used to identify them. The option CLASSVAR=FULL specifies that the input dataset contains classification variables explicitly, and that there is one record per level (or combination of levels) of the classification variables for which a parameter was estimated. The MODELEFFECTS statement lists the effects in the dataset for which the estimates need to be combined. Each effect is specified by a variable or a combination of variable names. For example, when combining the estimates of the LSM differences between treatments (contained in the dataset *lsmdiffs*), we specify the name of the treatment arm variable *trt*. When combining the estimates of the ANCOVA model parameters, we specify the effects of *Intercept*, *trt* and *tst_0*.

PROC MIANALYZE produces an ODS dataset PARAMETERESTIMATES, which has a similar structure to its input dataset (e.g., as shown in SAS Output 6.8), but which no longer contains the *_Imputation_* variable, because the results were pooled across all imputations. SAS Output 6.9 shows an example of the output dataset combining the estimates of LSM differences between treatments. It has one record per visit and variables that contain the combined LSM estimates, their standard errors, confidence interval limits, value of the *t*-statistic for the hypothesis test that the estimated parameter is equal to null value (zero in this case) and the corresponding *p*-value.

In the SAS Output 6.9, confidence interval limits, degrees of freedom, *t*-statistic and the *p*-value for Visit 1 are not provided. This is because there were no missing values of the TST at Visit 1, which results in between-imputation variance being

visit	Parm	trt	Estimate	Std Err	LCL Mean	UCL Mean	DF	t Value	Probt
1	trt	2	32.17	5.62	.	.	.	.	.
2	trt	2	16.74	5.62	5.72	27.76	717761	2.98	0.0029
3	trt	2	22.99	5.66	11.89	34.09	415445	4.06	<0.001
4	trt	2	22.46	6.10	10.50	34.42	116379	3.68	0.0002
5	trt	2	18.74	6.42	6.16	31.32	91674	2.92	0.0035

SAS Output 6.9   Overall (pooled) estimates of LSM differences between treatments from an ANCOVA analysis with multiply-imputed data for the insomnia example.

equal to zero. Since the between-imputation variance appears in the denominator of the degrees of freedom definition (see Equation 6.12), the value of the degrees of freedom is undefined and thus other quantities depending on it are not produced by SAS. In this case, the corresponding statistics have to be obtained from the complete-data analysis at Visit 1. The following warning is printed in the SAS log is this case:

```
WARNING: Between-imputation variance is zero for the effect trt.
NOTE: The above message was for the following BY group:
      visit=1
```

This type of warning message can also appear if MI resulted in all imputed values being equal. It is a very unlikely outcome if a large number of imputations are produced, but it is recommended always to investigate the cause of this message.

In the example of SAS Code Fragment 6.9, unadjusted degrees of freedom were used to perform hypothesis tests. We can see in the SAS Output 6.9 that the numbers of degrees of freedom are very large compared to the complete-data degrees of freedom (equal to 637, as shown in the SAS Output 6.8 for the analysis of each imputed dataset separately). As previously discussed, when the number of imputations is large we can use the adjusted degrees of freedom as defined in Equation 6.14. This can be done with the help of the EDF option in the PROC MIANALYZE statement, which allows us to specify the complete-data degrees of freedom, as shown in SAS Code Fragment 6.10.

Combined results, using the adjusted degrees of freedom are shown in SAS Output 6.10. Comparing these results to the ones presented in SAS Output 6.9, we can see that the confidence intervals are slightly wider and *p*-values are slightly larger.

SAS Code Fragment 6.11 illustrates the use of PROC MIANALYZE to combine the results of an MMRM analysis (longitudinal analysis model with repeated measures applied to imputed data). Since the results are produced by PROC MIXED in the same ODS output datasets as for the ANCOVA analysis, the invocations of PROC MIANALYZE are very similar, except that in this case, we can specify the *visit* variable in the CLASS statement because it would be one of the model effects. Similarly, the MODELEFFECTS statement now contains a *trt*visit* effect for which the LSMs of interest were obtained. Since the *visit* variable is now included in the CLASS statement, a BY *visit* statement is no longer used.

```
PROC MIANALYZE PARMS(CLASSVAR=FULL)=lsmdiffs EDF=637;
    CLASS trt;
    MODELEFFECTS trt;
    ODS OUTPUT PARAMETERESTIMATES=mian_lsmdiffs;
    BY visit;
RUN;
```

SAS Code Fragment 6.10   Combining results from ANCOVA analysis of multiply-imputed data using adjusted degrees of freedom for the insomnia example.

visit	Parm	trt	Estimate	Std Err	LCL Mean	UCL Mean	DF	t Value	Probt
1	trt	2	32.17	5.62	.	.	.	.	.
2	trt	2	16.74	5.62	5.70	27.79	610.8	2.98	0.0030
3	trt	2	22.99	5.66	11.86	34.11	602.99	4.06	<0.001
4	trt	2	22.46	6.10	10.47	34.44	573.34	3.68	0.0003
5	trt	2	18.74	6.42	6.14	31.34	565.21	2.92	0.0036

SAS Output 6.10   Overall (pooled) estimates and hypothesis tests using adjusted degrees of freedom for LSM differences between treatments from an ANCOVA analysis with multiply-imputed data for the insomnia example.

Table 6.4 summarizes the combined estimates of the LSM differences in the change from baseline in TST between the experimental and placebo treatments at Visit 5 (Week 8) resulting from the analyses discussed above.

Above, we provided an example of how to combine the estimates of model parameters and LSMs produced by PROC MIXED. Not all SAS procedures produce output datasets in the same format, so different options may need to be used when performing other types of analyses. For further details, we refer the reader to SAS User Guide (SAS Institute Inc., 2011) for PROC MIANALYZE, which includes numerous helpful examples for combining the results produced by different procedures. Below, we will explore one more example for the analysis of a multiply-imputed categorical outcome, using the mania example dataset described in Section 1.10.3.

```
PROC MIANALYZE PARMS(CLASSVAR=FULL)=lsmdiffs EDF=637;
   CLASS trt visit;
   MODELEFFECTS trt*visit;
   ODS OUTPUT PARAMETERESTIMATES=mian_lsmdiffs ;
RUN;

PROC MIANALYZE PARMS(CLASSVAR=FULL)=lsm EDF=637;
   CLASS trt visit;
   MODELEFFECTS trt*visit;
   ODS OUTPUT PARAMETERESTIMATES=mian_lsm;
RUN;
```

SAS Code Fragment 6.11   Combining results from an MMRM analysis of multiply-imputed data for the insomnia example.

6.4.3   Pooling analyses of categorical outcomes

6.4.3.1   Pooling logistic regression analyses

Recall that in the mania dataset, the primary endpoint is the treatment responder status assessed at five post-baseline visits with the primary endpoint being the response

Table 6.4   LSM estimates of the difference in the change from baseline to Week 8 in TST between experimental and placebo arms based on multiply-imputed data for the insomnia example.

Imputation method	Analysis method	Estimate	SE	95% CI	p-value
SAS Code Fragment 6.2	ANCOVA Unadjusted DF	18.74	6.42	6.16, 31.32	0.0035
SAS Code Fragment 6.2	ANCOVA Adjusted DF	18.74	6.42	6.14, 31.34	0.0036
SAS Code Fragment 6.4	MMRM Adjusted DF	19.44	6.38	6.90, 31.98	0.0024

at the last visit (study Day 28). We would like to adjust our analysis model for a baseline value of the YMRS score as well as country (the trial was conducted in three countries). In this dataset, the pattern of missingness is monotone, and we can use the monotone logistic regression method to perform MI. SAS Code Fragment 6.12 presents an invocation of PROC MI to perform this imputation using a model that

```
*** Impute missing responder status using monotone logistic
    regression;
PROC MI DATA=maniah SEED=883960001 NIMPUTE=1000 OUT=mania_logreg;
   VAR base_YMRS country trt resp_1-resp_5;
   CLASS country trt resp_1-resp_5;
   MONOTONE LOGISTIC;
RUN;


*** Analyze imputed responder status at visit 5 with logistic
    regression model;
PROC LOGISTIC DATA=mania_logreg;
   CLASS country trt(DESC);
   MODEL resp_5(EVENT="1") = base_ymrs country trt;
   ODS OUTPUT PARAMETERESTIMATES=lgsparms;
   BY _Imputation_;
RUN;


*** Combine results;
PROC MIANALYZE PARMS(CLASSVAR=CLASSVAL)=lgsparms;
   CLASS trt;
   MODELEFFECTS trt;
   ODS OUTPUT PARAMETERESTIMATES=mania_mian_logres;
RUN;
```

SAS Code Fragment 6.12   Combining results from a logistic regression analysis on multiply-imputed responder status at Visit 5 (study Day 28) for the mania example.

includes the effects for treatment arm, country, YMRS baseline score and previous responder status assessments as predictors for subsequent outcomes. The imputed responder status at the last time point (Visit 5) is then analyzed using PROC LOGISTIC with a model including treatments arm, country and baseline YMRS score.

In this example, the parameter estimates for the effects of the logistic regression model and their standard errors are captured in the ODS output dataset PARAMETERESTIMATES produced by PROC LOGISTIC. This datasets is subsequently passed as input to PROC MIANALYZE using the option PARMS (as in the case of the analysis performed with PROC MIXED) in order to obtain a combined estimate of the treatment effect parameter and the associated p-value for the significance of the treatment effect adjusted for baseline YMRS score and country. In this case, the option CLASSVAR=CLASSVAL is used, so that PROC MIANALYZE reads the levels for the classification effects from values of the variable ClassVal0 which is expected to be included in the input dataset. PROC LOGISTIC's ODS output dataset PARAMETERESTIMATES is generated using this type of structure.

6.4.3.2   Pooling results of the Cochran–Mantel–Haenszel and similar tests

The combination rules presented in this section assume that the parameter estimates $\hat{Q}^m$ are asymptotically normally distributed, which may not be the case with all parameters that we may wish to estimate based on imputed data. For example, the sampling distribution of Pearson's correlation coefficient is known to become increasingly skewed as the population correlation coefficient approaches 1 or -1. In this case, it is necessary to apply normalizing transformations to the estimates $\hat{Q}^m$ prior to combining them for the overall inference. Van Buuren (2012) provides some suggestions for normalizing transformations for several statistics. In the case of Pearson's correlation, Fisher's z transformation can be used (SAS Institute Inc., 2011, PROC MIANALYZE Example 57.10):

$$\widehat{z\rho}^m = \frac{1}{2} \log \left(\frac{\hat{\rho}^m + 1}{\hat{\rho}^m - 1} \right) \tag{6.16}$$

where $\hat{\rho}^m$ is an estimate of the correlation coefficient from the mth imputed dataset and $\widehat{z\rho}^m$ is a corresponding transformed (normalized) value. This transformed statistic is normally distributed with mean $\log([\rho + 1]/[\rho - 1])$ and variance $1/(n - 3)$ where ρ is the population correlation coefficient and n is the total number of observations in one imputed dataset. Variance $1/(n - 3)$ can then be used for the purposes of $\widehat{Var(Q)}^m$ in order to compute the combined variance, confidence intervals and to perform a hypothesis test for the estimated correlation coefficient.

A similar situation arises when performing certain analyses on multiply-imputed categorical data. For example, a Cochran–Mantel–Haenszel (CMH) test (Landis et al., 1978) is often used in the analysis of clinical trials for a complete-data analysis of the relationship between two categorical variables (e.g., treatment group and response to treatment) after controlling for one or more stratification variables (e.g., baseline disease severity) in a multi-way table. The CMH general association statistic has an asymptotic chi-square distribution with $(C_1 - 1)(C_2 - 1)$ degrees of freedom where C_1 and C_2 represent the number of categories assumed by each of the two categorical variables under the null hypothesis of no association. The chi-square distribution is highly skewed for smaller degrees of freedom, and thus obtaining a combined result of the CMH test from multiply-imputed data requires a transformation that would normalize the CMH statistic. For example, the Wilson–Hilferty transformation (Wilson and Hilferty, 1931; Goria, 1992) can be used for this purpose:

$$wh\_cmh^{(m)} = \sqrt[3]{cmh^{(m)}/df} \qquad (6.17)$$

where $cmh^{(m)}$ is the CMH statistic computed from the mth imputed dataset, df is the number of degrees of freedom associated with the CMH statistic and $wh\_cmh^{(m)}$ is the transformed value. The transformed statistic is approximately normally distributed with mean $1 - 2/(9 \times df)$ and variance $2/(9 \times df)$. We can standardize this transformed statistic to obtain a variable that is normally distributed with mean 0 and variance 1.

$$st\_wh\_cmh^{(m)} = \sqrt[3]{cmh^{(m)}/df} - \left(1 - \frac{2}{9 \times df}\right) \bigg/ \sqrt[2]{2/(9 \times df)} \qquad (6.18)$$

This transformed statistic can now be passed to PROC MIANALYZE in order to perform a combined CMH test.

SAS Code Fragment 6.13 illustrates the steps involved. First, analysis is performed using PROC FREQ to compute the CMH statistics in each of the imputed datasets, which are captured in the ODS output dataset CMH. Note that we performed a CMH test adjusting for the baseline YMRS score category (*basegrp_YMRS* variable) which takes a value of 0 if the subjects' baseline value is less than or equal to the overall baseline mean, and the value of 1 otherwise. We also adjusted for the country, similar to the analysis with the logistic regression model. A subsequent DATA step then performs a transformation and standardization of the CMH statistics. Then, a dataset containing the transformed statistics is passed to PROC MIANALYZE using a DATA option. With this option, the MODELEFFECTS statement contains the name of the variable that represents the statistic to be combined, and the STDERR statement contains the name of the variable that represents standard errors of that estimate. The combined results are captured in the ODS dataset PARAMETERESTIMATES. Finally, a p-value for the combined CMH test can be obtained as the upper-tailed p-value from the normal test produced by PROC MIANALYZE on the transformed statistic. This is done in the last DATA step of the SAS Code Fragment 6.13.

SAS Code Fragment 6.14 illustrates how to combine the Mantel–Haenszel (MH) estimate of the common odds ratio (Mantel and Haenszel, 1959; Agresti, 2002) computed by PROC FREQ for adjusted 2×2 tables (e.g., two levels of treatment arm and a binary response variable, as in our example). In this case, the estimated odds ratio values can be log-transformed to arrive at a normally distributed statistic, and the corresponding standard errors can be computed from the confidence interval

```
*** Perform CMH test;
PROC FREQ DATA=mania_logreg;
   TABLES basegrp_YMRS*country*trt*resp_5 / CMH;
   ODS OUTPUT CMH=cmh;
   BY _Imputation_;
RUN;


*** Apply Wilson-Hilferty transformation to the CMH statistic and
    standardize the resulting normal variable;
DATA cmh_wh; SET cmh(WHERE=(AltHypothesis="General Association"));
   cmh_value_wh=((VALUE/DF)**(1/3) - (1-2/(9*DF)))/SQRT(2/(9*DF));
   cmh_sterr_wh = 1.0;
RUN;


*** Combine results;
PROC MIANALYZE DATA=cmh_wh;
   ODS OUTPUT PARAMETERESTIMATES=mania_mian_cmh0;
   MODELEFFECTS cmh_value_wh;
   STDERR cmh_sterr_wh;
RUN;


*** Compute one-sided p-value;
DATA mania_mian_cmh; SET mania_mian_cmh0;
   IF tValue > 0 THEN Probt_upper = Probt/2;
   ELSE Probt_upper = 1-Probt/2;
RUN;
```

SAS Code Fragment 6.13   Combining results from a CMH test on multiply-imputed responder status at Visit 5 (study Day 28) for the mania example.

limits produced by PROC FREQ for the odds ratio. After the transformed estimates are pooled by PROC MIANALYZE, the combined values can be back-transformed to obtain an overall odds ratio and its confidence limits.

SAS Code Fragment 6.15 illustrates how to combine the estimates of binomial proportions of responders in each treatment arm and the difference between these proportions. For the proportions of responders in each treatment arm, the asymptotic standard errors provided by PROC FREQ for each imputed dataset are passed to PROC MIANALYZE along with the estimates of these proportions. For the difference between proportions in two arms, the standard error of the estimated difference is computed as the square root of the sum of squared standard errors for each proportion.

6.4.3.3   Summary of pooled analyses of binary responses in the mania example

Table 6.5 summarizes the results of all analyses discussed above for the responder rate at Visit 5 for the mania dataset. All analyses were performed on the same set of imputed data, and all of them lead to a conclusion that the difference between treatments in the response rate at Visit 5 is not statistically significant at the 0.05

```
*** Obtain Mantel-Haenszel estimate of the common odds ratio
    (Mantel-Haenszel Estimator);
PROC FREQ DATA=mania_logreg;
    TABLES basegrp_YMRS*trt*resp_5 / CMH;
    ODS OUTPUT COMMONRELRISKS=comrrout;
    BY _Imputation_;
RUN;


*** Apply log transformation to MH estimate of odds ratio and
    compute its standard error from the confidence interval;
DATA ormh; SET comrrout(WHERE=(StudyType="Case-Control"));
    log_or_mh_value=log(VALUE);
    log_or_mh_se=(log(UPPERCL)-log(LOWERCL))/(2*1.96);
RUN;


*** Combine transformed estimates;
PROC MIANALYZE DATA=ormh;
    ODS OUTPUT PARAMETERESTIMATES=mania_mian_orMH0;
    MODELEFFECTS log_or_mh_value;
    STDERR log_or_mh_se;
RUN;


*** Back-transform combined values;
DATA mania_mian_ormh; SET mania_mian_ormh0;
    Estimate_back = exp(ESTIMATE); *Overall odds ratio;
    LCL_back=Estimate_back*exp(-1.96*STDERR); *Overall lower limit;
    UCL_back=Estimate_back*exp(+1.96*STDERR); *Overall upper limit;
RUN;
```

SAS Code Fragment 6.14   Combining Mantel–Haenszel estimates of the common odds ratio for multiply-imputed responder status at Visit 5 (study Day 28) in the mania example.

significance level. This is consistent with the results of the longitudinal logistic regression analysis discussed in Chapter 6 for this dataset.

6.5   Required number of imputations

MI theory (Rubin, 1987) shows that MI is equivalent to maximum likelihood methods when $M = \infty$. However, in practice, an important question arises about how many imputations are sufficient to produce a reliable result in a statistically efficient manner.

A statistic that is useful for addressing this question is the fraction of missing information about the estimated parameter Q:

$$\hat{\lambda} = \frac{\left(r + {}^{2}\!/_{(v_M + 3)} \right)}{r + 1} \tag{6.19}$$

where v_M and r are defined as in (6.15) and (6.16).

```
*** Estimate proportions of responders in each treatment arm;
PROC FREQ DATA=mania_logreg;
   TABLES resp_5 / cl binomial(level=2);
   BY _Imputation_ trt;
   ODS OUTPUT BINOMIALPROP=prop;
RUN;


*** From ODS output dataset BINOMIALPROP, create a dataset
    containing estimated proportion of responders in each
    treatment arm and their standard errors;
DATA prop_trt;
   MERGE
     prop(WHERE=(Label1="Proportion")
          KEEP=_Imputation_ trt nValue1 Label1
          RENAME=(nValue1=prop))
     prop(WHERE=(Label1="ASE")
          KEEP=_Imputation_ trt nValue1 Label1
          RENAME=(nValue1=prop_se));
   BY _Imputation_ trt;
RUN;


*** Combine proportion estimates;
PROC SORT DATA=prop_trt; BY trt _Imputation_; RUN;
PROC MIANALYZE DATA=prop_trt;
   MODELEFFECTS prop;
   STDERR prop_se;
   BY trt;
   ODS OUTPUT PARAMETERESTIMATES=mania_mian_prop_trt;
RUN;


*** Compute estimates of the difference in proportions of
    responders between treatment arms and their standard errors;
DATA prop_diff;
   MERGE prop_trt(WHERE=(trt=1) RENAME=(prop=p1 prop_se=se1))
         prop_trt(WHERE=(trt=2) RENAME=(prop=p2 prop_se=se2));
   BY _Imputation_;

   prop_diff = (p2-p1);
   se_diff = sqrt(se1*se1 + se2*se2);
RUN;


*** Combine estimates of the proportion differences;
PROC MIANALYZE DATA=prop_diff;
   MODELEFFECTS prop_diff;
   STDERR se_diff;
   ODS OUTPUT PARAMETERESTIMATES=mania_mian_prop_diff;
RUN;
```

SAS Code Fragment 6.15 Combining estimates of responder proportions in each treatment arm and difference in proportions from multiply-imputed responder status at Visit 5 (study Day 28) in the mania example.

Table 6.5   Results of analyses on multiply-imputed categorical data for responder status at Visit 5 (study Day 28) in the mania example.

Test or statistic	Estimate	95% CI	p-value
Treatment effect from a logistic regression model adjusted for baseline YMRS score and country	0.13	−0.018, 0.276	0.0849
CMH test for general association, adjusted for baseline YMRS score category and country			0.1182
MH estimate of common odds ratio, adjusted for baseline YMRS score and country	1.26	0.935, 1.687	0.1302
Proportion of responders in the placebo arm	0.60	0.551, 0.649	
Proportion of responders in the experimental arm	0.66	0.617, 0.708	
Difference in proportions of responders between treatment arms	0.06	−0.004, 0.129	0.0680

Fraction of missing information $\hat{\lambda}$ is the basis for computing the relative efficiency of using the finite number of M imputations versus an infinite number (fully efficient imputation). It serves as an indicator of the number of imputations sufficient for the dataset at hand. Relative efficiency is defined as follows (Rubin, 1987):

$$RE = \left(1 + \frac{\hat{\lambda}}{M} \right)^{-1} \qquad (6.20)$$

As formula (6.20) suggests, when the amount of missing information is small, only a small number of imputations would be required, since relative efficiency is inversely proportional to the fraction of missing information. Theoretical results (Rubin, 1987) suggest that a small number of imputations (three to five) are sufficient to ensure satisfactory results. The default number of imputations in SAS PROC MI, for example, is set to 5.

In practice, the analyst can run the analysis with an increasing number of imputations and examine how the values of relative efficiency change. When relative efficiency does not appear to change significantly with the increasing number of imputations, it may serve as an indicator that the number of imputations is sufficient. Another aspect that may be examined in practice is the variability of the results produced with a fixed number of imputations but with different random seeds. Practical evidence suggests that it might be beneficial to use a higher number of imputations to reduce the variability due to randomness (Horton and Lipsitz, 2001).

Graham *et al.* (2007) conducted a simulation study in order to evaluate the variability in the estimation of standard errors and p-values for the regression coefficients, as well as statistical power for small effect sizes depending on the fraction of missing information $\hat{\lambda}$ and the number of imputations used. They observed that the estimated relative efficiency did not always adequately indicate the losses in power for diminishing number of imputations. They concluded that in practice, the fraction of missing information $\hat{\lambda}$, and consequently the relative efficiency, may not be accurately estimated unless M is rather large, and may provide a misleading impression that a small M stabilizes the relative efficiency. The simulation results suggested that a recommended number of imputations should rather be between 20 and 100, or even higher for data with very large fractions of missing information. Similar recommendations were provided in Bodner (2008), Von Hippel (2009) and White *et al.* (2011), where the authors proposed a rule of thumb that the number of imputations should be similar to the percentage of cases (subjects) that have missing data. In our experience, using the number of imputations even on the order of several thousand does not present any practical challenges with the current technology and produces results that are quite stable with respect to different random seeds used, as well as close to the results of the maximum likelihood analysis with an equivalent model.

PROC MIANALYZE produces the information on the within- and between-imputation variance, relative increase in variance, fraction of missing information and relative efficiency associated with the parameter estimates combined by the procedure. This information is printed in an active SAS output destination and can also be captured in the ODS output dataset VARIANCEINFO. SAS Output 6.11 shows the information printed by PROC MIANALYZE when combining the estimates of the LSM treatment differences in the change from baseline to Week 8 for the TST in the insomnia example using 1000 imputations (see also SAS Code Fragment 6.10). A row at the bottom of SAS Output 6.11 lists the references to the equations provided in this section and the previous section that contain the definitions of the corresponding statistics.

Table 6.6 provides an example of the variability in the results when a small number of imputations is used ($M = 5$) versus a large number ($M = 1000$). This table lists the

Variance Information							
		Variance				Relative Increase in Variance	Fraction Missing Information	Relative Efficiency
Parameter	trt	Between	Within	Total	DF			
trt	2	4.29308	36.86920	41.16658	565.2	0.116557	0.104409	0.999896
Refer to Equation		(6.9)	(6.8)	(6.10)	(6.14)	(6.13)	(6.17)	(6.18)

SAS Output 6.11 Variance information produced by PROC MIANALYZE for the ANCOVA estimates of LSM treatment difference in the change from baseline to Week 8 for the TST in the insomnia example based on multiply-imputed data with 1000 imputations.

Table 6.6   Example of variability in the estimates of LSM treatment difference in the change from baseline to Week 8 for the TST in the insomnia example based on multiply-imputed data with 5 and 1000 imputations. Each run was produced with a different random seed.

M	Run #	Relative efficiency	Estimate	SE	95% CI	p-value
5	1	0.992580	18.1269	6.1616	6.0454, 30.2084	0.0033
5	2	0.976936	18.4828	6.4257	5.8402, 31.1254	0.0043
5	3	0.958342	18.9577	6.7964	5.4712, 32.4442	0.0063
5	4	0.994210	19.5737	6.1175	7.5806, 31.5667	0.0014
5	5	0.977535	17.9992	6.3869	5.4354, 30.5630	0.0051
1000	1	0.999896	18.7399	6.4161	6.1644, 31.3154	0.0035
1000	2	0.999898	18.6897	6.4065	6.1330, 31.2464	0.0035
1000	3	0.999899	18.7583	6.4007	6.2129, 31.3036	0.0034
1000	4	0.999903	18.7651	6.3849	6.2508, 31.2795	0.0033
1000	5	0.999903	18.6332	6.3827	6.1231, 31.1433	0.0035

results obtained from five different runs of PROC MI (with different seed numbers) for each M. The results represent the estimates of LSM treatment difference in the change from baseline to Week 8 for TST (recall, TST = total sleep time in minutes), and the associated relative efficiency. As we can see, the variation due to random sampling is reduced with 1000 imputations, although even with $M = 5$ the observed variations are of the order of 2 min in the LSM treatment difference estimate and of the order of 0.005 in the p-value. For another examination of variability with varying numbers of imputations, see also Carpenter and Kenward (2007, p. 88).

6.6   Some practical considerations

6.6.1   Choosing an imputation model

Including ancillary variables that represent potential causes of missingness or are correlates of either missingness or the incomplete outcome variable can provide significant benefits for the quality of imputation. Recall that the MAR assumption is model dependent as it relies on the fact that all factors on which the missingness depends are included in the model. In other words, a MNAR scenario that we would have when using one imputation model may be converted to a MAR scenario with a more complete model, including additional relevant ancillary variables that are correlated with missingness (Schafer and Graham, 2002). These variables may represent baseline characteristics such as demographic factors, baseline value of the primary efficacy measure, or other important characteristics of baseline disease severity and a patient population subgroup. Various assessments collected post-baseline are also likely to be important predictors of dropout. Most notably, the value of the primary

```
*** Tests for no difference between baseline values in subjects
    who discontinued (disc=1) and completers (disc=0) by treatment;

*** t-test for continuous variables;
PROC TTEST DATA=sleep_base;
   CLASS disc;
   VAR age tst_0 mss_0;
   BY trt;
   ODS OUTPUT TTESTS=ttests;
RUN;


*** Chi-square test for a categorical variable;
PROC FREQ DATA=sleep_base;
   TABLES sex*disc / CHISQ;
   BY trt;
   ODS OUTPUT CHISQ=chisq;
RUN;
```

SAS Code Fragment 6.16 Tests for no difference in baseline characteristics between completers and dropouts for the insomnia example.

efficacy parameter at one or more visits prior to discontinuation is likely to be a significant predictor, especially for the group of subjects that discontinue due to lack of efficacy. In addition, other clinical assessments (e.g., secondary efficacy endpoints) are likely to reflect other important aspects of patient satisfaction with the treatment and their decision to remain in the trial.

The decision regarding which variables should be included in the imputation model can be done based on expert knowledge of the patient population and/or previous trials. Data from a given clinical trial can be used to inform such decisions either for an exploratory analysis of the same trial or for future ones using a similar patient population and treatment. Clinical data collected prior to a subject's discontinuation should be examined to get a better understanding of the factors that contribute to the subject's decision to withdraw from the trial.

For example, a simple way of testing whether a particular continuous variable observed prior to discontinuation is correlated with missingness is to perform a t-test for the difference of group means of this variable between subjects that dropped out and those who remained in the trial. To assess the relationship of categorical variables with missingness, a chi-square test may be performed in place of the t-test. SAS Code Fragment 6.16 illustrates how these tests can be performed for several baseline characteristics in the insomnia dataset.

The results of the t-test and chi-square test are presented in Table 6.7 for each treatment arm. From these results, it appears that in the placebo arm, baseline values of the TST were associated with dropout, whereas in the experimental arm, age and sex have significant p-values.

Another option for identifying significant predictors of missingness among baseline and post-baseline variables collected prior to discontinuation would be to use

Table 6.7 *P*-values from a test for no difference in the means or proportions of baseline characteristics between completers and dropouts by treatment arm in the insomnia example.

Variable (test)	*p*-value – Placebo arm	*p*-value – Experimental arm
age (t-test)	0.4395	<0.0001
tst_0 (t-test)	0.0375	0.9524
mss_0 (t-test)	0.6621	0.6624
sex (chi-square test)	0.3072	0.0105

logistic regression that models a binary missingness outcome based on a number of predictor variables. Standard model selection techniques (Burnham and Anderson, 2002) can be used to identify a set of variables that best predict missingness. It is also possible to use longitudinal logistic regression to model dropout across time points based on various baseline and post-baseline variables while accounting for the correlated longitudinal nature of the data. An example of applying such a model is provided in SAS Code Fragment 6.17, where the effects for treatment, sex, age, baseline values of the TST and MSS, as well as change from baseline to post-baseline visits in these parameters are included in the model. Variable *drop_out* on the left-hand side in the MODEL statement represents the fact whether the subject dropped out after a given visit or continued in the trial.

Parameter estimates and the corresponding *p*-values from this longitudinal model of dropout are presented in Table 6.8. These results suggest that treatment and baseline value of MSS do not have a significant effect on dropout, whereas other variables included in the model have significant *p*-values. Looking at the values of the parameter estimates, it appears that females are less likely to dropout than males; that the probability of dropout decreases with age; that subjects with larger values of baseline TST are less likely to discontinue; that larger values of change from baseline in TST (more favorable change in TST) reduce the probability of dropout and that larger values of change from baseline in MSS (less favorable change in MSS) increase the probability of dropout.

```
PROC GENMOD DATA=sleep(WHERE=(visit>=1)) DESCEND;
   CLASS trt(REF="1") sex(REF="MALE") subjid visit / PARAM=REF;
   MODEL drop_out=trt sex age tst_0 mss_0 tstc mssc /
       NOINT DIST=BIN;
   REPEATED SUBJECT=subjid / WITHINSUBJECT=visit CORR=UN PRINTMLE;
   ODS OUTPUT PARAMETERESTIMATES=Parms;
RUN; QUIT;
```

SAS Code Fragment 6.17 Longitudinal logistic model of dropout to explore the effects of baseline and post-baseline values on discontinuation in the insomnia example.

Table 6.8   Parameter estimates and p-values from a longitudinal logistic regression model of dropout exploring the effects of baseline and post-baseline values on discontinuation in the insomnia example.

Variable (level)	Estimate	p-value
TRT (=2)	0.2692	0.1587
sex (=FEMALE)	−0.5451	0.0073
AGE	−0.0374	<0.0001
tst_0	−0.0041	<0.0001
mss_0	0.0131	0.8010
tstc	−0.0029	0.0213
mssc	0.2056	0.0008

Approaches based on statistical tests such as those described above are prone to identifying spurious associations when testing many variables without any Type I error control. In theory, there is no harm in including ancillary variables uncorrelated with missingness, but with limited sample sizes, the succinctness of the imputation model would be important. On the other hand, if the number of discontinued subjects is not large, the above mentioned techniques may lack power and fail to identify some true correlates. If prior or expert knowledge suggests that a variable may be a correlate of missingness it is better to include it in the model regardless of the statistical significance of the above tests.

Graphical tools can also be very insightful. For example, figures shown in Section 1.10 to illustrate patterns of missingness of the example datasets used in this book were quite helpful for understanding possible relationships between change from baseline in the primary and secondary endpoints and early discontinuation.

In addition to considering variables that may be correlated with the event of withdrawal, one should consider any variables that may be correlated with the values of the missing outcome. Two scenarios may be of interest in this respect. There may be variables that are correlated with the outcome measure when assessed at the same time point. Including such ancillary variables may be beneficial for non-monotone missing data. For example, if in an HIV study, two parameters – the CD4 counts and plasma RNA viral load – are measured, and there are instances where CD4 results are available but viral load results are missing, including CD4 in the imputation model can greatly improve the accuracy of the imputations for the viral load in the populations of patients where the two tests are correlated (Bhatt et al., 2009). On the other hand, there may be variables that act as precursors to the primary clinical outcome in a sense that earlier measurements of these variables are predictive of the future values of the primary endpoint. For example, Boulware et al. (2006) found that depression symptoms were highly correlated with future cardiovascular outcomes. In this case, including measures of depression at earlier time points to predict missing cardiovascular events at later time points may positively impact the quality of imputations.

Finally, we note that the imputation model should contain interaction terms that will be included in the analysis model. Omitting these terms may result in imputed data that does not reflect the correlations between these interaction terms and the outcome variable and thus attenuate the effect of the interactions on the outcome in the analysis model. One example of an interaction term that is sometimes included in the analysis of clinical trial data is the interaction between baseline and treatment.

Another example is when an assumption is made that the correlations between outcomes at different post-baseline visits may differ depending on the treatment arm. This would correspond to allowing the correlation matrix in the MMRM analysis to differ by treatment arm, as discussed in Chapter 5 (recall the use of GROUP option in the REPEATED statement of PROC MIXED). In the imputation model, this assumption can be implemented by including interaction terms between treatment and post-baseline outcomes used as predictors. SAS Code Fragment 6.18 illustrates how this imputation model can be specified using the insomnia example, where the model is explicitly specified for each post-baseline visit outcome using multiple MONOTONE REGRESSION statements, and where interactions of *trt* with TST variables at previous visits are included. Subsequently, if the analysis of the imputed data is performed using an MMRM model, it is necessary to implement the assumption of heterogeneous correlations at the analysis stage as well (see the GROUP option in the PROC MIXED invocation that analyzes the imputed data in SAS Code Fragment 6.18).

Table 6.9 presents the results of insomnia example analyses using models with or without heterogeneous correlations. We can see that the results from the MI-based analysis using the imputation model without treatment by outcome interactions (Imputation Method 1) agree very closely with the results from the likelihood-based analysis using an equivalent MMRM model with a homogeneous correlation matrix (denoted MMRM Method 1 in Table 6.9). The MI result based on the imputation model including such interactions (denoted Imputation Method 4) differs slightly from the previous results, but agrees very well with the likelihood-based analysis using an MMRM model with a heterogeneous correlation matrix (denoted MMRM Method 2).

6.6.2   Multivariate normality

As previously discussed, many imputation methods discussed above (notably MCMC and regression-based method for monotone missingness) make an assumption of multivariate normality for variables included in the imputation model. In practice, this assumption is not always satisfied, so the question arises as to the ways of dealing with non-normality and performance of MI under such conditions.

Fortunately, many simulation studies provide evidence that normality-based imputations are still quite accurate for non-normal distributions (Rubin and Schenker, 1986; Schafer, 1997; Schafer and Olsen, 1998; Graham and Schafer, 1999; Bernaards *et al.*, 2007; Carpenter and Kenward, 2007; Demirtas *et al.*, 2008; Leite and Beretvas, 2010). The magnitude of the bias under non-normal distributions depends on the sample size and the proportion of missing data. It is difficult to establish reliable

```
PROC MI DATA=sleeph NIMPUTE=1000 SEED=883960001 OUT=tst_reg3;
VAR trt tst_0 - tst_5;
CLASS trt;
MONOTONE REGRESSION (tst_2 = trt tst_0 tst_1 tst_1*trt);
MONOTONE REGRESSION (tst_3 = trt tst_0 tst_1 tst_1*trt
                             tst_2 tst_2*trt);
MONOTONE REGRESSION (tst_4 = trt tst_0 tst_1 tst_1*trt
                             tst_2 tst_2*trt tst_3 tst_3*trt);
MONOTONE REGRESSION (tst_5 = trt tst_0 tst_1 tst_1*trt
                             tst_2 tst_2*trt tst_3 tst_3*trt
                             tst_4 tst_4*trt);
RUN;

*** Analyze imputed data using MMRM.
Imputed dataset tst_reg3 has been transposed into a vertical
structure (tst_reg3vc) to contain one record per subject and visit,
and change from baseline (tstc) has been computed on each record ***;

PROC MIXED DATA=tst_reg3vc;
    CLASS trt visit subjid;
    MODEL tstc = tst_0 tst_0*visit trt visit trt*visit/ DDFM=KR
                                                        SOLUTION;
    REPEATED visit / TYPE=UN SUBJECT=subjid GROUP=trt;
    LSMEANS trt*visit / CL DIFF=CONTROL("1" "5");
    ODS OUTPUT DIFFS=lsmdiffs2 LSMEANS=lsm2;
    BY _Imputation_ ;
RUN; QUIT;
```

SAS Code Fragment 6.18   Imputation using monotone regression with a model for each imputed variable corresponding to TST assessments in the insomnia example including treatment by outcome interactions for post-baseline visits used as predictors.

rules of thumb, but some simulation studies (Schafer, 1997; Graham and Schafer, 1999) reported good performance with a sample size of 100, while Demirtas *et al.* (2008) reported poor results with sample sizes of 40. The latter study also reported accurate parameter estimates with proportions of missing data as high as 25% with larger sample sizes.

The question of whether the non-normality needs to be addressed at the imputation phase by using normalizing transformations for some variables (e.g., logarithmic or square root) has been studied by some researchers. Unfortunately, there does not seem to be a consensus in the methodological literature at present, and if anything, it cautions rather against the use of such transformations (Demirtas *et al.*, 2008). There are various reasons for this. First of all, it is not easy to choose an appropriate transformation in advance as it depends on the magnitude of the skewness and kurtosis of data, which may not be known a priori. Moreover, assessing these

Table 6.9   LSM estimates of the difference in the change from baseline to Week 8 in TST between experimental and placebo arms based on multiply-imputed data and likelihood-based MMRM analyses for the insomnia example. Imputation Methods 1 and 4 represent the MI-based methods shown in SAS Code Fragments 6.2 and 6.18, respectively. MMRM methods 1 and 2 represent likelihood-based MMRM analyses (no imputation) using homogeneous and heterogeneous correlation matrices, respectively.

Analysis/Imputation Method	Estimate	SE	95% CI	p-value
Imputation Method 1 (no interactions with treatment)	18.74	6.42	6.14,31.34	0.0036
MMRM Method 1(no imputation) with homogeneous correlation structure	18.71	6.39	6.17,31.26	0.0035
Imputation Method 4 (interactions with treatment included)	19.84	6.40	6.26,32.4	0.0020
MMRM method 2 (no imputation) with heterogeneous correlation structure	19.72	6.38	7.19,32.25	0.0021

characteristics based on observed data only would not be accurate, especially if data are systematically missing from the tails of the distribution. Some researchers are not comfortable using transformed data, as analyzing them on an unfamiliar transformed scale makes the interpretation of the results more difficult. One possibility would be to perform transformation at the imputation phase and then back-transform the data for analysis. However, data transformations affect the covariance structure of the data, and for imputation methods such as regression (which rely heavily on the associations between variables) back-transformation can affect the accuracy of the imputation.

Certain measures for dealing with non-normality can be undertaken at the analysis stage as well. It appears that non-normality can differ in its impact on different parameter estimates. In particular, variance estimates tend to be more affected than estimates of the means and regression coefficients because they are more sensitive to the values in the tails of a distribution. This issue is not unique to MI, and corrective procedures exist for complete-data analysis methods to improve the accuracy of variance estimates. For example, a so-called sandwich estimator of the sampling variance (Huber, 1967; White, 1982; Freedman, 2006) is used to provide a correction for the standard errors depending on the kurtosis of the data for non-normal distributions. Another approach used to estimate standard errors with non-normal data is bootstrap re-sampling (Stine, 1989; Bollen and Stine, 1992; Efron and Tibshirani, 1993; Enders, 2002) which uses a Monte Carlo simulation technique to generate an empirical sampling distribution of each estimated parameter. In order to generate this sampling distribution, the method repeatedly forms new samples of size N with replacement from the original dataset and analyzes each such dataset to obtain the desired parameter estimates. The observed standard deviation of the parameter from this sampling distribution is used as the bootstrap standard error. The accuracy of the standard error estimates is not affected by non-normality because the bootstrap method does not make any distributional assumptions. See Chapter 8 for a fuller account of the bootstrap and an example of its use in the context of doubly robust estimation. Techniques like the sandwich estimator or bootstrap can be used to obtain more accurate standard errors when analyzing multiply-imputed datasets, and these standard errors can then be used in the pooling formulas of Rubin discussed in Section 6.4.

6.6.3   Rounding and restricting the range for the imputed values

Discrete measurements are often used in clinical trials resulting in binary or categorical variables. For example, responses to the questionnaire items are typically selected from a pre-fixed list of choices which can be coded into discrete ordinal categories. When the number of categories is relatively small and missingness is monotone, it is best to use logistic regression to impute such values. However, for non-monotone missing data, in order to use the MCMC method, the categorical variables would need to be coded with numerical values and treated as continuous variables. This may result in a number of issues, for example, the imputed values may be fractional, which makes it cumbersome to convert them to the original categorical scale.

Sometimes, the number of possible discrete values is large. For example, a total score for a questionnaire based on a sum of the individual items could range between zero and a few dozens, yet be restricted to integer values because the individual items are all coded to integers. Such assessments are often analyzed as continuous variables. Even when using a regression method for monotone missingness, imputed values may be fractional rather than integers. In these cases, imputed values do not look like real values and in order to make them more intelligible to the analyst, one possibility is to round them to the nearest integer.

In some cases, rounding imputed values is not a matter of taste but rather a necessity if the analysis model subsequently requires these variables to be categorical. However, if the analysis model that will be applied on the multiply-imputed data can treat these variables as continuous, recent empirical studies (Horton *et al.*, 2003; Allison, 2005; Bernaards *et al.*, 2007; Yucel *et al.*, 2008) suggest that it may be best to leave the imputed values as produced by the imputation method, that is, unrounded, in order to avoid bias. However, these studies focused mainly on the rounding of the binary variables and there is some evidence (Van Ginkel *et al.*, 2007a, 2007b) that rounding may be less problematic as the number of categories increases.

In summary, we suggest to follow the following guidelines. When categorical data need to be imputed and intended for subsequent analysis with categorical methods, logistic regression should be used for the imputation of monotone missing values. If the dataset contains some non-monotone values, the MCMC method should be used to perform only partial imputation to obtain a monotone pattern.

The values imputed by the MCMC should be rounded, and if the proportion of non-monotone data is not large, it would have a limited impact on the overall results. PROC MI can produce rounded values automatically when the option ROUND is used based on a simple rounding to the closest integer with a 0.5 threshold. However, using this simple rounding method can lead to bias and alternative methods have been explored in the literature, for example, adaptive rounding (Bernaards *et al.*, 2007) and calibration (Yucel *et al.*, 2008) for binary data, which seem to reduce bias. In adaptive rounding, instead of using a fixed threshold of 0.5, the threshold is based on the imputed data using a normal approximation for a binomial distribution. This threshold is defined as follows:

$$threshold = \hat{\mu}_{UR} - \Phi^{-1}\left(\hat{\mu}_{UR}\right)\sqrt{\hat{\mu}_{UR}(1 - \hat{\mu}_{UR})} \tag{6.21}$$

where $\hat{\mu}_{UR}$ is the mean of the imputed variable computed using unrounded values and $\Phi^{-1}\left(\hat{\mu}_{UR}\right)$ is the z value from a standard normal distribution (inverse of the standard normal cumulative distribution). With the threshold thus computed, imputed values that are greater or equal to this threshold are rounded to 1, and values that are smaller than the threshold are rounded to 0.

When a categorical variable with more than two categories is included in the imputation model with a method such as MCMC, a so-called dummy coding is often used (as described in Section 6.2.4). These dummy variables would be included in the imputation model and the MCMC method could fill the missing values with fractional values, including some smaller than 0 or greater than 1. After the imputation is produced for these dummy variables, rounding each dummy variable separately to 0 or 1 (either with a simple or adaptive rounding) may produce a set of incompatible values where more than one dummy variable would be rounded to 1 thus leading to multiple choices of the original C categories.

Allison (2002) suggested a procedure to deal with this problem. We summarize it here, although it should be noted that this approach does not appear to have been well studied in the literature. As the first step in this procedure, a new variable is computed as 1 minus the sum of unrounded values imputed for each dummy variable. We will denote this variable by $D_C = 1 - \sum_{c=1}^{C-1} D_c$ and consider it to represent the reference category, while $D_c, c = 1, \ldots, C - 1$ are the unrounded values corresponding to other categories. Then, a variable with the maximum value is identified among the variables $D_1, D_2, \ldots, D_C$, and the category corresponding to this variable is selected as a categorical value. For example, suppose we are imputing a variable that can take one of the three categories. In the imputation model, we would use two dummy variables, D_1 and D_2, coding the original value of category one with a combination of $D_1 = 1$ and $D_2 = 0$; category two with $D_1 = 0$ and $D_2 = 1$ and considering the third category as reference corresponding to values $D_1 = 0$ and $D_2 = 0$. Suppose that the imputation produces unrounded values $D_1 = -0.10$ and $D_2 = 0.52$. Using the procedure described above, we calculate $D_3 = 1 - (-0.10 + 0.52) = 0.58$. The value of D_3 is the largest of the three, and so we select the third category as the value for the original categorical variable.

On the other hand, when a variable takes a discrete but large range of values and is intended to be analyzed as a continuous variable in the analysis phase, the rounding is not necessary and generally is not recommended (Enders, 2010).

Another nuisance of working with the imputed values is that with certain imputation methods, they can fall outside of the clinically meaningful range. All clinical measurements have a lower and upper limit for possible values dictated by physiological constraints (e.g., blood glucose levels) or measurement design (e.g., questionnaire responses), whereas methods such as MCMC and regression-based imputation may sometimes produce a prediction from the imputation model that would be outside of this range. Possible effects of forcing the imputed values in the allowed range are not clear and formal methodological studies of this issue do not seem to exist in the current literature. On the one hand, having data with clinically impossible values may lead to estimates of variance that are unrealistic. On the other hand, forcibly moving the imputed values from one extreme of the Bayesian posterior predictive distribution closer towards the mean can effectively change the mean of the imputed data and introduce bias. If the proportion of out-of-range imputed values is small and if such values do not deviate significantly from the allowed range, the imputed data should probably be analyzed as is, but investigations of this aspect would be desirable.

If the analyst needs to enforce specific ranges on the imputed data, PROC MI provides options MIN and MAX intended to specify the desired limits. With these options, when the procedure obtains a sample of a value for imputation that is outside of the specified range, it attempts to obtain another sample. However, if after a limited number of such re-sampling attempts, an acceptable value is not found, the imputation is not performed and the MI procedure produces a warning statement. In such cases, it would not be possible to use MIN and MAX options, and the desired range limits will need to be enforced separately after the imputation is performed if necessary.

6.6.4   Convergence of Markov chain Monte Carlo

One problem that occurs occasionally with the data augmentation algorithm used to generate a Markov chain is that the chain does not converge to a stable stationary distribution. Theoretical convergence properties have been explored by Schafer (1997) but they are asymptotic in nature (i.e., they apply when the number of chain elements goes to infinity). Unfortunately, it is not easy to verify convergence in practice (Cowles and Carlin, 1996). We will only discuss the use of some graphical diagnostic tools that are readily available in software implementations for MI and which could provide an indication that convergence has not been achieved.

It can be helpful to examine a trace plot of the parameters $\theta(\eta)$ across iterations η of the data augmentation algorithm (see the description of the MCMC method in Section 6.2.4). If the process converges, this plot is expected to present random scatter around some mode of the distribution in a long run (remember, we are concerned with convergence to a distribution, and not to a single point in the parameter space). If this plot exhibits any systematic trends across hundreds of iterations, it would indicate

```
PROC MI DATA=sleeph NIMPUTE=1 SEED=883960001 OUT=sleep_mcmc_full;
   VAR trt age sexn tst_0 mss_0 tst_1 mss_1 tst_2 mss_2
                    tst_3 mss_3 tst_4 mss_4 tst_5 mss_5;
   MCMC TIMEPLOT (WLF)
        ACFPLOT  (WLF / CCONF=GREY WCONF=2 WNEEDLES=3 NLAG=200);
RUN;
```

SAS Code Fragment 6.19   Diagnostic plots of MCMC convergence for the insomnia example.

that successive iterations are highly correlated and that there is a lack of convergence to a stationary distribution. In SAS PROC MI, trace plots can be produced for variable means, variances and covariances, as well as their log-transformations.

Additionally, a trace plot can be produced for the worst linear function (WLF) of parameters (Schafer, 1997). The WLF is a scalar function of all parameters in the vector θ, simulated at each iteration of the data augmentation algorithm, that weights each parameter according to its convergence speed and it represents the "worst" convergence speed in a sense that this function's values converge more slowly than any individual parameter. So if the imputation model contains many variables (and thus many parameters), it is easier to examine a trace plot of the WLF to get an indication of the worst convergence.

SAS Code Fragment 6.19 provides an example of a PROC MI option TIMEPLOT that can be specified in the MCMC statement in order to generate a trace plot for the WLF.

The resulting trace plot is shown in Figure 6.3. In the SAS Code Fragment 6.19, we specified one imputation in the NIMPUTE option and used a default value of the NBITER option (equal to 200), which resulted in a plot presenting the WLF over the 200 iterations of a burn-in phase, after which one imputation was generated. There

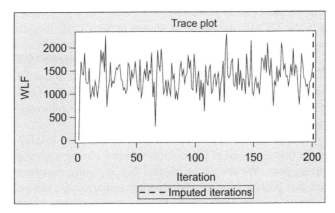

Figure 6.3 Trace plot for worst linear function generated by SAS Code Fragment 6.18.

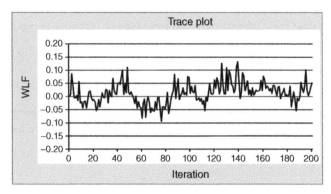

Figure 6.4   Trace plot for worst linear function with apparent systematic trends suggesting non-convergence of a Markov chain. Reproduced by permission of Guildford Press.

does not seem to be any systematic trend observed on this plot (the WLF seems to oscillate around some mean value, especially after 100 iterations). This plot does not seem to provide any evidence of non-convergence.

Figure 6.4, reproduced from Enders (2010), provides an example of a trace plot where some systematic trends, lasting approximately 60 iterations, can be observed.

Another useful graph to examine is the autocorrelation function plot. Autocorrelation at lag τ is the correlation between parameter estimates at the iteration η and $(\eta + \tau)$ for $\eta \geq 1$. Autocorrelation function can also be computed for the WLF. This type of plot depicts autocorrelation values on the y-axis and lag values on the x-axis. If it appears that strong serial dependencies persist even as the lag increases, it indicates a problem with convergence. If autocorrelations are initially large but then stabilize around a small value with an increased lag, then this information is helpful in order to determine the required number of burn-in iterations as well as number of iterations to skip on a single Markov chain between using the draws for MI.

Autocorrelation plots can be generated from PROC MI with the use of the ACF-PLOT option in the MCMC statement, as shown in SAS Code Fragment 6.19. As can be observed from Figure 6.5, autocorrelations between the values of WLF (and thus parameter estimates) quickly become very small, especially for lag values larger than 150. Based on this plot, it appears that it would be best to use NITER option (number of iterations skipped between generating imputed datasets) equal to a value larger than 150, although even with a default value of 100, the autocorrelations seem to be quite small and would be acceptable.

In order to assess convergence and its speed, it may be helpful to examine diagnostic graphs discussed above for multiple Markov chains, each generated from a different starting point. We already mentioned that, typically, maximum-likelihood parameter estimates generated by the EM algorithm are used as a starting point for a Markov chain. Exploring the chains from different starting points can help to assess whether different points in the parameter space influence the behavior of a chain, for example, whether it can get trapped in some local region for a large number

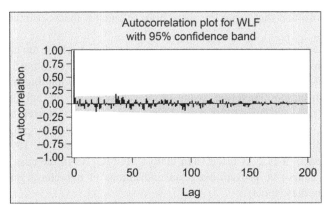

Figure 6.5   Autocorrelation plot for worst linear function generated by SAS Code Fragment 6.18.

of iterations. Even when the chain is started from the EM estimate, it may visit these other points in the space on certain runs, and thus it is helpful to explore the parameter space as much as possible. If it is observed that convergence speed is significantly slower for some starting points then one could increase the number of burn-in iterations in order to increase the chances that convergence will be attained on any run. One method that can be used to obtain alternative starting points is a bootstrap procedure that performs simple random sampling with replacement from the input dataset prior to computing the EM estimates (Gelman and Rubin, 1992). One can also use a smaller bootstrap sample than the original dataset to increase the noisiness of the bootstrap procedure and obtain a more diverse set of starting points (Schafer, 1997). This approach produces what is referred to as over-dispersed starting points. In PROC MI, this can be done using the option INITIAL=EM(BOOTSTRAP= b) with the MCMC statement, where b is the proportion of the observations in the original dataset to be included in the bootstrapped sample.

Convergence problems may also occur because there is insufficient data to estimate certain parameters. This may arise when too many variables are included in the imputation model so that the number of parameters to be estimated is very large compared to the number of available observations. Linear dependencies between the variables may also cause convergence issues. Systematic patterns of missingness, for example, when two variables are always missing together, can make it difficult to estimate certain elements of the covariance matrix. When convergence problems are suspected, the analyst can try to remove certain variables from the model or use a composite index combining multiple variables that may be highly correlated.

If convergence problems are observed when using a non-informative prior, the analyst can try to specify a ridge prior. Using the ridge prior may be viewed as adding a small number of artificial observations from a hypothetical population where variables are uncorrelated, thus introducing some bias towards zero values for the covariance matrix. This can help stabilize the estimation process but the analyst should bear in mind that using the ridge prior attenuates the associations between variables.

As a final note, sometimes it may appear from the plots that there are no systematic trends and thus no issue with convergence, but it may just be the case that the algorithm is trapped for some finite time in a local region instead of sampling from a stable posterior distribution. Therefore, using graphical tools may be helpful to get an indication of non-convergence but cannot be used as a proof of convergence.

Convergence of the FCS algorithm can be assessed using similar graphical tools. Experimental evidence (Brand, 1999; van Buuren and Oudshoorn, 1999) suggests that convergence of FCS is faster than that of MCMC. As in the case of MCMC, convergence cannot be proven, but some indications of non-convergence may be detected using these tools.

6.7   Pre-specifying details of analysis with multiple imputation

As with any analysis used in clinical trials, be it the primary or sensitivity analysis, it is very important to pre-specify all details in advance, in the protocol and/or statistical analysis plan prior to study unblinding. Leaving a possibility of choosing between various alternative options in the model or computational settings may leave the door open for post-study unblinding manipulation aimed at finding the settings that produce the most favorable results, and could therefore undermine confidence in the integrity of the study conclusions, especially in situations where the results are border-line significant. When using MI methodology, the following aspects should be fully pre-specified.

- Imputation model should be fully described in terms of the following aspects:
  - type of the model or non-parametric method that will be used (e.g., regression for monotone missingness for continuous variables);
  - predictors (explanatory variables), including all ancillary variables, to be included in the imputation model for each variable that will be imputed, including any interaction terms;
  - user-defined parameters that may be associated with the chosen imputation method, for example, a number of groups used in the propensity score method;
  - transformations, if any, applied to the explanatory variables prior to imputation.

- Full specification of the imputation model/method should be provided both for the non-monotone missing data and for monotone missing data, if different methods are used.

- The order of variables that will be used to establish monotone patterns of missingness should be specified. This is particularly important when ancillary variables include outcomes collected post-baseline, and thus several variables have to be ordered within each time point.

- If the MCMC method is used, either for partial imputation with the non-monotone missingness or for a full imputation, the following options need to be specified: single versus multiple chains, number of burn-in iterations, number of iterations between imputations for a single Markov chain, a method of choosing starting points for multiple Markov chains (e.g., over-dispersion), and a form of prior distribution for the parameters. Tools that will be used to examine convergence of the MCMC process should ideally be mentioned along with the planned actions to be taken if a lack of convergence is observed.

- Number of imputations needs to be specified.

- Random seed(s) need to be specified for each planned invocation of the multiple-imputation procedure (e.g., one for the partial imputation with MCMC, and one for a subsequent imputation of the remaining monotone missing data).

- An analysis model (complete-data method used for the analysis of each imputed dataset) needs to be specified with the same level of detail as the imputation model.

- For the pooling phase, some options may also need to be specified. For example, one should describe the use of adjusted degrees of freedom if applicable, the mean value for the null hypothesis, any transformations or additional calculations needed on the parameters/statistics estimated from imputed datasets prior to combining them, for example, as in the case of the correlation coefficient or the CMH test.

Any deviations from the planned specifications after study unblinding should be discussed and justified in the Clinical Study Report.

Prior specification of these details will not only increase confidence in the impartiality of the analyses but also allow for a rigorous quality control process. Specifying such options as the exact number of imputations and random seeds would allow an exact reproduction of the results by independent reprogramming.

Appendix 6.A: Additional methods for multiple imputation

In addition to the imputation methods described in Section 6.2.4, several other methods are available in SAS PROC MI and are briefly summarized below.

Predictive mean matching method

Predictive mean matching (Heitjan and Little, 1991; Schenker and Taylor, 1996) is another parametric method that can be used to impute continuous variables in a sequential imputation strategy. It is very similar to the regression method, as it uses the same linear regression model as described in Equation 6.1 and involves two steps to generate each of M imputed datasets: (a) draw a new sample of the parameters of the regression model from the Bayesian posterior distribution; (b) generate imputations from the regression model instance. It is the latter step that is carried out in a different manner in the predictive mean matching method. Step (b) is performed as follows.

(b.1) For each subject i with an **observed** value of Y_j, use this subject's available values of the predictor variables to generate a prediction for Y_j from the regression model instance:

$$y_{j,i}^{(m)} = \beta_0^{(m)} + \beta_1^{(m)} w_{1,i} + \beta_2^{(m)} w_{2,i} + \cdots + \beta_{K_j}^{(m)} w_{K_j,i} \qquad (6.22)$$

(b.2) For each subject q with a **missing** value of Y_j, also obtain a predicted value from the same regression model:

$$y_{j,q^*}^{(m)} = \beta_0^{(m)} + \beta_1^{(m)} w_{1,q} + \beta_2^{(m)} w_{2,q} + \cdots + \beta_{K_j}^{(m)} w_{K_j,q} \qquad (6.23)$$

Find a set of N_j subjects whose corresponding predicted values $y_{j,i}^{(m)}$ from step (b.1) are closest to the predicted value $y_{j,q^*}^{(m)}$. Randomly draw one subject, i^*, out of these N_j subjects, and use this subject's observed value $y_{j,i}$ to fill in the missing value of subject q.

Obviously, this method generates imputed values from the values that are actually observed in other subjects. Thus, such imputed data will always be "plausible" and will never be out of range of possible values for a given variable. This feature cannot be guaranteed by the regular regression method discussed above, because predictions from a regression model may not always be constrained to a set of practically plausible values, for example, a limited range of values corresponding to a total score from a questionnaire. More discussion regarding limiting the range of the imputed values is provided in Section 6.6.3.

The predictive mean matching method depends on a user-specified parameter N_j that determines a pool of "similar" subjects from whom an observed value is sampled in order to fill in a missing value. A smaller N_j would have a tendency to increase the correlation among the multiple imputations and result in a higher variability of point estimators obtained based on multiply-imputed data. On the other hand, a larger N_j would tend to lessen the effect from the imputation model and may result in biased estimators (Schenker and Taylor, 1996).

In PROC MI, predictive mean matching method is invoked with the REGPMM keyword specified in the MONOTONE statements, as shown in SAS Code Fragment 6.20. An option K is used to pass the parameter N_j discussed above, and its default value is 5. This example also illustrates that it is possible to specify one imputation method for some variables, and another method for other variables using the

```
PROC MI DATA=sleeph NIMPUTE=1000 SEED=883960001 OUT=tss_mss_rp;
   VAR trt tst_0 mss_0 tst_1 mss_1 tst_2 mss_2
           tst_3 mss_3 tst_4 mss_4 tst_5 mss_5;
   MONOTONE REGPMM      (mss_1 / K=5);
   MONOTONE REGRESSION  (tst_2);
   MONOTONE REGPMM      (mss_2 / K=5);
   MONOTONE REGRESSION  (tst_3);
   MONOTONE REGPMM      (mss_3 / K=5);
   MONOTONE REGRESSION  (tst_4 );
   MONOTONE REGPMM      (mss_4 / K=5);
   MONOTONE REGRESSION  (tst_5 );
   MONOTONE REGPMM      (mss_5 / K=5);
RUN;
```

SAS Code Fragment 6.20   Imputation using monotone regression and predictive mean matching methods for TST and MSS in the insomnia example.

syntax with one MONOTONE statement per imputed variable with the appropriate method keyword. In our case, the TST variables are imputed with the regression method, while the MSS variables are imputed with the predictive mean matching method.

It may appear that predictive mean matching is more appropriate for the MSS parameter than regression because the real MSS are limited to the 0–10 range, and this method will ensure that the imputed values always fall within this range as they are sampled from the observed values. SAS Outputs 6.12 and 6.13 present the minimum and maximum values obtained for the MSS variables with the regression and predictive mean matching methods, respectively. We can see that in the case of regression, there are values outside of the 0–10 range, whereas this does not happen

STAT	mss_1	mss_2	mss_3	mss_4	mss_5
MIN	−1.955	−3.281	−3.371	−4.090	−3.995
MAX	11.434	12.701	11.374	11.419	12.687

SAS Output 6.12   Range of MSS values imputed by regression method for the insomnia example.

STAT	mss_1	mss_2	mss_3	mss_4	mss_5
MIN	0	0	0	0	0
MAX	10	9.627	9.101	8.44	8.447

SAS Output 6.13   Range of MSS values imputed by predictive mean matching method for the insomnia example.

Table 6.10 LSM estimates of the difference between experimental and placebo arms for the change from baseline to Week 8 in TST for the insomnia example. Imputation Method 5 represents the method shown in SAS Code Fragment 6.20.

Imputation Method	Estimate	SE	95% CI	p-value
Imputation Method 5	19.3863	6.3835	6.8747, 31.8980	0.0025

with the predictive mean matching imputation. This issue was also discussed in Section 6.6.3.

Finally, the results of the analysis based on the imputed data with this method are shown in Table 6.10, and demonstrate that the results are very close to those using the regression method for all variables (see Imputation Method 3 in Table 6.2).

Propensity score method

Once again, we will focus on one step aimed at imputing missing values of the variable Y_j. In this method, a so-called "propensity score" (Rosenbaum and Rubin, 1983) is generated for each subject i as the estimated probability that Y_j is missing. We will use an indicator variable A_j to represent the fact that Y_j is missing ($A_j = 0$) or that it is observed ($A_j = 1$). A conditional probability of missingness given observed covariates $p_j = \Pr(A_j = 0 | W_1, W_2, \dots, W_{K_j})$ is estimated using a logistic regression model:

$$logit(p_j) = \beta_0 + \beta_1 W_1 + \beta_2 W_2 + \cdots + \beta_{K_j} W_{K_j} \qquad (6.24)$$

where $W_j, j = 1, \dots, K_j$ represent model effects constructed from variables $X_1, \dots, X_S, Y_1, \dots, Y_{j-1}$, similar to the regression method.

This model is fitted using available values of $W_1, \dots, W_{K_j}$ (based on $X_1, \dots, X_S, Y_1, \dots, Y_{j-1}$) and A_j indicators for all subjects. Once this model is estimated, a propensity score is generated for each subject i as probability $p_{j,i}$ from (6.24) (Lavori et al., 1995). Then all subjects are divided into a number of groups based on similarity of their propensity scores. In each group, imputed values are generated using approximate Bayesian bootstrap (Rubin, 1987), which can be summarized as follows. Let $y_{k(\mathbf{obs})}$ represent a set of n_1 values from subjects with observed values of Y_j within that group. Let $y_{k(\mathbf{mis})}$ represent a set of n_0 missing values of Y_j from subjects within the same group. Then the following random sampling steps are performed:

(a) Draw n_1 values randomly with replacement from $y_{k(\mathbf{obs})}$ to create a new set $y_{k(obs)}^{(m)}$. This is a non-parametric analog of drawing samples from a Bayesian posterior distribution of the imputation model.

(b) Draw n_0 values randomly with replacement from the set $y^{(m)}_{k(obs)}$ and use them to impute n_0 missing values of Y_j.

Steps (a)–(b) are carried out in each of the groups formed based on subjects' propensity scores and are repeated M times to generate M imputed datasets. Then the entire process is repeated for each variable with missing values.

This method has a user-defined parameter for the number of groups to be formed based on the calculated propensity scores. The default value in SAS is 5. In PROC MI, the propensity score imputation can be performed using the PROPENSITY keyword in the MONOTONE statement.

The propensity score method uses only covariate information associated with missingness but not the correlation among variables (i.e., it models missingness indicators A_j as opposed to modeling the missing variable Y_j itself). Because of this, it can be effective for subsequent inferences about the distributions of individual imputed variables using univariate analyses (e.g., ANCOVA at the final time point), but it is not appropriate for analyses that involve relationships among variables, such as a repeated measures models (Schafer, 1999). In some settings, this method may also produce highly biased results (Allison, 2000). For example, if missingness is truly MCAR (i.e., not related to any variable), the grouping based on the propensity score is absolutely random. Thus each imputation is equivalent to a random draw of a variable's value from the set of observed values and not adjusted for any covariates.

Discriminant function method

Discriminant function method (Brand, 1999) can be applied to impute categorical variables for monotone missing patterns, but it is limited to the cases where all predictor variables are continuous and satisfy the assumptions that the predictor variables are approximately multivariate normal and the within-group covariance matrices are approximately equal. Because of the limitation of continuous predictor variables, it seems that this method would not be generally useful in the context of clinical trials. A first problem with using this method in clinical trials is that treatment arm is typically represented by a binary or categorical variable. Also, if a categorical endpoint needs to be imputed, we generally wish to include values of this endpoint from previous time points as predictors, but because they are categorical, we would not be able to do so. This method may be useful in some limited scenarios where a missing baseline categorical covariate needs to be imputed based on a set of some other continuous baseline characteristics. We refer the reader for more details regarding this method to Brand (1999) and SAS Institute Inc. (2011).

Fully conditional specifications

FCS is a method which, similar to the MCMC method, can be used both with monotone and non-monotone missing patterns. This approach has been explored by many researchers and is known under several different names, including "chained equations" or "chained regression." The FCS method uses univariate models similar to those for monotone missingness and provides a strategy for applying them even in the context of non-monotone patterns. Works by Brand (1999) and van Buuren (2007) provide a good foundation and overview of this topic.

This approach has not been widely used in practice so far, but is starting to gain some popularity. An implementation of this method has been recently included in SAS version 9.3 as an experimental option (available with the FCS statement in PROC MI). We will briefly describe the general principles of this strategy below.

Contrary to the use of a multivariate normal model in the MCMC method, the FCS strategy uses a sequence of univariate models (one for each variable with missing data), similar to methods for monotone missingness. Producing each of the M imputations involves two distinct steps referred to as fill-in and imputation. The fill-in step resembles very much the imputation process used for the monotone missing data, where a model is fit for each variable Y_j using variables $X_1, \ldots, X_S, Y_1, \ldots, Y_{j-1}$ as predictors. During this process, the FCS algorithm relies on a specific ordering of variables that is specified by the analyst, for example, $X_1, \ldots, X_S, Y_1, \ldots, Y_J$. Initial filled-in values are generated in the same manner as they would be for the monotone missing data, however, they are not used for the actual imputation. After the fill-in step, the imputation step is carried out, which itself employs an iterative process to generate each of the M imputations. On any given iteration, each variable with missing data is refilled with new values using a sequence of univariate models, but in this case, each univariate model for Y_j can include as predictors any other variables $X_1, \ldots, X_S, Y_1, \ldots, Y_{j-1}, Y_{j+1}, \ldots, Y_J$ and not just those that precede Y_j in the chosen ordering. When fitting such a model, subjects with observed values of Y_j are used, including their values of all other variables that may be either observed or filled-in on the previous steps. One iteration consists of a cycle through all variables $Y_j, j = 1, \ldots, J$. A number of such iterations are performed in order to achieve convergence and simulate an approximately independent draw of the missing values for the entire dataset, similarly as in the case of the MCMC method. It is only after a certain number of such burn-in iterations of the imputation step that the refilled values are used for the actual imputation. The entire process, including the initial filled-in step and the iterative imputation step, is repeated in order to generate another imputed dataset.

If the joint probability distribution $P(X_1, \ldots, X_S, Y_1, \ldots, Y_j | \theta)$, defined by conditional distributions $P(Y_j | X_1, \ldots, X_S, Y_1, \ldots, Y_{j-1}, Y_{j+1}, \ldots, Y_J)$ used for individual variables exists, then this process is a Gibbs sampler (Casella and George, 1992). Theoretical properties of the FCS method are not known, in general. The main issue is that of possible incompatibility of the conditional distributions, in a sense that no corresponding multivariate density exists. In other words, it is not known to which multivariate distribution the algorithm converges and this convergence may depend on the order of variables used in the univariate fill-in steps. The impact of incompatibility on the quality of imputation is not yet well understood. However, simulation studies conducted so far provide some experimental evidence that this strategy works well in practice and has good operational characteristics even under some strongly incompatible models (van Buuren *et al.*, 2006).

As with sequential MI for monotone missing data, an advantage of the FCS over MCMC method is its modeling flexibility. With the FCS approach, distinct models can be used for each imputed variable, including appropriate methods for modeling categorical ones. Some researchers, for example, Gelman and Raghunathan (2001) and van Buuren (2007) noted that using separate conditional models helps maintain consistencies in the imputed data and reduce bias that may result from modeling binary and categorical variables within the multivariate normal distribution in MCMC. Others, for example, Lee and Carlin (2010), observed similar results with both the FCS and multivariate normal distribution-based methods in analyses involving variously scaled and non-normally distributed variables.

References

Agresti A (2002) *Categorical Data Analysis*, 2nd ed. John Wiley & Sons, New York.

Allison PD (2000) Multiple Imputation for Missing Data: A Cautionary Tale. *Sociological Methods and Research* **28**: 301–309.

Allison PD (2002) *Missing Data*, Sage, Newbury Park, CA.

Allison PD (2005) Imputation of Categorical Variables with PROC MI. Proceedings of the Thirtieth Annual SAS® Users Group International Conference, available at http://www2.sas.com/proceedings/sugi30/113-30.pdf, accessed 7 July 2013.

Barnard J, Rubin DB (1999) Small-sample degrees of freedom with multiple imputation. *Biometrika* **86**: 948–955.

Bernaards CA, Belin TR, Schafer JL (2007) Robustness of multivariate normal approximation for imputation of incomplete binary data. *Statistics in Medicine* **26**: 1368–1382.

Bhatt NB, Gudo ES, Semá C, Bila D, Di Mattei P, Augusto O, Garsia R, Jani IV (2009) Loss of correlation between HIV viral load and CD4+ T-cell counts in HIV/HTLV-1 co-infection in treatment naïve Mozambican patients. *International Journal of STD and AIDS* **20**(12): 863–868. DOI:10.1258/ijsa.2008.008401

Bodner TE (2008) What improves with increased missing data imputations? *Structural Equation Modeling* **15**(4): 651–675.

Bollen KA, Stine RA (1992) Bootstrapping goodness of-fit measures in structural equation models. *Sociological Methods and Research* **21**: 205–229.

Boulware LE, Liu Y, Fink NE, Coresh J, Ford DE, Klag MJ, Powe NR (2006) Temporal relation among depression symptoms, cardiovascular disease events, and mortality in end-stage renal disease: contribution of reverse causality. *Clinical Journal of American Society of Nephrology* **1**: 496–504.

Brand JPL (1999) *Development, Implementation and Evaluation of Multiple Imputation Strategies for the Statistical Analysis of Incomplete Data Sets*. Ph.D. dissertation, Erasmus University, Rotterdam.

Burnham KP, Anderson DR (2002) *Model Selection and Multimodel Inference*, 2nd edn. Springer-Verlag, New York.

Carpenter JR, Kenward MG (2007) *Missing data in randomised controlled trials – a practical guide*, available at http://missingdata.lshtm.ac.uk/downloads/rm04_jh17_mk.pdf, accessed 7 July 2013.

Carpenter JR, Kenward MG (2013) *Multiple Imputation and its Application*. John Wiley & Sons, Ltd., West Sussex.

Casella G, George EI (1992) Explaining the Gibbs sampler. *The American Statistician* **46**: 167–174.

Collins LM, Schafer JL, Kam CM (2001) A comparison of inclusive and restrictive strategies in modern missing data procedures. *Psychological Methods* **6**: 330–351.

Cowles MK, Carlin BP (1996) Markov chain Monte Carlo convergence diagnostics: a comparative review. *Journal of the American Statistical Association* **91**: 883–904.

Demirtas H, Freels SA, Yucel RM (2008) Plausibility of multivariate normality assumption when multiple imputing non-Gaussian continuous outcomes: a simulation assessment. *Journal of Statistical Computation and Simulation* **78**: 69–84.

Dempster AP, Laird NM, Rubin DB (1977) Maximum likelihood from incomplete data via EM algorithm. *Journal of the Royal Statistical Society, Series B* **39**: 1–38.

Efron B, Tibshirani RJ (1993) *An introduction to the bootstrap*. Chapman & Hall, New York.

Enders CK (2002) Applying the Bollen-Stine bootstrap for goodness-of-fit measures to structural equation models with missing data. *Multivariate Behavioral Research* **37**: 359–377.

Enders CK (2010) *Applied Missing Data Analysis*. The Guilford Press, New York.

Freedman DA (2006) On the so-called "Huber sandwich estimator" and "robust standard errors." *The American Statistician* **60**: 299–302.

Gelman A, Raghunathan TE (2001) Discussion of Arnold *et al.* 'Conditionally specified distributions'. *Statistical Science* **16**: 249–274.

Gelman A, Rubin DB (1992) Inference from iterative simulation using multiple sequences. *Statistical Science* **7**: 457–472.

Goria MN (1992) On the fourth root transformation of chi-square. *Australian Journal of Statistics* **34**(1): 55–64.

Gottschall AC, West SG, Enders CK (2012) A comparison of item-level and scale-level multiple imputation for questionnaire batteries. *Multivariate Behavioral Research* **47**(1): 1–25.

Graham JW, Olchowski AE, Gilreath TD (2007) How many imputations are really needed? Some practical clarifications of multiple imputation theory. *Prevention Science* **8**: 206–213.

Graham JW, Schafer JL (1999) On the performance of multiple imputation for multivariate data with small sample size. In: R Hoyle (ed.), *Statistical Strategies for Small Sample Research*. Sage, Thousand Oaks, CA.

Hartley HO, Hocking RR (1971) The analysis of incomplete data. *Biometrics* **27**: 783–808.

Heitjan F, Little RJA (1991) Multiple imputation for the fatal accident reporting system. *Applied Statistics* **40**: 13–29.

Horton NJ, Lipsitz SR (2001) Multiple imputation in practice: comparison of software packages for regression models with missing variables. *The American Statistician* **55**: 244–254.

Horton NJ, Lipsitz SR, Parzen M (2003) A potential for bias when rounding in multiple imputation. *The American Statistician* **57**: 229–232.

Huber P (1967) The behaviour of maximum likelihood estimates under nonstandard conditions. In *Proceedings of the 5th Berkeley Symposium on Mathematical Statistics and Probability* **1**: 221–233.

Landis RJ, Heyman ER, Koch GG (1978) Average partial association in three-way contingency tables: a review and discussion of alternative tests. *International Statistical Review* **46**: 237–254.

Lavori PW, Dawson R, Shera D (1995) A multiple imputation strategy for clinical trials with truncation of patient data. *Statistics in Medicine* **14**: 1913–1925.

Lee KJ, Carlin JB (2010) Multiple imputation for missing data: fully conditional specification versus multivariate normal imputation. *American Journal of Epidemiology* **171**(5): 624–632.

Leite WL, Beretvas N (2010) The performance of multiple imputation for Likert-type items with missing data. *Journal of Modern Applied Statistical Methods* **9**(1): 64–74.

Little TD, Howard WJ, McConnell EK, Stump KN (2011) *Missing Data in Large Data Projects: Two methods of missing data imputation when working with large data projects*, available at http://crmda.ku.edu/resources/kuantguides/11_ImputationWithLargeDataSets.pdf, accessed 7 July 2013.

Little RJA, Yau L (1996) Intent-to-treat analysis in longitudinal studies with dropouts. *Biometrics* **52**: 1324–1333.

Mantel N, Haenszel W (1959) Statistical aspects of the analysis of data from retrospective studies of disease. *Journal of the National Cancer Institute* **22**: 719–748.

Meng X-L (1994) Multiple imputation inferences with uncongenial sources of input. *Statistical Science* **9**: 538–558.

Molenberghs G, Kenward MG (2007) *Missing Data in Clinical Studies*. John Wiley & Sons Ltd, West Sussex.

National Research Council, Panel on Handling Missing Data in Clinical Trials, Committee on National Statistics, Division of Behavioral and Social Sciences and Education (2010) *The Prevention and Treatment of Missing Data in Clinical Trials*. The National Academies Press, Washington, DC.

Oudshoorn CGM, van Buuren S, Rijckevorsel JLA (1999) Flexible Multiple Imputation by Chained Equations of the AVO-95 survey. *TNO Prevention and Health, TNO Report* G/VGZ/99.045.

Raghunathan TE, Lepkowski JM, Van Hoewyk J, Solenberger P (2001) A multivariate technique for multiply imputing missing values using a sequence of regression models. *Survey Methodology* **27**(1): 85–95.

Rosenbaum PR, Rubin DB (1983) The central role of the propensity score in observational studies for causal effects. *Biometrika* **70**: 41–55.

Rubin DB (1978) Multiple imputation in sample surveys - a phenomenological Bayesian approach to nonresponse. *Proceedings of the Survey Research Methods Section of the American Statistical Association* **1**: 20–34.

Rubin DB (1987) *Multiple Imputation for Nonresponse in Surveys*. John Wiley and Sons, New York.

Rubin DB (1996) Multiple imputations after 18+ years. *Journal of the American Statistical Association* **91**(434): 473–489.

Rubin DB, Schenker N (1986) Multiple imputation for interval estimation from simple random samples with ignorable response. *Journal of the American Statistical Association* **81**: 366–374.

SAS Institute Inc. (2011) *SAS/STAT® 9.3 User's Guide*. SAS Institute Inc., Cary, NC.

Schafer JL (1997) *Analysis of Incomplete Multivariate Data*. Chapman and Hall, New York.

Schafer JL (1999) Multiple imputation: a primer. *Statistical Methods in Medical Research* **8**: 3–15.

Schafer JL, Graham JW (2002) Missing data: our view of the state of the art. *Psychological Methods* **7**: 147–177.

Schafer JL (2003) Multiple imputation in multivariate problems when the imputation and analysis models differ. *Statistica Neerlandica* **57**: 19–35.

Schafer JL, Olsen MK (1998) Multiple imputation for multivariate missing-data problems: a data analyst's perspective. *Multivariate Behavioral Research* **33**: 545–571.

Schenker N, Taylor JMG (1996) Partially parametric techniques for multiple imputation. *Computational Statistics and Data Analysis* **22**: 425–446.

Stine R (1989) An introduction to bootstrap methods: Examples and ideas. *Sociological Methods and Research* **18**: 243–291.

Tanner MA, Wong WH (1987) The calculation of posterior distributions by data augmentation (with discussion). *Journal of the American Statistical Association* **82**: 528–550.

Thijs H, Molenberghs G, Michiels B, Verbeke G, Curran D (2002) Strategies to fit pattern-mixture models. *Biostatistics* **3**: 245–265.

van Buuren S (2007) Multiple imputation of discrete and continuous data by fully conditional specification. *Statistical Methods in Medical Research* **16**: 219–242.

van Buuren S (2012) *Flexible Imputation of Missing Data*. Chapman & Hall/CRC Press, Boca Raton, FL.

van Buuren S, Brand JPL, Groothuis-Oudshoorn CGM, Rubin DB (2006) Fully conditional specification in multiple imputation. *Journal of Statistical Computation and Simulation* **76**: 1049–1064.

van Buuren S, Oudshoorn CGM (1999) Flexible multivariate imputation by MICE. TNO-rapport PG 99.054. TNO Prevention and Health, Leiden, available at http://www.stefvanbuuren.nl/publications/Flexible%20multivariate%20-%20TNO99054%201999.pdf, accessed 7 July 2013.

van Ginkel JR, Van der Ark LA, Sijtsma K (2007a) Multiple imputation for item scores when test data are factorially complex. *British Journal of Mathematical and Statistical Psychology* **60**: 315–337.

van Ginkel JR, Van der Ark LA, Sijtsma K (2007b) Multiple imputation of test and questionnaire data and influence on psychometric results. *Multivariate Behavioral Research* **42**: 387–414.

Von Hippel PT (2009) How to impute interactions, squares, and other transformed variables. *Sociological Methodology* **39**(1): 265–291.

White, H (1982) Maximum likelihood estimation of misspecified models. *Econometrica* **50**: 1–26.

White IR, Royston P, Wood AM (2011) Multiple imputation using chained equations: issues and guidance for practice. *Statistics in Medicine* **30**: 377–399.

Wilson EB, Hilferty MM (1931) The distribution of chi-squared. *Proceedings of the National Academy of Sciences, Washington* **17**: 684–688.

Yucel RM, He Y, Zaslavsky AM (2008) Using calibration to improve rounding in imputation. *The American Statistician* **62**: 1–5.

Table of SAS Code Fragments

7

Analyses under missing-not-at-random assumptions

Michael O'Kelly and Bohdana Ratitch

Key points

- Pattern-mixture models (PMMs) allow assumptions about missingness to differ across subsets of subjects (patterns) in a clinical trial.

- PMMs are a straightforward and transparent way of modeling a wide variety of assumptions about missing data, and are particularly suited to implementing missing-not-at-random (MNAR) assumptions.

- The MNAR assumption – the assumption that missingness is dependent on the unobserved data – may be reasonable for a primary analysis, but is most frequently used for sensitivity analyses.

- We describe how to implement a variety of MNAR assumptions via a sequence of models that use selected subsets of data – the modeling and imputation can be performed in a number of steps (e.g., separately for each visit) – we call this *multiple imputation (MI) using sequential modeling*.

- We also describe how to implement MNAR assumption using a joint model estimated just once – here various functions of model's regression coefficients

---

Clinical Trials with Missing Data: A Guide for Practitioners, First Edition. Michael O'Kelly and Bohdana Ratitch.
© 2014 John Wiley & Sons, Ltd. Published 2014 by John Wiley & Sons, Ltd.

can be used to implement different MNAR assumptions – we call this *MI using joint modeling*.

- Both of the above implementations are publicly available as SAS macros, but we also give fragments of SAS code to implement PMMs using sequential modeling.

- The two PMM methods can implement reference-based (often, control-based) imputation, which imputes missing values from the experimental arm with a model using values from some reference arm, usually a control arm.

- The PMM methods can also implement statistically appropriate versions of last observation carried forward (LOCF) and baseline observation carried forward (BOCF) assumptions by accounting for uncertainty associated with missing data.

- Delta adjustment, which can be used to "penalize" imputed values to make them less favorable, may also be implemented by PMMs.

- We illustrate the use and impact of a variety of MNAR assumptions by plotting the mean outcomes for a selection of simple PMMs for our three illustrative datasets.

- We then illustrate the use of PMMs in practice by implementing primary and sensitivity analyses as they might be done in a real study, for each of our three illustrative datasets, and assess the resulting test statistics and p-values.

7.1   Introduction

This chapter discusses ways of implementing the assumption that data are not missing at random ("missing not at random," or MNAR), with an emphasis on using PMMs to do this. We have seen in Sections 4.2.2.1 and 4.2.2.2 that one might consider a primary analysis that assumed that outcomes are MNAR in, for example, studies in Parkinson's disease (PD) or insomnia. Sensitivity analyses often assume MNAR also, and most of the analyses in this chapter are designed to investigate sensitivity to assumptions about missing data. We make extensive use of PMMs for MNAR analyses because the assumptions of such PMMs can be stated clearly, their results are usually easy to interpret by non-statisticians, and their implementation transparent and capable of quality control (QC) and review by a typical statistical study team. This chapter first discusses the background to sensitivity analyses and PMMs. Two methods that use MI to implement sensitivity analyses with PMMs are then described and compared. We will use one of these methods in the rest of this chapter, but will note how the other may be used also.

The second part of the chapter is a "toolkit" indicating via SAS code fragments how to implement a variety of sensitivity analyses, using illustrative clinical trial data in the three example indications described in Chapters 1 and 4: Parkinson's disease, insomnia and mania. Most of the sensitivity analyses featured in the "toolkit" section can also be implemented using macros available at the Drug Information Association (DIA) Scientific Working Group (SWG) on Missing Data web page in the www.missingdata.org.uk site (Roger, 2012; Ratitch, 2012a, 2012b). Even though publicly accessible macros are available, we think it is also useful to show the analyses implemented using relatively simple SAS code, for a number of reasons. First, the reader oriented towards statistical programming may find the code useful as showing the logical steps performed in detail in working code. Second, if these sensitivity analyses are carried out in trials aimed at regulatory submission, and the primary analysis implemented via a downloaded macro, a QC check may be required via an independent implementation using straightforward SAS "open code." Such code could be written using the code fragments in the "toolkit" section as a template. Study analyses using easily readable SAS code (as opposed to using a complex SAS macro) will also be extremely useful to the regulator who may wish to scrutinize the workings of the method in detail. The "homemade" SAS code could form an appendix to the statistical analysis plan (SAP) reviewed by the regulator.

In the final section of the chapter, the strategies suggested in Chapter 4 for three indications are implemented as they might have been for a real clinical trial, and the results discussed. Appendices provide further, fuller code examples. Additionally, Appendix 7.I and 7.J give short descriptions of the implementation of selection models and shared parameter models, which are also sometimes used as sensitivity analyses. See Chapter 4 for some discussion of why we generally favor PMMs over selection models and shared parameter models for implementing sensitivity analyses.

7.2   Background to sensitivity analyses and pattern-mixture models

7.2.1   The purpose of a sensitivity analysis

We believe that, for the most part, the implied question answered by sensitivity analyses should be "If we take a clinical view of what happens to withdrawals that is plausibly unfavorable to the experimental arm, is the conclusion from the primary statistical test still credible?"

Sensitivity analyses may also be required to explore robustness to other assumptions of the primary analysis such as robustness to outliers and more generally robustness to the assumption about the distribution of the outcome. We have noted these briefly in Section 4.5; doubly robust estimation (Chapter 8) may provide some assurance of robustness to these kinds of assumptions also. However, the current chapter is focused on analyses of sensitivity to the assumptions made about the unknown, missing outcomes of subjects.

Trialists have only recently started to use sensitivity analyses routinely to assess the robustness of trial results against missing data. The idea of the sensitivity analysis is not to test a range of assumptions, in order to find the assumption about missing data that fits the best – we do not have the missing data, so we will never know what assumption is nearest the truth. Rather, it is to assess to what degree the conclusion we make from the primary trial result is dependent on the assumptions about missing data of the primary statistical test. We devise sensitivity analyses that are of clinical interest and which make some kind of clinical sense, whose assumptions about missing data are different from those of the primary analysis, and are usually less favorable to the experimental arm. The reasoning is that if, under these unfavorable assumptions, the conclusion from the primary analysis is not undermined to an important degree then that conclusion may be credible to patients, clinicians and regulators, even though some data are missing.

If we wish to draw conclusions about a general treatment policy of including an experimental treatment in a regime, compared to a general treatment policy of using the control treatment, then we may need to include post-withdrawal data in order to assess the treatment regimes fairly (see the discussion in Section 4.2.1). However, we believe that for most objectives with an efficacy endpoint, the assumption of missing at random (MAR) mechanism will give an acceptable working estimate of the outcome *for subjects in the control group* at least. If withdrawals from the control arm are expected to have worse outcomes than those who remain in the study, in most cases it will still be acceptable to regulators, clinicians and patients to estimate the effect of control *as if* subjects continued on the control treatment, that is, assuming MAR. If, on the other hand, withdrawals from the control arm are expected to have better outcomes than those who remain on treatment, but the objective is to compare the effect attributable to experimental treatment versus that attributable to control treatment, it may still be acceptable to estimate the effect of control *as if* subjects continued on the control treatment, that is, assuming MAR, (again see Section 4.2.1). Often, though, withdrawals will receive a treatment similar to the control treatment, and this can be reasonably well modeled assuming MAR.

Because of this, the sensitivity analyses we propose generally stress test the primary result by challenging its assumptions about *the experimental arm*, and use a working assumption of MAR for the control group. We think that this approach makes it more straightforward to interpret the sensitivity analyses – the reader of the clinical study report has to juggle with only one set of assumptions at a time in viewing the results.

To be helpful in assessing the credibility of a result, a sensitivity analysis should be based on assumptions that are unfavorable enough to the study treatment to constitute a convincing stress test of the primary analysis. On the other hand, we do not recommend sensitivity analyses with assumptions that are so unfavorable to the experimental arm as to be clinically implausible. Such sensitivity analyses do not answer a clinically useful question, and run the risk of appearing to undermine the conclusions of the trial report, when there are in fact no *clinical* grounds to doubt its credibility. An exception to this is the "tipping point" analysis, (see Section 4.2.3.1, Section 3.6.2 and Section 7.4.7.3, later in this chapter), where the degree of clinical implausibility of the assumptions that overturn the primary conclusion is itself used as a measure of the credibility of the result of the trial.

7.2.2   Pattern-mixture models as sensitivity analyses

PMMs were first suggested by Glynn *et al.* (1986, pp. 115–142). Little (1993) added the word "pattern" to Glynn *et al.*'s "mixture model" and came up with a number of practical uses for PMMs, which in turn gave rise to many of the methods for sensitivity analyses that we describe in this chapter.

We first briefly present a general mathematical formulation of PMMs.

Denote the entire matrix of outcome data as Y and decompose it into two parts: Y_{obs}, representing observed outcomes and Y_{mis}, representing missing (unobserved) outcomes. Let X denote a set of observed covariates. Finally, let R represent a matrix of indicators of missingness at scheduled time points, which can also be interpreted as a representation of different patterns of missingness. PMMs decompose the joint probability of outcome and missingness, conditional on observed covariates, in the following way:

$$p(Y_{obs}, Y_{mis}, R|X) = p(R|X)\, p(Y_{obs}, Y_{mis}|R, X) \qquad (7.1)$$

Probability distribution $p(R|X)$ is the conditional probability distribution of R based on observed covariates, and can be viewed as representing a conditional distribution over the patterns of missingness. The probability distribution $p(Y_{obs}, Y_{mis}|R, X)$ for a complete outcome data matrix $Y = (Y_{obs}, Y_{mis})$ is a model based (conditioned) on the possible missingness patterns represented by R and can potentially accommodate different sub-distributions for each pattern.

The main objective of a clinical trial is to provide an overall assessment of treatment effect on clinical outcome for all subjects regardless of their trial completion status and availability of data. Usually, it is not the pattern-specific models $p(Y_{obs}, Y_{mis}|R, X)$ that are of interest in themselves, but rather the overall model, from which one can derive a summary statistic such as the (weighted) average across the patterns. This summary of outcome for a PMM allows us to arrive at a general conclusion about the distribution of outcome, observed and unobserved, after taking into account the likelihood of different missingness patterns. Nevertheless, one builds a PMM by first estimating the individual components of $p(Y_{obs}, Y_{mis}|R, X)$ within each pattern; then one "mixes" them together using $p(R|X)$.

Unfortunately, some parameters of the distribution $p(Y_{obs}, Y_{mis}|R, X)$ cannot be estimated exclusively from the available data due to incomplete data within patterns – one cannot derive a relationship between Y_{mis} and X from data because, of course, there are no observed Y_{mis}. Because of this, PMMs are said to be under-identified. However, it is still possible to estimate such models by imposing some explicit assumptions regarding parameters inestimable from data alone. Such assumptions are known in the PMM terminology as "identifying restrictions" (Little, 1993). The necessity to be explicit about these additional assumptions can, in fact, be viewed as one of the advantages of the PMMs, as it forces the analyst to be very clear about what is being done about the model components affected by missing data and how they are similar or different from model components estimated directly from available data.

There are several methodologies for imposing these identifying restrictions. We focus on one of them that essentially links the model of missing data to the model of observed data across different patterns. The probability distribution in Equation 7.1 can be further decomposed as follows:

$$p(Y_{obs}, Y_{mis}, R|X) = p(R|X)\,p(Y_{obs}, Y_{mis}|R, X)$$
$$= p(R|X)\,p(Y_{obs}|R, X)p(Y_{mis}|Y_{obs}, R, X) \qquad (7.2)$$

In this formulation, $p(Y_{obs}|R, X)$ represents a model for available data within each pattern, and $p(Y_{mis}|Y_{obs}, R, X)$ represents a model for missing data conditioned on observed data within each pattern. In pattern-mixture modeling, a link can be defined between the two, so that the model $p(Y_{obs}|R, X)$ from one pattern could be used to identify $p(Y_{mis}|Y_{obs}, R, X)$ in the same or another pattern.

As mentioned previously, the notion of pattern that is used in the context of clinical trials is related to various characteristics of monotone missingness (dropout) that a group of subjects defined by R and X may exhibit and share in a given trial. For example, patterns can be defined based on the timing of dropout so that all subjects that discontinue after the same study visit belong to the same pattern. It can often be sensible to take the time of withdrawal into account in defining patterns of missingness, because most indications are expected either to worsen or to improve over time in their symptoms. The picture of a subject's health we get from observed data would therefore be expected to change with the timing of withdrawal. Patterns can also be defined based on the reasons for discontinuation, or even simply on the treatment arm to which the subject was randomized. Similarly, any combination of the aforementioned and other characteristics can serve to distinguish patterns. The group of trial completers also constitutes a pattern.

Information contained in the form of a model derived from observed data can be used as a basis for assumptions about subjects with a certain pattern of missing data, for whom parameters could not otherwise be estimated. The imposed assumptions are often of a form which defines the similarities or specific differences of the inestimable parameters compared to the estimable ones. In such cases, the selected observed data with estimable parameters can be regarded as lending information to subjects with selected patterns of missing data, to furnish assumptions about inestimable parameters so that the latter can be identified. As noted above, these imposed assumptions should not be regarded as approximating some "true" conclusion given the missing data, but as plausible hypotheses or scenarios having the status of "what ifs," which allow the reader of the clinical trial report to assess the robustness of results given the missing data. The information flow from the observed data to the imputed missing data occurs according to a link function which specifies which observed data are linked to which missing data patterns; what information is provided by the observed data; and how it is incorporated by the recipient pattern. The transfer of information can be done by estimating a statistical model within the selected observed data, and then using this model to obtain imputations for the missing data in the recipient pattern. Imputations from the observed-data model can be used as is (if the distributions are assumed similar), or they can be modified in a specific way according to the imposed assumptions about the differences between the selected observed data and the particular missing data. The National Research Council (NRC) report on missing data (2010) refers to this imputation model as a predictive distribution of missing outcomes, "given the observed outcomes and whatever modeling assumptions are being used for inference." Imputation of missing data in the recipient patterns and subsequent analysis can be done in a principled way using the MI methodology of Rubin (1987, 1996) and Glynn *et al.* (1993).

7.2.2.1 Traditional identifying restrictions: Complete cases, neighboring cases, available cases

In his 1993 paper, Little noted the need to make assumptions about the missing data in a pattern-mixture model, in order to make inferences about those data: "the models require restrictions or prior assumptions to identify the parameters." He gave examples of these "identifying restrictions" that could implement such assumptions. "*Complete-case restrictions* tie unidentified parameters to their (identified) analogs in the stratum of complete cases … . Alternative types of restriction tie unidentified parameters to parameters in other missing value patterns or sets of such patterns." Little's complete case restriction assumes that a missing value at a given time point *j* can be imputed from similar subjects who have completed the trial. This assumption is now often referred to as complete case missing values, or CCMV. Little also describes more generally how distributions of selected observed data could be used to impute missing values. Neighboring case missing value (NCMV) is a second commonly used "identifying restriction" with a similar structure to CCMV. The NCMV restriction imputes visit *j* based on subjects who are observed up to visit *j* + 1 but no further. The idea here is that such subjects may be most similar to the subjects who withdrew at visit *j*. A third case is that of available case missing values (ACMV), which combines information from all subjects with available data at visit *j*, and is a PMM analogy to a direct likelihood approach such as mixed models for repeated measures (MMRM), or MI under MAR assumption.

We believe that while CCMV, NCMV and ACMV may be of interest as demonstrating the versatility of PMMs, these PMM approaches will not be very helpful as sensitivity analyses to test the robustness of a trial result. We have seen in Chapter 1 that complete cases tend to give a rather favorable estimate of efficacy score for a treatment, because complete cases tend to have better efficacy scores than subjects who discontinue early. In the context of an intention-to-treat (ITT) estimand, therefore, CCMV is biased and of limited interest for clinical trials. (Note: "estimand" means "that which is to be estimated"). As to NCMV, it may be intuitively attractive to use subjects who withdraw at visit *j* + 1 to impute visit *j*. However, (a) withdrawals at some visit *j* + 1 may be scarce or non-existent, making this strategy difficult to implement; (b) the NCMV approach makes no use of potentially valuable information from subjects very similar to those who withdrew at visit *j*, but who withdrew later than visit *j* + 1, which seems wasteful. It may be expected that the NCMV estimate for treatment will be close to the MAR one, but with higher variance. We believe that the NCMV approach will generally cast limited additional light on the nature of the missingness in a trial. It could act as a mild sensitivity analysis to the MAR assumption, likely to be inconclusive, but is not clearly aimed to answer a question about the robustness of the trial result to missing data with substantially less favorable assumptions regarding withdrawals from the experimental arm. Finally, ACMV is an analogue to MAR estimation, and thus cannot be used as a sensitivity analysis to an MAR analysis, or to answer any question about robustness of trial results that could not be answered more easily by an MAR analysis implemented via MI or a direct likelihood approach such as MMRM. (We note, however, that MI assuming MAR could be regarded as a kind of ACMV analysis, and in this limited sense ACMV can be said to be useful to the statistician, either as a primary analysis, or as an analysis to "bridge" between a primary MMRM analysis and other MI-based sensitivity analyses).

7.2.2.2   The versatility of pattern-mixture models

Little, in that same 1993 paper, went on to describe how patterns of missing data could be imputed very flexibly by applying models derived from any defined group of trial data to any pattern of missing data – "the possibilities seem almost endless," Little noted. In a development of that idea of flexible imputation from in-study data, Little and Yau (1996) made some concrete suggestions for PMMs that are very useful in estimating treatment effect under a variety of "what ifs" that are often clinically plausible and may be less favorable towards the experimental arm than MAR. Some distinguish the CCMV, NCMV and ACMV approaches from Little's more general use of PMMs by calling the latter "controlled imputation" (Mallinckrodt, 2013).

In 2008–2012, James Roger came up with a series of implementations of Little–Yau-type "controlled imputation" PMMs (Roger *et al.*, 2008; Roger, 2010; Carpenter and Kenward, 2013; Carpenter *et al.*, 2013). Others in the pharmaceutical industry followed Roger's work with a variety of implementations inspired by Roger's (e.g., Ratitch and O'Kelly, 2011; Mallinckrodt, 2013; Ratitch *et al.*, 2013).

7.3   Two methods of implementing sensitivity analyses via pattern-mixture models

7.3.1   A sequential method of implementing pattern-mixture models with multiple imputation

In Chapter 4 on planning for missing data, we have recommended some "controlled imputations" as sensitivity analyses, and even for the primary analysis. In this section, we will use an example to show how to implement these using the method of Ratitch and O'Kelly (2011) (see also Ratitch *et al.*, (2013)). Ratitch *et al.* estimate a sequence of models, each model implementing the assumptions desired for a missing data pattern. We will refer to this method as the *sequential modeling* approach. In the next section, we will outline a very useful and flexible alternative modular implementation of "controlled imputations" that in effect uses a single joint mixed model (implemented via Markov Chain Monte Carlo (MCMC) methods) developed by Roger with support from GlaxoSmithKline. We will refer to this method as the *joint modeling* approach. We will compare the two approaches later in this chapter. SAS macros for both approaches are available at the web page of the DIA SWG for missing data, on the www.missingdata.org.uk website. In subsequent sections, we will describe in detail a variety of "controlled imputations," again using the sequential modeling approach with SAS code fragments and show the results of these "controlled imputations" when used with illustrative clinical data. We will also indicate how MI with joint modeling can be used to obtain similar results or other useful ones.

We saw in Chapter 6 how in MI we can impute missing values using the posterior distribution of the parameters from a model based on study data. In standard MI where we assume MAR, if we are using the regression method, we then use all appropriate study data to estimate the regression parameters that will impute the values that are missing. This model could have such explanatory variables as the subject's previous post-baseline outcomes, plus perhaps a baseline measurement, some demographic variables, and of course the treatment group variable. In his 1993 paper, Little noted how well suited MI would be to implement PMMs. In fact, we have noted that MI assuming MAR as described in Chapter 6 implements a PMM using a version of Little's ACMV identifying restriction.

How could we use MI with sequential modeling to implement CCMV? In other words, how could we use only complete cases to impute missing values for subjects who withdraw? Consider a trial with two post-baseline visits, Visit 1 and Visit 2. Assume that the outcome is continuous, and all baseline measurements were observed. Assume also that missingness was monotone, that is, missingness was solely due to withdrawal from the trial. Assume that we wish to model Visit 1 missing outcome using baseline and treatment; and Visit 2 missing outcome using baseline, treatment, and the Visit 1 outcome. If we include all subjects in the MI, then Visit 1 will be modeled using

- study completers and
- subjects who withdrew after Visit 1.

This uses available data from all subjects, and is ACMV, not CCMV. We can implement CCMV by performing MI sequentially as follows.

To impute Visit 1 missing outcomes under CCMV, include only data from subjects with missing Visit 1 and subjects who completed the trial – omit data from subjects who withdrew after Visit 1, because they are not "CC" – not complete cases. MI will now estimate regression parameters for Visit 1 using completers' data only. Draws from the posterior distribution of those regression parameters will then be used to impute Visit 1.

To impute Visit 2, perform a second imputation, this time including only subjects who completed the trial and subjects with missing Visit 2. If you are reading this carefully, you will see that this means we are including all subjects for this last imputation. Subjects with missing Visit 1 and Visit 2 contribute no information about

Visit 2; their missing values will be imputed using a model estimated from complete cases. Draws from the posterior distribution of those regression parameters will then be used to impute Visit 2, for all subjects who have missing data at Visit 2.

It turns out that this sequential MI is a very flexible tool in the statistician's armory for implementing sensitivity analyses. As an exercise, see if you can write out the steps to implement NCMV, noting which subjects are to be included in each MI step. Our description of the steps for NCMV can be found in Appendix 7.A at the end of this chapter.

7.3.2   Providing stress-testing "what ifs" using pattern-mixture models

We have argued that CCMV, NCMV and ACMV are not very useful as stress tests of an MAR primary analysis. However, the sequential modeling method illustrated in the previous section can implement a wide variety of other assumptions useful for a more comprehensive stress testing of MAR-based analyses.

Anticipating Section 7.4 where we will discuss in detail the implementation of various PMMs, let us look at how we might use this sequential method to implement the assumption that subjects who withdraw from the experimental arm have correlations like similar subjects from the control arm (i.e., have approximately the slope of the control arm – a version of the analysis posited by Little and Yau (1996)).

To multiply impute subjects under this assumption, we first impute Visit 1 missing outcomes. For this step, we include all subjects with missing Visit 1, plus subjects from the control arm with Visit 1 observed. We omit subjects from the experimental arm with outcomes observed at Visit 1. MI will now estimate regression parameters for Visit 1 using data from the control arm only, because control subjects are the only ones available to MI that have Visit 1 data with which to estimate the regression parameters to model Visit 1. Draws from the posterior distribution of those regression parameters will then be used to impute Visit 1. The imputed data for Visit 1 for a subject from the experimental arm will look similar to the imputed data for a similar subject from the control arm. If the between-visit correlation is strong and positive (which it usually is), then the trajectory of the outcome from baseline to Visit 1 will be similar to that of the observed data in the control arm. Note that if the correlation between baseline and Visit 1 for control subjects is weak, then missing values for both treatment groups will with this method be imputed to drift towards the mean for the control group at that time point.

To impute Visit 2, the final visit, perform a second imputation, this time including all subjects with missing Visit 2, plus completers only from the control group. In this step, MI will estimate regression parameters for Visit 2 using only subjects from the control group, because they are the only subjects who have available values at Visit 2. Draws from the posterior distribution of those regression parameters will then be used to impute Visit 2, for all subjects with Visit 2 missing – from experimental or control arm. Again, if the correlation for the control group between visits is strong and positive, the trajectory of the outcome across visits for the experimental arm subjects with missing data will be close to that of subjects from the control group. If the correlations at this later visit are somewhat weaker, as often happens in later visits, then imputations for subjects in the experimental arm will drift somewhat towards the mean of the control arm.

7.3.3   Two implementations of pattern-mixture models for sensitivity analyses

We have noted that two methods of implementing "controlled imputations" via MI are available as SAS macros, the sequential modeling method and the joint modeling method. Before we discuss the differences between the two methods, it may be useful to keep in mind that PMMs make use of two models: (1) the model estimated from observed data and (2) a model used for imputation, where model (2) may be the same or may be different from (1), depending on MNAR assumptions.

In the *sequential modeling method* (Kenward and Carpenter, 2009; Ratitch and O'Kelly, 2011; Ratitch, 2012a, 2012b; Ratitch *et al.*, 2013), which we have been illustrating in the previous section, a single model is used for both (1) and (2). This is the case for most standard MI applications – the analyst estimates and imputes in a single step. However, that modeling-and-imputation step may be performed for different patterns separately, allowing the analyst to model and impute using different assumptions about missingness for selected subsets of subjects. Each time a model-and-impute step is performed, the analyst can vary the model by changing the explanatory variables as well as by selecting a different subset of available data which is designated as the best basis for modeling missing values in a given missing pattern. If missing pattern is assumed to have a model different from that of the group that was used to estimate the model, typically the imputations obtained from the estimated model are subsequently modified in a controlled way to implement these differences. One way of accomplishing such controlled differences is by adding to or subtracting from the imputed values a pre-specified amount δ – "delta adjustment."

In the *joint modeling method* (Roger, 2012; Carpenter and Kenward, 2013; Carpenter *et al.*, 2013), a single joint model (or rather a Bayesian posterior distribution for parameters of such a joint model) is estimated from all available trial data, where "joint" means that all time points and all explanatory variables, including treatment, are simultaneously included in a (mixed effects) MMRM-like longitudinal model. Then from this posterior distribution, model parameters can be sampled and used to construct an imputation model (model (2) above) that can be different from the estimated model, so as to reflect a variety of MNAR assumptions.

In summary, in the sequential modeling method, MNAR assumptions are imposed by (a) selecting a particular subset of data to estimate the imputation model for a particular pattern of missing data; (b) manipulating imputations from the estimated model in a controlled and transparent way, for example, by adding an amount δ to selected imputations so as to make them quantifiably "worse"; (c) carrying out steps (a) and (b) for all patterns of missing data with distinct assumptions. In the joint modeling method, first a joint model is estimated from all available data, and then MNAR assumptions are imposed by manipulating the parameters sampled from the posterior of this model in order to construct an imputation model for each missing pattern; as with sequential modeling method, the joint modeling method can also perform controlled and transparent manipulations of the imputed values.

The macro due to Roger that uses the joint modeling approach offers a greater variety of "packaged" choices for sensitivity analyses than the macros due to Ratitch (2012a, 2012b) that use the sequential modeling approach. The joint modeling approach also makes subtly different assumptions in its regression model, although we shall see that its results in the examples we analyze can be close to those of the sequential modeling approach, when similar MNAR assumptions are implemented. We list the characteristics and limitations of the two methods in Sections 7.3.4 and 7.3.6, describe the methods of estimation of the joint modeling method in Section 7.3.5 and summarize the statistical differences between the two methods in Section 7.3.7.

Because of the simplicity and transparency of the sequential modeling method illustrated in the previous section, we will use that method to show in detail in this chapter how a variety of "controlled imputations" may be implemented. We also find the sequential modeling method useful in practice because the simplicity and brevity of its SAS implementation makes it feasible to perform independently programmed quality control for these sensitivity analyses, which in turn makes it easy for regulators to review. However, we will also indicate in this chapter the analyses for which the joint modeling macro may be used.

The joint modeling and the sequential model approaches have similar assumptions when imputing non-monotone missing data. Intermediate or non-monotone missing data are imputed assuming MAR. An argument for doing this is that intermediate missing data may often have no connection to the missing outcome, but may rather be caused by logistical problems (subject has clashing appointment or was busy) or administrative issues (measuring instrument was not functioning), which would be expected to give rise to MCAR or MAR missingness. Thus, while our main objective may be to implement an MNAR assumption for those who withdrew, that objective will not usually be hindered by assuming MAR for intermediate missing data that occur before withdrawal. Note, though, that the issue of how to handle non-monotone missingness is vehemently debated (see Sections 3.4 and 3.5).

7.3.4   Characteristics and limitations of the sequential modeling method of implementing pattern-mixture models

We have indicated in Section 7.3.1 how MI implementations available in common software such as SAS could be used to implement a variety of assumptions about missing data. Instead of processing all trial data in a single MI step, as we would under MAR, we could use subsets of trial data to model iteratively, for example, visit-by-visit, the distribution of the missing values under a variety of assumptions other than MAR. Here we note the selected characteristics of this sequential modeling method, some of which differ from Roger's implementation of the joint modeling method which is described in the next section.

Non-monotone missing data: intermediate or non-monotone missing data are imputed assuming MAR. In the DIA macros that implement sequential modeling, the explanatory variable for investigational site (clinic) entered via the *poolsite=* parameter, usually a multi-category variable, is omitted from the MCMC step that models and imputes non-monotone missing data. An additional point regarding the DIA macros for sequential MI is that the user may choose to model the non-monotone missing data either across all treatment groups or separately for each treatment group.

How regression parameters are estimated: the regression parameters for the MNAR imputations at each visit will often be estimated using only a subset of the observed trial data, selected to reflect a specific MNAR assumption regarding a group of subject/visit data that should serve as a basis for modeling values in a given missing pattern. A disadvantage of this is that we might achieve a more precise estimate of certain parameters, for example, the association between baseline and the outcome, if we used more trial data or indeed all trial data related to this association. On the other hand, an advantage is that parameters of all explanatory variables in the regression will be estimated in a way that is consistent with the particular MNAR assumption we are implementing. For example, if we want to implement the assumption that withdrawals from the experimental arm have correlations similar to the control arm, then it may be regarded as consistent to estimate the association between baseline and outcome using only the control arm. Note also that for the sequential modeling method, the correlations between a subject's observed post-baseline outcomes and the missing outcome will also be estimated using only the control arm.

Interaction of explanatory variables with time: when the definition of patterns includes visit of discontinuation (i.e., subjects discontinuing at different visits are included in different patterns), imputation models are estimated separately for each visit – the statistician has no choice in this matter. Thus, if it is desired to match such a sequential modeling analysis with an equivalent direct likelihood ("MMRM") approach, one should include a by-visit interaction in the direct likelihood model for any factor included in the sequential models. As with sequential modeling, the direct likelihood approach can also imply interactions that are not immediately obvious. MMRMs include a treatment-by-visit interaction, so the mean of each treatment group is allowed to vary by visit. But recall (Section 5.4.2.1) that, with MMRMs, outcomes prior to withdrawal contribute to inference via the within-subject correlations that are modeled. Thus the correlations in MMRM can be thought of as doing the same work as post-baseline covariables in sequential MI with regard to withdrawals. In "standard" MMRM one may choose to estimate the variance–covariance matrix across the treatment groups, or separately for each treatment group (see again Section 5.4.2.1). When covariances are estimated separately for each treatment group, the relationship between data observed prior to withdrawal and the modeled (missing) outcome is allowed to differ by treatment group. Therefore, if it is desired to have a sequential modeling approach that is consistent with MMRM with such separate covariance estimates, the MI modeling should include an interaction with treatment for post-baseline outcomes at each relevant visit. To see this, let us take a simple example. Consider a longitudinal study with treatment group variable *trt* and efficacy score variables *score_j* for visit *j*. Suppose that in a sequential modeling procedure we impute outcomes for Visit 3 using the code in SAS Code Fragment 7.1.

```
* Perform MI using regression-based MI;
PROC MI DATA=monotone OUT=imputed NIMPUTE=1 SEED=34535499;
   BY _Imputation_;
   VAR trt score_1-score_3;
   CLASS trt;
   MONOTONE REG(score_3=trt score_1 score_2);
RUN;
```

SAS Code Fragment 7.1   Simplified MI model to illustrate interaction by visit.

The regression coefficients for *trt* and *score_1* are, as noted above, estimated afresh here to impute *score_3*, and would differ from those estimated in an earlier step when *trt* and *score_1* were used in the model to impute *score_2*. We might expect the estimate of the outcome for Visit 3 to be consistent with a direct likelihood MMRM model with separate covariances for each treatment group such as that in SAS Code Fragment 7.2.

```
PROC MIXED DATA=infile;
CLASS trt visit subjid;
MODEL score=visit*trt/ ddfm=KR;
EPEATED visit /SUBJECT=subjid TYPE=UN GROUP=trt;
RUN;
```

SAS Code Fragment 7.2   Simplified direct likelihood MMRM model to illustrate interaction by visit.

The option "GROUP=*trt*" specifies that the model defined by SAS Code Fragment 7.2 uses separate correlations for each treatment group. This allows partially observed outcomes to contribute differently to the estimate of Visit 3, depending on their assigned treatment. Thus if outcomes at Visit 1 for subjects in the control treatment group tend to be weakly negatively correlated with Visit 3, while outcomes in the experimental arm data tend to be strongly positively correlated, this will be honored in the estimate of Visit 3 outcomes, by the model defined by SAS Code Fragment 7.2, because the correlations between each visit are allowed to vary by the treatment group *trt*. The MI model in SAS Code Fragment 7.1, on the contrary, allows for the mean outcome at Visit 3 to vary by treatment group (the model includes *trt* as a factor), but does not allow the estimate of the relationship between Visit 1 and Visit 3 to differ by treatment group (there is no *trt**score_1 factor in SAS Code Fragment 7.1). To be consistent with the MMRM just described, a sequential modeling approach will need to include an interaction between treatment and each visit's outcome. In the context of MNAR, when assumptions about missing data often vary by treatment group, it may be sensible to allow this interaction between treatment group and visit outcomes. We will see examples of such interactions included in code in later sections, for example, SAS Code Fragment 7.5.

Interactions with treatment arm: we discussed in the previous paragraph the interaction between treatment group and visit; any other variable (e.g., baseline) may also have an interaction with treatment arm, if desired.

Missing covariates: missing covariates can be imputed as part of the approach.

Categorical explanatory variables: categorical covariates with missing data (e.g., ancillary post-baseline categorical variables) can be "correctly" modeled using logistic regression – we do not have to treat categorical variables as "approximately" normally distributed.

Categorical outcomes: binary and categorical outcomes can be imputed using MNAR assumptions in a manner similar to that described above for continuous outcomes. We will show in the subsequent section that it is straightforward to implement "controlled imputations" for a binary/categorical outcome using this sequential modeling approach.

Ancillary variables: one can easily include ancillary variables (e.g., related measurements, including post-baseline measurements) when using the sequential approach – such variables can reduce bias in the imputation of the missing values.

Flexibility: the sequential modeling method can be used to implement versions of most of the assumptions about missing data that are possible using the joint modeling method. As with the joint modeling method, a variety of pre-planned delta adjustments can also be applied as part of the process, and the δs can vary based on, say, reason for discontinuation. However, the sequential modeling approach uses a single step in which it accomplishes both modeling and imputation. The analyst can implement a number of different assumptions for different groups (patterns) of withdrawals for a single visit, by performing a number of sequential imputations, one per assumption/pattern. Note that sequential modeling assumes a different model for each step of the imputation (often, for each visit) and so draws of the regression parameters are taken from different models to create the multiply imputed datasets. (An exception would be with a delta-adjusting approach where different δs need to be applied to different groups of withdrawals, which can sometimes be implemented in a single step.)

7.3.5   Pattern-mixture models implemented using the joint modeling method

It will be useful to clarify that by "explanatory variable" in this section we mean any baseline or demographic variable; "outcome" means a post-baseline outcome.

We are indebted to documentation by available at www.missingdata.org.uk by Roger (2012), of which we make use in the following account of his implementation of the joint modeling method for "controlled imputation," together with many helpful communications with Roger.

To enable the reader to cross-refer to Roger's own documentation, for this discussion we adopt Roger's parameterization as shown in Table 7.1.

Roger's implementation of "controlled imputation" has two stages.

Table 7.1   Notation for the description of the joint modeling method implementation by Roger (2012).

Index letter	Range	Function
i	$1 \ldots n$	Subject
j	$1 \ldots q$	Treatment allocated to the individual subject
k	$1 \ldots t$	Time or visit number
r	$1 \ldots q$	Reference treatment
p	$0 \ldots t$	Withdrawal visit: the visit at which the last observation is made (0 for those with no observed data and t for those with complete data)
s		Indexes the covariates

In its first stage, as noted earlier, the method estimates regression parameters for the outcome using a single joint model – "effectively the MMRM model" (Roger, 2012), though implemented via SAS PROC MCMC. Thus, as in standard MMRM, there is no straightforward way to make use of ancillary post-baseline variables as there would usually be with MI. That is, post-baseline variables, other than the outcome variable, cannot be used to reduce bias and increase the precision of the imputation of the missing values.

Any explanatory variable can either be crossed with visit or the interaction can be omitted from the model, as the analyst decides. As in standard MMRM, all explanatory variables are required to be fully observed (otherwise, the entire subject record is omitted from the modeling process). All parameters corresponding to explanatory variables other than treatment group are estimated across treatment groups, rather than separately for each treatment group. This assumes that the association of explanatory variables with outcome does not vary by treatment group. Such an assumption is often sensible, although some trialists like to include an investigator-by-treatment or baseline-by-treatment effect in the model, for example. The variance–covariance matrix for the outcomes across visits is assumed to be "unstructured," that is, no particular scale or type of relationship is assumed between outcomes at different time points. The method allows the variance–covariance matrix to be estimated either across treatment groups, or separately for each treatment group. The latter is the usual choice. It is also possible to specify that between-visit correlations be set to zero. This will ignore subject's previous post-baseline values when imputing. This facility allows the analyst to compare the joint modeling approach with other MI approaches that may not take subject's observed post-baseline outcomes into account when imputing missing outcomes.

After estimating the MMRM model, the Roger approach makes draws based on the posterior distributions of the outcomes at each time point that have just been estimated. To understand what is meant by "posterior distributions of the outcomes at each time point," a rather technical aspect of the approach must now be described. Usually we write a longitudinal model as follows:

$$E\left[Y_{ik}\right] = A_{jk} + \sum_s X_{iks}\beta_s \qquad (7.3)$$

where subjects are independent and the vector Y_i for the ith subject is distributed with a multivariate normal distribution with variance–covariance matrix Σ_j, A_{jk} denotes the visit-by-treatment interaction term, and the β are the regression coefficients for explanatory variables X (baseline or demographic factors). The rightmost term can be thought of as a subject's individual covariate offset from the general visit-by-treatment intercept Λ_{jk}. However, parameterized in this way, the elements of A are not invariant to the constraints applied in the definition of the covariate design matrix X. For example, if for a categorical explanatory variable the regression coefficient is constrained to be zero for a particular category, A will then include the estimate for the relationship between that category and the outcome. A constraint can be arbitrary, and A is therefore not invariant to such constraints.

Now the heart of this method of implementing "controlled imputations" is to allow the statistician to specify "what if" assumptions in terms of the A component. To do this in an interpretable way, A must be made invariant to the design of X. This is done by reconfiguring the model as follows:

$$E\left[Y_{ik}\right] = A_{jk}^* + \sum_s X_{iks}\beta_s - \frac{1}{n}\sum_{is} X_{iks}\beta_s \tag{7.4}$$

This is the MMRM-like estimation model. The term $\frac{1}{n}\sum_{is} X_{iks}\beta_s$ has now been "silently" added to A_{jk} in Equation 7.3, giving A_{jk}^*, to balance that same quantity which has been subtracted from the last term in Equation 7.3. The last term in Equation 7.4 is the average subject covariate offset. The last two terms now quantify a subject's difference from the average covariate offset. The A_{jk}^* can now be thought of as the visit-by-treatment intercept for a subject, *plus* the average covariate offset. Note that this A_{jk}^* estimates the mean outcome *for treatment* at a time point, plus the mean covariate offset estimated *across treatments* at that time point. It is this A_{jk}^* that estimates the mean of the "posterior distribution of the outcomes at each time point." It is in terms of the A_{jk}^* that the "what ifs" are specified in Roger's macro, which can now be used to construct an imputation model. For simplicity, we will now drop the asterisk from A_{jk}^*, and A_{jk} will be used to represent the "posterior distribution of the outcomes at each time point."

The imputation model looks similar,

$$E\left[Y_{ik}\right] = B_{pjk} + \sum_s X_{iks}\beta_s - \frac{1}{n}\sum_{is} X_{iks}\beta_s \tag{7.5}$$

but the first term on the right-hand side, B_{pjk}, may vary by missingness pattern p and may be a linear combination of the components of A. Missing values are imputed as in "standard" MI: a new sample of the parameters on the right-hand side of the model in Equation 7.5 is drawn from a Bayesian posterior distribution of Equation 7.4 for each imputed dataset, and the imputed values are generated based on that instance of the imputation model. Each draw gives a vector of means μ for the outcome at all time points for a subject. A subject's outcomes Y can be split into Y_1 (observed) and Y_2 (unobserved or missing). The vector μ can be similarly split into μ_1 and μ_2. The variance–covariance matrix Σ is derived from sampled parameters that are obtained from Equation 7.4, and likewise splits into four components Σ_{11}, Σ_{12}, Σ_{21} (the transpose of Σ_{12}) and finally Σ_{22}. When the imputed values are sampled they are drawn from the distribution of Y_2 conditional upon the observed value of Y_1. This distribution is multivariate normal:

$$Y_2|Y_1 \sim N(\mu_2 + \Sigma_{21}\Sigma_{11}^{-1}(Y_1 - \mu_1), \Sigma_{22} - \Sigma_{21}\Sigma_{11}^{-1}\Sigma_{21}) \tag{7.6}$$

The mean in Equation 7.6 is the usual mean of a set of normally distributed variables conditional on other variables with which they are correlated. The μ_2 is the vector of means for the missing values of a subject, as estimated by Equation 7.5. The $Y_1 - \mu_1$, quantifies how "different" the observed values for a particular subject are from the mean for all subjects of that treatment group. To the extent that a particular subject is "different" (e.g., more improved or in worse health) than others, the conditional mean of the missing values is estimated to be different too, but only insofar as the time points in μ_2 are correlated with those of μ_1 (hence $\Sigma_{21}\Sigma_{11}^{-1}$). We will illustrate a variety of assumptions as implemented via MI using Figures 7.1, 7.2, 7.3, 7.4 and 7.5, which were devised by James Roger and are used here with his permission. Figure 7.1 illustrates how a subject's residual at observed post-baseline visits (i.e., the difference between the subject's observed and model-predicted values) can be reflected, given positive correlations between visits, in the standard MAR imputations using the joint model. As is often the case with withdrawals, the example subject in Figure 7.1 has poor observed responses, compared with the mean of

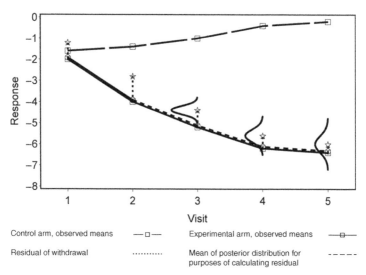

Figure 7.1   MAR: schematic plot showing likely imputations for a subject from the experimental arm who withdraws after Visit 2. Lower values of the response are better. The stars represent the subject's observed values and, post-withdrawal, the mean of the posterior distribution of the subject's imputed values, which reflect the subject's residual at observed visits. The sideways bell curves indicate the posterior distribution.

his/her treatment group. Notice how the mean of the posterior distribution of the imputations for the subject reflects earlier relatively poor response, but drifts towards the mean of that subject's treatment group, as the correlations with earlier observed outcomes become weaker; notice also that the variance of the posterior distribution of the imputations increases with time. Both these phenomena are typical of MAR imputations. We will see in Figures 7.2, 7.3 and 7.4 that similar phenomena generally also occur in MNAR imputation.

One of the assumptions that can be implemented by the joint modeling method is known as "copy reference" (CR) (Roger, 2012). For "copy reference," a mean and variance based on the reference group (often the control group) is assumed for the population of observations belonging to subjects who withdrew, so $B_{pjk} = A_{rk}$ for all p, j and k, (r here denotes the reference or control treatment). This means that under CR, for purposes of imputing Y_2 in Equation 7.6 the mean μ will always be that of the reference group. This seems strange at first, since the mean for the reference arm may be quite different from that of the experimental arm, but note that the observed values prior to withdrawal are honored, so that if the mean of the reference group is distant from that of the experimental treatment group (as it may often be), the subject's missing observations when imputed will look like those of a rather successful subject in the reference group. That is, the $(Y_1 - \mu_1)$ term in the mean of the imputed distribution will often be large, since the μ_1 will be that of the reference arm, while the Y_1 will be the observed values for the subject from the experimental arm. This will honor any health gain achieved up to the point of withdrawal, but the correlation $\Sigma_{21}\Sigma_{11}^{-1}$ will be that of any similar subject from the reference arm. Figure 7.2 sketches how the CR assumption is calculated for the subject plotted in Figure 7.1. For CR the subject, who has a rather poor response relative to

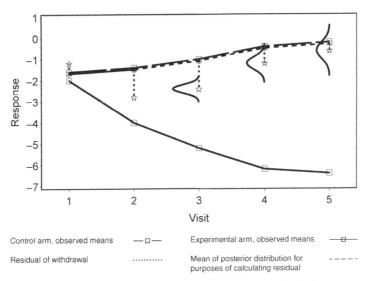

Figure 7.2   Copy reference (CR): schematic plot showing likely imputations for a subject from the experimental arm who withdraws after Visit 2.

the experimental treatment group, now "looks like" a subject with reasonably good response from the control treatment group. As in Figure 7.1, the sketch shows a drift towards the mean of the control group and an increase of variance in the posterior distribution of the imputations with time. Thus the "copy reference" assumption is very similar to assuming that subjects who withdraw from the experimental arm have correlations like similar subjects from the reference arm. This in turn is an assumption very similar to that of the sensitivity analysis whose implementation we described in Section 7.3.1 earlier in this chapter for the sequential modeling method. In fact, we find that Roger's "copy reference" assumption tends to give estimates of treatment effect close to the sequential modeling method of section 7.3.1. The main difference is that in the joint modeling approach the regression parameters of explanatory variables are estimated across all treatment groups, while in sequential modeling the regression parameters are estimated based on the subset of subjects on which the missing values are modeled. Thus, the sequential modeling version of CR bases its estimate of regression parameters only on the reference group.

Roger's macro implements another assumption that he calls "copy increment from reference" (CIR). This variant helps us to understand how the joint modeling method can differ in its assumptions (and its mechanics of calculation) from those of the sequential method. With CIR, $B_{pjk} = A_{jk}$ for $k \le p$, but $B_{pjk} = A_{jp} + A_{rk} - A_{rp}$ for $k > p$. That is, *for purposes of imputation*, at visits before withdrawal ($k \le p$), the subject is assumed to have the mean of his/her own treatment group. Thus when it comes to imputation of missing visits, the $(Y_1 - \mu_1)$ term in the mean of the imputed distribution (i.e., the residuals from observed values for the subject) will be calculated as for a member of the withdrawer's own treatment group, and the correlation with past visits in $\Sigma_{21}\Sigma_{11}^{-1}$ will be that of any similar subject from the withdrawer's own treatment arm. However, the μ_2 term – the mean attributed to the unobserved visits – will be a function of both the withdrawer's own treatment group means (A_{jp}) and those of the reference group (A_{rk} and A_{rp}). That μ_2 term will have the value you would get if you plotted a line from the treatment-by-time intercept for the withdrawer's own treatment group at time of withdrawal (A_{jp}) to the imputed time point, using the slope of the reference group ($A_{rk} - A_{rp}$). Notice the dashed line in Figure 7.3 between the lines for the control and experimental arms. This line joins the means relative to which the subject's observed residuals are applied via the modeled between-visit correlations. The line has been calculated to match the slope of the control group exactly. As in Figures 7.1 and 7.2, the sketch shows a drift towards the means indicated by the middle dashed line that matches the slope of control; and also shows the expected increase of variance in the posterior distribution of the imputations with time.

In CR, the imputed change from previous visit is estimated via the correlation among the reference treatment group time points $\Sigma_{21}\Sigma_{11}^{-1}$, while in CIR the imputed change is calculated via the difference between time point intercepts. We can see that CR and CIR calculate imputations that could be quite similar (if the correlations between visits strongly determined the slope of the reference group outcome), but do so in rather different ways. With CR, withdrawals are assumed to have efficacy trajectory of the reference group insofar as this is detectable via the correlations between time points in the reference group. Therefore, if correlations between time points are not strong, the withdrawals will tend to be imputed as tending to drift towards the mean of the reference group, that is, in Equation 7.6, Σ_{21} will minimize the contribution of $(Y_1 - \mu_1)$, and the imputation will be dominated by μ_2, the mean of the reference arm. It can be argued that this is clinically realistic: weak correlations over time could reflect that the indication does not have a distinct trajectory over time and this should be reflected in assumptions about withdrawals from the treatment group. On the other hand, CIR simply calculates the difference between the reference-arm means for time points, and imposes this same increment on withdrawals from the experimental arm, taking into account the subject's covariate offset relative to his/her own treatment arm. Under CIR, therefore, the analyst is "guaranteed" that the trajectory of imputed values follows that of the reference arm, other things being equal. This control over the trajectory could be attractive to some, but may be regarded by others as less clinically realistic, CR being consistent with the estimated correlations in the reference arm.

Another useful kind of assumption for sensitivity analyses is that withdrawals from the experimental arm immediately change to have the distribution of the reference arm. Roger has called this the "jump to reference" (J2R) assumption (Roger, 2012). With the joint modeling approach, the analyst can choose to estimate J2R imputations taking account of the subject's "differentness" in observed post-baseline outcomes relative to that subject's own treatment group, by making imputations have the mean of the reference arm but which take account of the subject's residual relative to that of his/her own treatment group, prior to withdrawal. Since withdrawals often have worse outcomes than average for their treatment group, this makes the default joint modeling J2R relatively harsh in its assumption about the experimental arm:

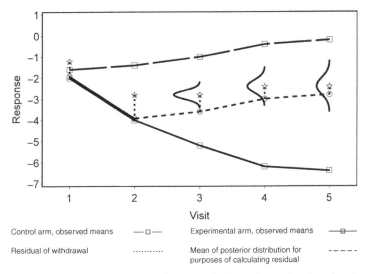

Figure 7.3   Copy increment from reference (CIR): schematic plot showing likely imputations for a subject from the experimental arm who withdraws after Visit 2.

withdrawals are in effect assumed to have outcomes worse than the mean for the reference arm. This can be seen in the posterior distribution of the imputations at Visits 3–5 in Figure 7.4.

On the other hand, sequential modeling implements J2R for a visit by estimating parameters using only baseline covariables and reference-arm outcomes for the visit – see SAS Code Fragment 7.11 for an illustration of this. Since this model includes no post-baseline outcomes, only "differentness" at baseline, which under randomization has expectation zero, will be taken into account when imputing, and subjects from the experimental arm will look very much like subjects from the reference arm in their residuals. As a result, imputations for withdrawals from the experimental arm at a visit will have a mean very close to the mean for the reference arm for the visit. Figure 7.5 illustrates this. As in Figures 7.1, 7.2, 7.3 and 7.4, the subject has observed outcomes at Visits 1 and 2 that are somewhat worse than the mean for the subject's treatment group. But for this version of "jump to reference," that post-baseline "differentness" is ignored when modeling the subject's imputations – Figure 7.5 depicts the mean of the posterior distribution of the subject's imputations as almost identical to the observed mean of the control group. Note that since sequential approach uses only baseline covariables to model the imputations, the variance of the posterior distribution is rather large; the variance increases with time, but not as dramatically as in Figures 7.1, 7.2, 7.3 and 7.4, because the relationship between baseline covariables and outcome tends not to weaken over time to quite the same extent as the relationship between post-baseline outcomes.

The upshot is that the default implementation of J2R by the joint modeling approach is in practice harsher to the experimental arm than the implementation by

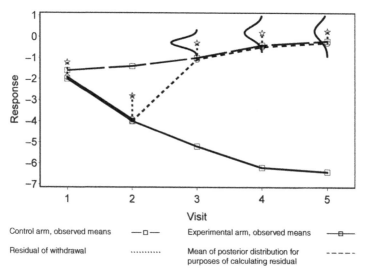

Figure 7.4   Jump to reference (J2R) implemented via joint modeling: schematic plot showing likely imputations for a subject from the experimental arm who withdraws after Visit 2.

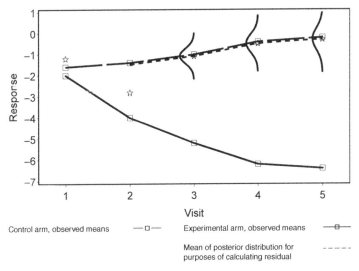

Figure 7.5   Jump to reference implemented via sequential modeling: schematic plot showing likely imputations for a subject from the experimental arm who withdraws after Visit 2.

the sequential modeling approach. We have noted that the joint modeling approach has inherent flexibility with regard to the calculation of residuals. In fact, in the DIA macro to implement this approach, the analyst can choose to ignore post-baseline outcomes for withdrawals in calculating residuals, and thus in this respect the joint modeling approach can be made consistent with the sequential modeling approach, if desired.

Table 7.2 shows the sensitivity analyses options offered by Roger's macro and the consequent values of *A* taken by *B* for each of the Roger analyses. The separation of the two stages (estimation of parameters *A*, followed by imputation using "modified" parameters *B*) allows great flexibility in manipulation of the missing study outcomes, and as noted enables all observed trial data to be used in estimating model parameters. The macro even allows the statistician to implement completely new sensitivity analysis assumptions, by writing her own assignment of the *A*s to the *B*s, in a special module of the macro. The analyst needs to be well versed in the interpretation of the parameters of a mixed model and SAS macro programming in order to translate clinical assumptions into mathematical language and thence into programming code.

7.3.6   Characteristics of the joint modeling method of implementing pattern-mixture models

Here, under the same headings as for the sequential method, we summarize the characteristics of the joint modeling method of implementing PMMs as implemented by Roger (2012).

Table 7.2   Sensitivity analyses offered by Roger's macro and consequent values of A taken by B from Roger (2012).

Assumption for discontinuations from the experimental arm	Roger abbreviation	Value for $B_{pjk}{}^a$	Similar analysis available via sequential MI?
Missing at random	MAR	A_{jk} for all patterns p, j and k	Yes
Copy increment from reference	CIR	$A_{jp} + A_{rk} - A_{rp}$ for $k > p$	No
Jump to reference	J2R	A_{rk} for $k > p$	Yes
Copy reference	CR	A_{rk} for all patterns p, j and k	Yes
Average last mean carried forward	ALMCF	A_{jp} for $k > p$	Yes
Own last mean carried forward	OLMCF	See Roger (2012) for details	Yes

$^a B_{pjk} = A_{jk}$ for $k \leq p$ unless otherwise specified. Roger draws attention to the fact that CR is a special case, in that, for CR, only the estimated mean of the distribution from which the subject comes is taken to be that of the reference arm, although the subject's values up to discontinuation are honored. The variance–covariance matrix Σ is generated on the same basis as the B_{pjk} for each imputed dataset, that is, it is sampled from a Bayesian posterior of the parameters from the appropriate treatment arm.

Non-monotone missing data: as with the sequential modeling approach, intermediate or non-monotone missing data are imputed assuming MAR, with all baseline and demographic explanatory variables estimated across treatment groups.

How regression parameters are estimated: all trial data are used to estimate the regression parameters for explanatory variables to be used in the imputation model.

Interactions of explanatory variables with time: the statistician may specify whether an explanatory variable should be crossed with visit or not.

Interactions with treatment arm: the interaction between treatment and visit is included as a factor in the model. However, with this approach no other explanatory variables may have an interaction with treatment – model factors are estimated across treatment groups. If an explanatory variable such as, say, gender, differs by treatment group in its association with the outcome, that is, if there is a true gender by treatment interaction, then the joint modeling method cannot reflect this in its model of the missing data. However, such interactions are not often included in practice in analysis of clinical trials, except for exploratory analyses. As noted in Section 7.3.4, the correlations in the MMRM-type model used in the joint modeling approach do the same work as the covariables in sequential MI. In the joint-modeling approach, to allow the imputation to take account of the relationship between visits separately for each treatment group – in effect a treatment-by-visit interaction for the imputations – the statistician may specify that the variance–covariance matrix of the MMRM-like model is estimated separately for each treatment arm.

If the variance–covariance matrix is estimated across treatment arms, no difference in the between-visit correlations is assumed between treatment arms. This is not to be confused with the fact that MMRM does include a treatment-by-visit interaction as a factor among the fixed effects. What this means is that, although a subject's residual is calculated given a treatment-by-visit interaction, the imputations themselves are modeled assuming that correlations between visits post-discontinuation are similar across treatment arms.

Missing covariates: no covariates can be missing.

Binary/categorical covariates: binary/categorical covariates are treated similarly to normally distributed covariates.

Binary/categorical responses: binary/categorical responses cannot be imputed.

Ancillary variables: ancillary variables cannot be included in a straightforward manner.

Flexibility: the joint modeling method allows the statistician flexibility in specifying which elements of the statistical model estimated from the trial data should be used to impute missing data. The same method and software facilitates imputations using a variety of assumptions that base imputations on the outcomes of subjects on the reference treatment (CR, CIR and J2R); on a subject's own last observed mean (OLMCF); and on the average mean of the last observed visit (ALMCF). Furthermore, the analyst can specify the assumption to be used for any subgroup or indeed for any given subject. This facilitates assumptions about missing data differing by, say, reason for discontinuation. A single draw of the regression parameters is used for each of the multiply imputed datasets, even when a variety of assumptions are made. Delta adjustment can also be implemented.

7.3.7   Summary of differences between the joint modeling and sequential modeling methods

Sections 7.3.4 and 7.3.6 list attributes that characterize the sequential and joint modeling methods. There are also subtle differences of a more technical nature inherent in the fact that joint modeling uses a single model to estimate parameters while sequential modeling uses a sequence of models. Drawing on Sections 7.3.4, 7.3.5 and 7.3.6, we summarize here key differences between joint modeling and sequential modeling approaches, with regard to the estimation of model parameters and residuals:

1. Using the terminology of "identifying restrictions" for PMMs, the joint modeling method imposes restrictions directly at the level of parameters previously estimated from all data, while sequential modeling method imposes restrictions at the level of data subsets used for the estimation of these parameters.

2. The joint modeling approach uses separate steps (a) to estimate model parameters from the observed data and (b) to use these parameters in a flexible way

to construct a separate model in order to obtain imputed values. The joint modeling method calculates the extent to which subject's covariate effects differ from the average in their contribution to the model-imputed outcome (Roger calls this the "average subject covariates offset"); then, for a given time point, values are imputed using an imputation model with a new specified mean and variance (e.g., the mean and variance of the reference group), plus the subject's original covariate offset, so as to preserve each subject's deviation from average efficacy as modeled by the MMRM-type model. The sequential modeling approach estimates a model and imputes values using that model for a given missing pattern, all in a single step, modeling the subject to be imputed as if that subject had become one of the group of subjects selected for model estimation (e.g., the reference group). Thus, the sequential modeling method specifies assumptions in terms of designation of subgroups of subjects with available data that are considered to be similar, or different in specific ways, to subgroups of subjects with missing data. Once such subgroups are designated and similarities/differences are specified, model estimation and imputation is confined within these subgroups.

3. Both joint modeling and sequential modeling approaches take account of a subject's "differentness" – the subject's residual – relative to the observations of other subjects, and reflect that residual in imputations. The residual depends upon the model, however. The joint modeling method first estimates parameters, and then in a separate step uses functions of those parameters to impute outcomes. This separation of imputation in the joint modeling approach allows the estimation of a subject's "differentness" to be independent of the assumption about missingness that is being implemented. Thus, as noted in the previous point, the joint modeling approach can calculate a subject's residual from the MMRM-type joint model, and then use the residual together with the estimate of a mean drawn from some other treatment group and/or visit to implement a wide variety of assumptions about withdrawals. Joint modeling allows the analyst to specify whether a subject's residual is calculated relative to the model mean for the subject's own treatment group or, for example, the model mean for a reference treatment group. Sequential modeling does not have the flexibility of the joint modeling approach in its estimation of a subject's "differentness" or residual. The sequential modeling approach calculates a subject's "differentness" or residual relative to the model mean of the outcomes selected to implement the particular MNAR assumption, often the model mean of the control group. In the case of the reference-based assumption known as copy reference (CR), a subject's "differentness" or residual at each visit is estimated similarly by the default joint modeling and sequential modeling approaches – both estimate the residual relative to the model mean of the reference treatment group. However, this will not always be the case. We have seen in Section 7.3.5 that for the J2R assumption, the joint modeling approach by default calculates a subject's residual taking into account that subject's difference in post-baseline outcomes relative to his/her own treatment group; while sequential modeling calculates the residual based only on

differences in baseline covariables, thus estimating imputed values very similar to the "average" subject in the reference group.

4. With the joint modeling approach, all baseline data and all observed instances of the outcome may be used to estimate the model parameters. With the sequential modeling method, subsets of data may be used to estimate a model intended for imputation of a given missing pattern, a corollary of this is that if explanatory variables do interact with treatment or other characteristics of a missing pattern, this interaction cannot be accounted for in the joint modeling method, whereas it is naturally done in the sequential modeling method. On the other hand, if such interaction is not present/assumed, then the joint modeling method will provide a more precise estimation of the corresponding model parameters by using more data.

5. With the joint modeling implementation, ancillary post-baseline variables cannot in practice be used to help the imputation of missing variables – using sequential modeling, ancillary variables can be used as in "ordinary" MI.

6. With the joint modeling implementation, the outcome variable – the one to be imputed – is assumed continuous; the sequential modeling method can model binary outcomes with the appropriate binary or binomial distribution.

7. The joint modeling method draws regression parameters once for each imputed dataset, while the sequential modeling method may draw from more than one model for a dataset.

Finally, we would like to point out that the features of sequential modeling approach highlighted in points 1 and 2 above, namely that the identifying restrictions are imposed at the level of data subsets used for the estimation of imputation model parameters and that imputation model estimation and filling in missing values are done in a single step, are artifacts of the particular implementation we chose which takes advantage of the PROC MI functionality to a full extent. It would be possible to devise an implementation that would still use sequential regression, but where identifying restrictions could be applied at the level of estimated parameters of the imputation model, similar to joint modeling. In order to do this, one would need to separate the task of estimation and drawing samples of imputation model parameters from their posterior distribution and the task of drawing samples for imputed values using a model with given parameters, just as it is done in joint modeling approach. PROC MI's monotone imputation methods that we used for sequential modeling capture, in an ODS dataset, imputation model parameter draws for each imputed dataset. These parameters can thus be retrieved, a new imputation model can be constructed using any function of these parameters to reflect identifying restrictions, as in the joint modeling, and then drawing samples for imputation from this new model can be implemented "by hand" in a separate step. This approach would be somewhat more programmatically demanding, as we would discard the imputed values provided by PROC MI and implement the filling-in part separately on our own. Nevertheless, this could certainly be done.

7.4   A "toolkit": Implementing sensitivity analyses via SAS

7.4.1   Reminder: General approach using multiple imputation with regression

We start with a brief review of the approach to implement MI using regression. The reader is referred to Chapter 6 for detailed background on MI.

MI and subsequent analysis of the imputed data can be performed in SAS by following a three-step process.

1. PROC MI is used to impute missing values, which results in creation of multiple copies of the original input dataset. All copies contain identical values of the non-missing data items, but different values imputed for missing items.

2. Each of these imputed datasets is then analyzed using a standard SAS procedure, for example, PROC GLM, PROC LOGISTIC and so on.

3. Results from the analysis of all imputed datasets are then combined together for overall inference using PROC MIANALYZE.

One of the advantages of MI is that it permits usage of an imputation model that is different from the analysis model applied to the imputed data (although certain considerations are needed to ensure that the two models are compatible, as described in Chapter 6). This allows one to account for factors that are potentially correlated with missingness, but are not of interest for the inference regarding the treatment effect on the primary efficacy outcome. When MI is used under MAR assumptions, the requirement is that the imputation model should be at least as complex as the subsequent analysis model. Thus, the imputation model may contain factors not included in the analysis model, but it should not omit terms included in the latter. This is required to ensure that the relationships between the efficacy outcome and other factors of interest are treated in a consistent way by the imputation model and the analysis model. However, when used under MNAR assumptions, we may, in fact, want to dilute or change some relationships to reflect various assumptions, and so this requirement will not always be adhered to in the same way as under MAR assumption. We will see an example of this below in the control-based imputation method.

If a dataset has some subjects with non-monotone missingness, the most frequently used imputation method in PROC MI is based on the MCMC methodology and assumes a multivariate normal distribution over all variables included in the imputation model, which may not always be appropriate. For datasets with monotone missingness, a number of different methods are available for continuous as well as categorical variables, including some parametric and non-parametric methods. We use the MCMC method to impute data only partially – just enough to obtain a dataset with monotone missingness. Then the remaining missing items can be imputed using other available methods if deemed more suitable. Thus our use of step 1 above in

```
* make dataset monotone missing;
PROC SORT DATA=updrsh;
   BY trt;
RUN;
PROC MI DATA=updrsh OUT=monotone nimpute=1000 SEED=34535499;
   BY trt;
   VAR base_UPD UPD_1-UPD_8;
   MCMC CHAIN=MULTIPLE IMPUTE=MONOTONE;
RUN;
```

SAS Code Fragment 7.3   Use MCMC to impute non-monotone missing values.

practice has two parts, one to impute enough observations to make the dataset monotone missing, and the second to impute the remaining monotone missing data. This two-part imputation is illustrated here using the example dataset of UPDRS scores from Chapter 1. See Section 1.10.1 for a description of the variables in this dataset.

It is assumed that the UPDRS dataset is in a "horizontal" format (one record per subject), with UPDRS for Visits 1–8 available as variables *upd_1-upd_8*. Baseline UPDRS variable is *base_upd*, and the treatment variable *trt* takes value 1 for the control group and 2 for the experimental treatment group. Assume that this "horizontal" dataset is called *updrsh*.

First, the MCMC method in PROC MI is used to partially impute non-monotone missing data (as requested by IMPUTE=MONOTONE option in the MCMC statement in SAS Code Fragment 7.3).

Note that SAS Code Fragment 7.3 estimates imputations separately for each treatment group. If it is judged appropriate to estimate non-monotone imputations across treatment groups, the "BY *trt*" statement may be omitted, and *trt* included in the VAR statement. Both options are available in the DIA macros to implement imputation via sequential modeling.

MCMC estimates for a key variable such as *upd_j* (where *j* is the ID of any study visit that was imputed by this partial procedure) should be checked for a variety of values of the MCMC parameters NBITER (the number of MCMC updates allowed for the sampler to converge to a stationary distribution) and NITER (the number of MCMC iterations between each saved draw from the posterior). Values for NBITER and NITER may need to be increased from the default if, based on the diagnostic graphs for the worst linear function of parameters, there is a concern about convergence of the MCMC algorithm (see Section 6.6.4 for further details of the checks and tuning that may be required).

Now, methods for monotone missingness can be applied to impute the rest of the missing data using the output dataset *monotone* as input to a subsequent call to PROC MI (SAS Code Fragment 7.4). Since dataset *monotone* already contains 1000 copies of the data with partial imputations, the subsequent call to PROC MI will use a BY _Imputation_ statement and request one imputed dataset (NIMPUTE = 1 option) within each BY group. This second call will fill in the remaining missing items in each of the 1000 copies stored in *monotone*. If we wished to be consistent with an

```
PROC MI DATA=monotone OUT=imputed NIMPUTE=1 SEED=34535499;
    BY _imputation_;
    VAR trt base_UPD UPD_1-UPD_8;
    CLASS TRT;
    MONOTONE REGRESSION;
RUN;
```

SAS Code Fragment 7.4   Use regression imputation to complete the MAR imputation, to match an MMRM where covariances are estimated across all treatment
groups.

MMRM analysis that estimated covariances across all treatment groups, SAS Code
Fragment 7.4 would create appropriate MAR imputations.

Often, especially in the context of a sensitivity analysis, it will be desirable to
obtain an MAR-based estimate in a manner that would be consistent with an MMRM
that estimated covariances separately for each treatment group. To achieve this with
PROC MI, the analyst must specify the model for each post-baseline outcome "by
hand" including interactions of treatment with previous post-baseline outcomes.

In SAS Code Fragment 7.5, MI models the missing data for all subjects using
all observed UPDRS data, and assumes MAR. Note that the model for each visit
includes an interaction for the treatment arm variable *trt* and the outcome. This MAR
model thus assumes that the correlations across visits may differ by treatment group
and thus is equivalent to an MMRM that estimates the variance–covariance matrix
separately for each treatment arm.

Figure 7.6 presents the means of the resulting imputed values. As often is the
case in clinical trials, subjects who discontinue tend to have relatively poor efficacy

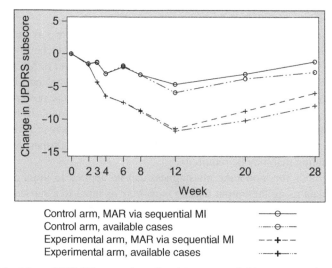

*Figure 7.6   Mean UPDRS score for all subjects, available cases and with missing
values imputed assuming MAR.*

```
* perform standard (MAR) MI using regression-based MI;
PROC MI DATA=monotone OUT=imputed NIMPUTE=1 SEED=34535499;
   BY _imputation_;
   VAR trt base_upd upd_1-upd_8;
   CLASS TRT;
   MONOTONE REG(upd_1=trt base_upd);
   MONOTONE REG(upd_2=trt base_upd upd_1 trt*upd_1);
   MONOTONE REG(upd_3=trt base_upd upd_1 trt*upd_1
                          upd_2 trt*upd_2);
   MONOTONE REG(upd_4=trt base_upd upd_1 trt*upd_1
                          upd_2 trt*upd_2
                          upd_3 trt*upd_3);
   MONOTONE REG(upd_5=trt base_upd upd_1 trt*upd_1
                          upd_2 trt*upd_2
                          upd_3 trt*upd_3
                          upd_4 trt*upd_4);
   MONOTONE REG(upd_6=trt base_upd upd_1 trt*upd_1
                          upd_2 trt*upd_2
                          upd_3 trt*upd_3
                          upd_4 trt*upd_4
                          upd_5 trt*upd_5);
   MONOTONE REG(upd_7=trt base_upd upd_1 trt*upd_1
                          upd_2 trt*upd_2
                          upd_3 trt*upd_3
                          upd_4 trt*upd_4
                          upd_5 trt*upd_5
                          upd_6 trt*upd_6);
   MONOTONE REG(upd_8=trt base_upd upd_1 trt*upd_1
                          upd_2 trt*upd_2
                          upd_3 trt*upd_3
                          upd_4 trt*upd_4
                          upd_5 trt*upd_5
                          upd_6 trt*upd_6
                          upd_7 trt*upd_7);
RUN;
```

SAS Code Fragment 7.5 Use regression imputation to complete the MAR imputation; the inclusion of interactions with treatment is consistent with an MMRM where covariances are estimated separately for each treatment group (as with the GROUP=*trt* option in PROC MIXED).

before discontinuation, and an MAR model will tend to reflect this by imputing mean UPDRS scores for the missing subjects that are higher (worse) than the means for completers.

In a standard way of using PROC MI with the MONOTONE statement under MAR assumptions, one would make a single call to PROC MI, as illustrated in SAS Code Fragment 7.5, while including all explanatory variables and all time points that need to be imputed in the VAR statement. The input dataset would contain all trial subjects and all relevant assessments/time points. Variables *upd_1* through *upd_8* contain missing values for some subjects, which PROC MI imputes using linear regression models as requested in the MONOTONE statements. PROC MI imputes each variable conditional on the others that are specified before that variable in the VAR statement or the model explicitly specified in a MONOTONE statement for the corresponding variable.

For non-monotone missing data, a variant of the regression imputation called fully conditional specification is now becoming available in standard software such as SAS version 9.3 (see Chapter 6).

Each copy of the imputed data (dataset *monotone*, records grouped by *_Imputation_* variable) can now be analyzed by any standard SAS analysis procedure. The results of analysis from multiply-imputed datasets can be combined using PROC MIANALYZE. Point estimates and variances are calculated by PROC MIANA-LYZE using Rubin's rules (Rubin, 1987) which take into account the variability in results from the multiple imputed datasets, reflecting the uncertainty associated with the missing values. Overall inferences are obtained by averaging over the estimates obtained from the multiple filled-in datasets and accounting for the between-imputation variance (see Chapter 6 for more details).

7.4.2   Sensitivity analyses assuming withdrawals have trajectory of control arm

In the Little and Yau (1996) paper that suggested reference-based analyses, the idea was to impute missing values after a subject's discontinuation from the trial using an "as-treated" model, with data based on an actual dose after dropout if it were known, or some plausible assumptions if unknown. In most clinical trials, subjects stop taking study medication after discontinuation. If this can be assumed, the as-treated model for discontinued subjects could be based on the notion that subjects are taking a zero dose of the experimental treatment, or are reverting to a standard-of-care treatment that will often feature as the control in a clinical trial. Therefore, it might often be reasonable to assume that after withdrawal from the trial, subjects from the experimental treatment arm (no longer receiving the experimental treatment) will exhibit the same future evolution of the disease as subjects on the control treatment (who are also not exposed to the experimental treatment). Note that, as argued in Section 4.2.3.1, even if it were known that some withdrawals from the experimental arm change to a treatment with better efficacy than the control arm, it may still be reasonable to impute a control-like trajectory to these withdrawals. Such an imputation in effect adopts as an efficacy estimand the efficacy *attributable to* the experimental arm.

However, if subjects who discontinue from the control arm are expected to change to a treatment that may be more effective for them, then the assumption that all withdrawals follow the pattern of the control completers may be less plausible clinically and may be argued not to be sufficiently conservative for intent-to-treat analysis. It is also important to examine the number and pattern of control group dropouts to assure that completers from the control group do not constitute a strong "placebo responder" group, to use which in imputing the experimental arm might not be sufficiently conservative. This possibility should be borne in mind when interpreting control-based imputation. Such bias will be diminished as the data in the control group tends to MAR. See also the discussion in Section 4.2.2.3, **Sources of bias in primary analyses**, the section on **Control-based or reference-based imputation**.

MAR assumes that withdrawals from the experimental arm will tend to have efficacy similar to subjects from the experimental arm who remain in the trial. Control-based imputation assumes on the contrary that subjects on the experimental treatment who withdraw will tend to have an efficacy trajectory similar to subjects on the control treatment. Thus, it will tend to provide a reduced estimate of treatment effect for experimental treatment. We have seen (Section 7.3.5) that a control-based assumption such as J2R can even impute values that tend to be somewhat worse than the mean for the control group, by taking account of a withdrawal's poor performance relative to his/her own treatment group. However, for a withdrawal who had been benefitting from the experimental treatment, control-based approaches do not push the assumption to the more extreme scenario where a withdrawal with average outcomes in the experimental arm is imputed to have outcomes worse than the mean for the control arm. Such a scenario could be appropriate, for example, if the experimental treatment interferes with the effect of the control drug and reduces its efficacy in a sub-population of subjects that discontinue. Subjects from the experimental arm could then do worse than control subjects with a similar history, and the control-based pattern imputation would underestimate this negative effect.

We present first a method that uses sequential modeling to implement the assumption that after discontinuation withdrawals from the experimental arm have correlations similar to those of subjects in the control arm. This is like the CR assumption sketched in Figure 7.2.

We will again use the Parkinson's disease illustrative dataset. We assume that, as in Section 7.4.1, the dataset has been rendered monotone missing.

In order to impute missing data at the first post-baseline Visit 1, in step 1 (SAS Code Fragment 7.6) prepare a dataset for the imputation that contains only

(a) records for subjects from both treatment arms with data to be imputed at Visit 1 and

(b) records for subjects from the control arm that have data observed at Visit 1.

PROC MI will then have only control group data with which to estimate a model of outcome at Visit 1.

In step 2 (see SAS Code Fragment 7.7), call PROC MI to impute missing data at Visit 1 using dataset IMPUTE1.

Note that treatment arm is not included as an effect in the model (it is not included in the VAR statement). Since subjects from the experimental arm with non-missing values at Visit 1 are not included in the input dataset, they will not contribute to the estimation of an imputation model for time point 1. The imputation model will be estimated using control subjects only, while this call to PROC MI will impute missing data at Visit 1 for all subjects who need imputation at that time point. This way, subjects from experimental arm will be imputed based on the control subjects' model.

```
* Step 1. Create dataset IMPUTE1 to impute Visit 1 using only
information from control (trt=1);

* name dataset appropriately as input for Visit 1;
DATA strtimp1;
  SET monotone;
RUN;
* select observations to be imputed (lastvis<1), plus the
control observations (trt=1)to be used to estimate the imputation
model ;
DATA impute1 rest1;
  SET strtimp1;
  * Put to one side subjects from experimental arm (trt=2) that
have data at time point 1;
  IF trt = 2 AND lastvis >=1
  THEN
      OUTPUT rest1;
  * Select all other subjects for the time point 1 imputation step;
  ELSE
      OUTPUT impute1;
RUN;
```

SAS Code Fragment 7.6   Select observations so as to impute Visit 1 using model based on control arm.

```
* Step 2. Call PROC MI to impute missing data at Visit 1 using
dataset IMPUTE1;
PROC MI DATA=impute1 OUT=imputed1 NIMPUTE=1 SEED=34535499;
  BY _imputation_;
  VAR trt base_upd upd_1;
  MONOTONE REGRESSION(upd_1 = base_upd);
RUN;
```

SAS Code Fragment 7.7   Impute Visit 1 using model based on control arm.

In step 3 (see SAS Code Fragment 7.8), re-assemble the dataset, now with Visit 1 imputed for all subjects:

```
* Step 3.  Re-assemble the dataset, now with Visit 1 imputed;
DATA strtimp2;
  SET rest1 imputed1;
RUN;
PROC SORT DATA=strtimp2;
  BY _imputation_;
RUN;
```

SAS Code Fragment 7.8   Re-assemble the dataset to impute missing values at the next visit.

```
PROC MI DATA=impute2 OUT= imputed2 NIMPUTE=1 SEED=34535499;
    BY _imputation_;
    VAR base_upd upd_1-upd_2
    MONOTONE REGRESSION(upd_2=base_upd upd_1);
RUN;
```

SAS Code Fragment 7.9   Impute Visit 2 using model based control arm.

Repeat steps 1–3 for all other visits sequentially using a reconstructed dataset as a starting point in place of the *monotone* dataset in step 1 (i.e., using *strtimp2* as a basis for the imputation of Visit 2). For example, to impute Visit 2, split *strtimp2* into *impute2* which holds all control arm records and those experimental arm records whose last observed visit is Visit 2; the PROC MI step for the next time point is given in SAS Code Fragment 7.9.

The final imputed dataset can be analyzed by standard SAS procedures and the results can be combined using PROC MIANALYZE.

Figure 7.6 showed means for available data and those imputed under MAR, and illustrated how, at least for the experimental arm, MAR imputes somewhat worse efficacy scores to early withdrawals compared to completers, as might be expected. Withdrawals in each treatment arm were imputed using the correlations of that treatment arm and followed closely the trajectory (slope) of their own arm after discontinuation. Control-based analyses can be seen as deviations from MAR that tend to favor the control group. Accordingly, Figure 7.7 compares the above control-based imputation with MAR: it presents mean UPDRS sub-score for all subjects

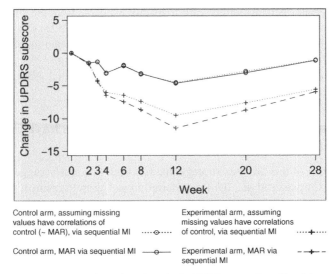

Figure 7.7   Mean change from baseline in UPDRS score for all subjects, assuming MAR versus assuming missing values have correlations of the control arm.

assuming MAR versus assuming that after withdrawal subjects in the experimental arm have correlations modeled by the control arm. Note that for the control arm, imputations from the two methods are almost the same, as should be expected, because both methods assume MAR for the control subjects. Small differences may arise due to the fact that the regression model for MAR imputations is estimated from all subjects, while the regression model for this control-based analysis are estimated using only subjects from the control group; some small differences may also be due to stochastic nature of the method and the fact that a different sequence of random numbers is used in the implementation of the two methods. For the experimental arm, on the other hand, we can see that the control-based method is less optimistic compared to MAR. The control arm trajectory is often somewhat less favorable than that of the experimental arm. The 44% of subjects from the experimental arm who withdrew early are then assumed to have this less favorable correlation. In Figure 7.7, we again plot means calculated from all subjects (observed and imputed), and, as expected, the means for the experimental arm that are somewhat higher (worse) than under MAR. The reader comparing Figure 7.7 to Figure 7.6 should note that the MAR estimates in Figure 7.6 are represented by dotted lines, but in Figure 7.7 are represented by the solid and dashed lines – those same line types will be used for plots of MAR imputations hereafter in this chapter.

As noted above, an attraction of this kind of control-based sensitivity analysis is that the stress test can be planned in advance (so avoiding "data dredging"), by making use of control arm study data to derive a distribution for the experimental arm that is likely to be considerably more pessimistic than that assumed by MAR, but not unreasonably so. See Section 4.2.2.3, for a discussion of arguments for and against control-based imputation.

See Appendix 7.B for complete SAS code to implement the above analysis. Appendix 7.B also includes sample calls to macros available from the DIA web page on missingdata.org.uk: one call to the macro due to Ratitch (2012a) that implements a sequential modeling analysis identical to the one above, and one to the macro due to Roger (2012) that implements the analysis via joint modeling.

We note that in the code above both control and experimental arms are imputed in the same imputation step.

7.4.3   Sensitivity analyses assuming withdrawals have distribution of control arm

Another variant of this analysis strategy that has been previously suggested (Roger *et al.*, 2008; Carpenter *et al.*, 2013) is referred to as "jump to control" or "jump to reference" (see Figure 7.4 for sketch of the default implementation via joint modeling). In the sequential-modeling version of this analysis, post-baseline outcomes prior to withdrawal are not used as explanatory variables in the imputation, and the missing outcome of a withdrawal is assumed to be similar to that of subjects from the reference treatment arm who have similar baseline characteristics (see Figure 7.5). This assumption therefore ignores any mean improvement in health that subjects may have gained due to experimental treatment up to the time of withdrawal. This strategy

```
PROC MI DATA=monotone OUT=imputedctrl NIMPUTE=1 SEED=34535499;
  BY _imputation_;
  VAR trt base_upd upd_1-upd_8;
  CLASS TRT;
  MONOTONE REG(upd_1=trt base_upd);
  MONOTONE REG(upd_2=trt base_upd upd_1 trt*upd_1);
  MONOTONE REG(upd_3=trt base_upd upd_1 trt*upd_1
                                   upd_2 trt*upd_2);
  MONOTONE REG(upd_4=trt base_upd upd_1 trt*upd_1
                                   upd_2 trt*upd_2
                                   upd_3 trt*upd_3);
  MONOTONE REG(upd_5=trt base_upd upd_1 trt*upd_1
                                   upd_2 trt*upd_2
                                   upd_3 trt*upd_3
                                   upd_4 trt*upd_4);
  MONOTONE REG(upd_6=trt base_upd upd_1 trt*upd_1
                                   upd_2 trt*upd_2
                                   upd_3 trt*upd_3
                                   upd_4 trt*upd_4
                                   upd_5 trt*upd_5);
  MONOTONE REG(upd_7=trt base_upd upd_1 trt*upd_1
                                   upd_2 trt*upd_2
                                   upd_3 trt*upd_3
                                   upd_4 trt*upd_4
                                   upd_5 trt*upd_5
                                   upd_6 trt*upd_6);
  MONOTONE REG(upd_8=trt base_upd upd_1 trt*upd_1
                                   upd_2 trt*upd_2
                                   upd_3 trt*upd_3
                                   upd_4 trt*upd_4
                                   upd_5 trt*upd_5
                                   upd_6 trt*upd_6
                                   upd_7 trt*upd_7);
RUN;

* create file for first run of J2R;
DATA strtimp1;
  SET monotone;
RUN;
```

SAS Code Fragment 7.10   Create dataset with missing values for reference treatment imputed assuming MAR, as preparation for J2R. (*Continued*)

may be appropriate where historic data suggest that patients who discontinue from the experimental treatment are likely to have an immediate worsening of outcomes. The "jump to reference" strategy may also be appropriate for subjects who discontinue from the experimental arm due to adverse events/drug toxicity, where it may

```
* select data for imputation of Visit 1;
DATA impute1 rest1;
   SET strtimp1;
   * Put to one side subjects from experimental arm (trt=2) that
have data at time point &visit;
   IF trt = 2 and LASTVIS >=&visit
   THEN
      OUTPUT rest1;
   * Select all other subjects for the time point &visit
imputation step;
   ELSE
      OUTPUT impute1;
RUN;


* impute Visit 1;
PROC MI DATA=impute1 OUT=imputed1 NIMPUTE=1 SEED=34535499;
   BY _Imputation_;
   VAR base_upd upd_1;
   monotone regression(upd_1 = base_upd);
RUN;


* re-assemble data for imputation of next visit;
DATA strtimp2;
   SET rest1 imputed1;
RUN;
PROC SORT DATA=strtimp2;
   BY _imputation_;
RUN;
```

SAS Code Fragment 7.10   (*Continued*)

be unreasonable to attribute any (even partial) benefit to the experimental treatment for subjects that clearly cannot complete the entire course of treatment. In some therapeutic areas, a BOCF method has sometimes been recommended for this purpose. However, BOCF cannot account for a trial (placebo) effect and the natural course of disease, to follow which would be more clinically plausible for many indications than a simple return to baseline severity. The "jump to control" assumption, on the other hand would allow the analyst to do so, while ignoring any positive effect of an incomplete experimental treatment that the subject was not able to tolerate.

As noted, sequential modeling can implement a "jump to control" assumption using an algorithm very similar to the one in the previous section, but with an MI step that models missing visits for the experimental arm with baseline covariables only. To implement the assumption, first impute the control arm using a standard MAR-based MI. SAS Code Fragment 7.10 will do this for the PD example dataset, using as input the same monotone dataset with which we started the previous algorithm. Note that, as in SAS Code Fragment 7.5, an interaction with treatment group (*trt*) is included at each visit, so the MAR here assumes that the correlations across visits may differ by treatment group.

Imputation of subsequent visits can be illustrated by SAS Code Fragment 7.11 for Visit 2:

```
* select data for imputation of Visit 2;
DATA impute2 rest2;
   SET strtimp2;
   * Put to one side subjects from experimental arm (trt=2) that
have data at time point &visit;
   IF trt = 2 and LASTVIS <=&visit
   THEN
      OUTPUT rest2;
   * Select all other subjects for the time point &visit
imputation step;
   ELSE
      OUTPUT impute2;
RUN;

* impute Visit 2;
PROC MI DATA=impute2 OUT= imputed2 NIMPUTE=1 SEED=34535499;
   BY _imputation_;
   VAR base_upd upd_2;
   monotone regression(upd_2 = base_upd);
RUN;
```

SAS Code Fragment 7.11   Impute distribution of control to Visit 2 value in experimental arm with baseline as the only covariable.

Only baseline values *base_upd* are used in the model as explanatory variable to impute Visit 2 values; values from Visit 1 (*upd_1*) are not used in this method. The PROC MI step for other visits will be similar, with for example, "*upd_j*" replacing "*upd_2*" for Visit *j*.

Figure 7.8 shows the means of imputed values for study withdrawals in each treatment arm over time under the MAR assumption and when "jump to reference" is assumed. A comparison with Figure 7.7 shows that the difference between the estimates is small. Recall that a withdrawal's outcomes are very likely poor, and may not be much better than those of the control arm. The sequential modeling implementation of "jump to reference" ignores such poor post-baseline outcomes. It may be seen that the change from poor outcomes in the experimental arm to outcomes close to the mean of the control arm may not always be such a very harsh or conservative one. See Section 7.3.5 for a discussion of the relative harshness of imputing the correlations of the control group (Figure 7.2) compared with imputing the distribution of the control group (Figure 7.5).

Table 7.3 shows that, for the illustrative PD dataset, when experimental arm imputations have the distribution of the control arm, (Figure 7.5), the treatment difference estimate is slightly smaller than that of MAR. The estimate becomes smaller when

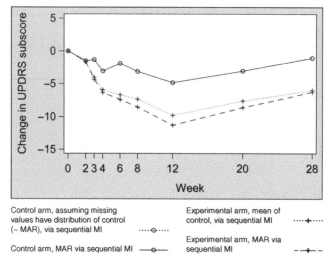

Control arm, assuming missing
values have distribution of control
(~ MAR), via sequential MI   ····◇····

Control arm, MAR via sequential MI   ——◇——

Experimental arm, mean of
control, via sequential MI   ····+····

Experimental arm, MAR via
sequential MI   –—+—–

Figure 7.8   Mean change from baseline in UPDRS score, assuming MAR versus assuming missings have distribution of the control arm. The lines for control overlap.

we assume that the correlations of control pertain, (Figure 7.2), and are smallest for the joint-modeling J2R assumption of Figure 7.4. However we emphasize that, while a sensitivity analysis should in some sense stress test the assumptions of the primary analysis, clinical plausibility rather than degree of harshness to the experimental arm should guide the strategy for missing data. If a control-based assumption seems to suit the trial and indication, the analyst and clinician should aim to select the control-based assumption that makes clinical sense be it CIR, CR, J2R with sequential modeling, or J2R with joint modeling. Appendix 7.B also includes a sample call to macros

Table 7.3   Estimates of the treatment difference in UPDRS for a variety of assumptions.

Analysis	Treatment difference, LSMEANS estimate	Standard error	p-value	95% CI, lower	95% CI, upper
MAR, sequential modeling	−4.7	2.6	0.0657	−9.7	0.31
Trajectory of control (~"CR"), sequential modeling	−3.7	2.5	0.1327	−8.7	1.1
"Jump to control," sequential modeling	−4.4	2.6	0.0893	9.4	0.67
"Jump to control," joint modeling	−2.8	2.4	0.2333	−7.4	1.8

available from the DIA web page on missingdata.org.uk, one call to the macro due to Ratitch (2012a) that implements a sequential modeling analysis identical to the one assuming that experimental arm withdrawals have correlations of the control group above, and one to the macro due to Roger (2012) that implements the analysis via joint modeling.

See Appendix 7.B for a sample call of the macro due to Roger (2012) available from DIA web page on missingdata.org.uk that implements the "J2R" analysis via joint modeling; with, in addition, a macro (also due to Roger and available from the same web site) to plot the results.

7.4.4   Baseline-observation-carried-forward-like and last-observation-carried-forward-like analyses

If it is clinically plausible to assume that withdrawals revert to their baseline disease severity after treatment discontinuation (as could be the case, for example, in chronic diseases), the subject's own baseline can of course be used to impute the missing values. We have noted in Section 1.4 that an objection to using such a single imputation is that it fails to reflect the uncertainty of the missing data. However, it is possible to use a pattern-mixture model to implement via MI the assumption that, after withdrawal, a subject's outcome reverts to a *distribution* similar to baseline values of the primary efficacy measure of the trial population. We can model baseline distribution using as covariates, for example, demographic variables such as age, sex, medical history and the baseline values of other disease-related variables. Then we assume that a baseline value estimated for a subject by this model can be used to impute a missing post-withdrawal outcome. The use of MI allows this BOCF-like method to reflect the variability inherent in the distribution of baseline values, and thus overcomes the objection noted in Section 1.4 to single BOCF imputation, namely that it may underestimate variance.

We will implement this analysis for the illustrative insomnia dataset – see Section 1.10 for a description. Recall that the insomnia dataset has three measures of efficacy. The primary efficacy variable of interest is total sleep time (tst) measured in minutes. The other two measures are a sleep quality score (sqs, range 1–10 with higher score indicating better quality sleep) and a score for morning sleepiness (mss, also range 0–10 with higher score indicating more sleepiness). Along with the observed baseline tst values, the baseline sqs and mss variables can be used to help impute a set of baseline-distributed tst values for each subject with missing post-baseline TST outcome. We do not have such variables as age, sex, time since diagnosis and medical history (e.g., presence of comorbid depression) in our dataset, but they might also be good candidates to use as covariates if available.

Insomnia is expected to improve over time. With such an indication, BOCF would be expected to "penalize" to an important degree treatments that lead to early withdrawal, since a subject's baseline can be expected often to be their worst score. Such penalizing may be most appropriate for a treatment with side effects that lead to discontinuation. While not necessarily reflecting true efficacy score and natural disease trajectory at the end of the trial for an indication such as insomnia,

```
* BOCF-like analysis;
* step 1. Impute control group (trt=1) assuming MAR;
* use all records for this imputation -
  but the imputations will only be used for the control group;
*ods Listing close;
* assumes baseline is always observed;
PROC MI DATA=monotone OUT=imputedmar NIMPUTE=1 SEED=883960001;
    BY _imputation_;
    VAR trt base_mss base_sqs base_tst tst_1 mss_1 tst_2 mss_2 tst_3
mss_3 tst_4 mss_4 tst_5 mss_5;
  CLASS trt;
  MONOTONE REG(tst_1=trt base_mss base_sqs base_tst);
  MONOTONE REG(mss_1=trt base_mss base_sqs base_tst
  tst_1 trt*tst_1);
  MONOTONE REG(tst_2=trt base_mss base_sqs base_tst
  tst_1 trt*tst_1 mss_1 trt*mss_1);
  MONOTONE REG(mss_2=trt base_mss base_sqs base_tst
  tst_1 trt*tst_1 mss_1 trt*mss_1
  tst_2 trt*tst_2);
  MONOTONE REG(tst_3=trt base_mss base_sqs base_tst
  tst_1 trt*tst_1 mss_1 trt*mss_1
  tst_2 trt*tst_2 mss_2 trt*mss_2);
  MONOTONE REG(mss_3=trt base_mss base_sqs base_tst
  tst_1 trt*tst_1 mss_1 trt*mss_1
  tst_2 trt*tst_2 mss_2 trt*mss_2
  tst_3 trt*tst_3);
  MONOTONE REG(tst_4=trt base_mss base_sqs base_tst
  tst_1 trt*tst_1 mss_1 trt*mss_1
  tst_2 trt*tst_2 mss_2 trt*mss_2
  tst_3 trt*tst_3 mss_3 trt*mss_3);
  MONOTONE REG(mss_4=trt base_mss base_sqs base_tst
  tst_1 trt*tst_1 mss_1 trt*mss_1
  tst_2 trt*tst_2 mss_2 trt*mss_2
  tst_3 trt*tst_3 mss_3 trt*mss_3
  tst_4 trt*tst_4);
  MONOTONE REG(tst_5=trt base_mss base_sqs base_tst
  tst_1 trt*tst_1 mss_1 trt*mss_1
  tst_2 trt*tst_2 mss_2 trt*mss_2
  tst_3 trt*tst_3 mss_3 trt*mss_3
  tst_4 trt*tst_4 mss_4 trt*mss_4);
  MONOTONE REG(mss_5=trt base_mss base_sqs base_tst
  tst_1 trt*tst_1 mss_1 trt*mss_1
  tst_2 trt*tst_2 mss_2 trt*mss_2
  tst_3 trt*tst_3 mss_3 trt*mss_3
  tst_4 trt*tst_4 mss_4 trt*mss_4
  tst_5 trt*tst_5);
RUN;
```

SAS Code Fragment 7.12   Perform the MI assuming MAR for the control arm.

```
ODS LISTING;

* only use the MAR imputed values for the control group (trt=1):
restore missings in the experimental arm;
DATA strtimp1;
   SET monotone(WHERE=(trt=2))
       imputedmar(WHERE=(trt=1));
RUN;
proc sort data=STRTIMP1;
  by _Imputation_ subjid;
run;
```

SAS Code Fragment 7.12 (*Continued*)

```
* step 2. Create a temporary input dataset that contains records with
  observed baseline values that  will be used to estimate the
  imputation model, and records that will receive imputed values;
DATA imputebl; SET strtimp1;
  LENGTH subjid_ $10;
  subjid_=subjid;

  * Create new variables with baseline values that will be used on
    the left-hand side of the imputation model specification in
    PROC MI;
  * Create records with non-missing baseline values to be used for
    estimation of the imputation model;
  ibase_tst=base_tst;
  OUTPUT;

   * Create records with missing values of the newly created
     variables corresponding to each time point that has
     missing value for discontinued subjects. They will be
     imputed by PROC MI. On these records, subject number is
     transformed with a concatenation of a number
     representing a time point that needs to be imputed;
  * for testing, make it BOC for all trt=2;
  IF trt = 2 AND lastvis < 5
  THEN
  DO;
     DO I=(lastvis+1) TO 5;
        subjid_=TRIM(LEFT(subjid)) || "_" || PUT(I,1.0);
        ibase_tst=.;
        OUTPUT;
     END;
  END;
RUN;
```

SAS Code Fragment 7.13   Prepare to model the distribution of baseline values for
BOCF-like imputation.

this approach can be regarded as facilitating a kind of risk-benefit assessment (see Section 4.2.2.3 on how regulators can favor BOCF). On the other hand, the assumption of reverting to baseline severity is most clinically plausible for chronic diseases where treatment is intended to relieve the symptoms only while it is being taken.

LOCF is an assumption that is rarely clinically plausible. Nevertheless, some have regarded it as useful for indications that tend to improve over time – for such indications, LOCF tends to penalize the treatment group with earlier or more frequent withdrawals. However, in cases where an LOCF-like or BOCF-like method would be applied in both treatment arms (and not just the experimental arm), the relative proportions of withdrawals in the two arms need to be taken into consideration – as discussed in Section 4.2.2.3 these methods may introduce bias in favor of experimental treatment if the proportion of withdrawals is larger in the control arm for indications that naturally improve with time. For trials where BOCF or LOCF assumptions are reasonable, these assumptions can be implemented using MI in a more statistically principled way compared to their single-imputation variants.

We show here example SAS code fragments to indicate how BOCF can be implemented using MI. We will then show how the LOCF assumption can be implemented similarly.

A complete SAS macro code to apply LOCF-like analysis to a dataset similar to the insomnia dataset is given in Appendix 7.C.

As before, we assume that the dataset has been rendered monotone missing, and is called *monotone*.

Control arm missing data will be imputed assuming MAR (SAS Code Fragment 7.12), while the experimental arm will be imputed assuming BOCF-like values. The MAR imputation should be done as normal, as if no BOCF imputation was planned. As before, interactions between treatment group and result at each visit are included, and it is thus assumed that correlations across visits may differ by treatment group. All data should be included in the MAR imputation of the control arm, including the experimental arm. The MAR imputations for the experimental arm will not be used.

We will use study baseline values to model the distribution of baseline values that will be carried forward for selected withdrawals (SAS Code Fragment 7.12). Note that we here select all withdrawals from the experimental arm ("IF $trt = 2$ AND $lastvis < 5$"), but we could, for example, impose BOCF only on subjects from the experimental arm who withdrew due to an adverse event (AE). We show an example of the use of such a restriction in SAS Code Fragment 7.20 below.

In Table 7.4 we can see how the data step in SAS Code Fragment 7.13 creates extra records with a blank *ibase_tst* for selected subjects. Extra records can be distinguished by a value for the working variable i which indexes the visit for which imputed value is needed, and the presence of "_i" at the end of *subjid_* variable. Extra records are created only for subjects from the experimental treatment group ($trt=2$) and correspond to their missed visits.

The "*ibase_tst*" variables in the *imputebl* dataset contain baseline values from those observed in the trial, but we have also made some records with values of the "*ibase_tst*" variables missing (one record per missing time point for discontinuing subjects). The records with missing "*ibase_tst*" values will now be imputed for later use as filled-in post-withdrawal values.

Table 7.4   Sample of typical records and variables from *imputebl* dataset after SAS Code Fragment 7.13.

subjid	subjid_	trt	lastvis	i	base_tst	ibase_tst
1	1	1	3	.	303	303
2	2	2	4	.	233	233
2	2_5	2	4	5	233	.
3	1	1	2	.	190	190
4	4	2	2	.	360	360
4	4_3	2	2	3	360	.
4	4_4	2	2	4	360	.
4	4_5	2	2	5	360	.

Subjects who withdraw have as many records with filled-in *ibase_tst* pseudo-baselines as they have post-baseline visits to be imputed (SAS Code Fragment 7.14). Using PROC TRANSPOSE, we convert the imputed baseline-distributed variables into imputations for the required number of missing post-baseline visits for each subject (SAS Code Fragment 7.15).

```
* step 3. Call PROC MI to impute baseline-distributed values;
PROC MI DATA=imputebl OUT=imputedbl NIMPUTE=1 SEED=883960001;
     BY _imputation_;
     VAR base_mss base_sqs agegrp sex ibase_tst;
     CLASS agegrp sex;
   * Model for the distribution of baseline MSS scores;
     MONOTONE REGRESSION(ibase_tst = agegrp sex base_mss base_sqs);
RUN;
```

SAS Code Fragment 7.14   Impute baseline-like values for the subject visits with missing outcomes.

```
* From the output dataset imputedbl, isolate records imputed above
and store the imputed values in the variables representing
post-baseline visits;
PROC TRANSPOSE DATA=imputedbl(WHERE=(INDEX(subjid_, "_")>0))
OUT=imputedtst PREFIX=tst;
          BY _imputation_ subjid;
          * IMPUTED tst;
          VAR ibase_tst;
          ID i;
RUN;
```

SAS Code Fragment 7.15   Transpose imputed values to obtain a dataset with one record per subject with all imputed values for a subject on the same record.

```
* Step 4. Merge imputed tst totals scores with the original dataset;
DATA imputed;
  MERGE imputedbl(WHERE=(INDEX(subjid_,"_")=0))
       imputedtst
       ;
     BY _imputation_ subjid;

  * imputed values;
     ARRAY tsto(5) tst_1 - tst_5;
     * original post-baseline variables;
     ARRAY tst(5) tst1 - tst5;

     DO j=1 TO 5;
           IF tsto [j]=. THEN tsto[j]=tst[j];
     END;
RUN;
```

SAS Code Fragment 7.16   Use baseline-distributed values for imputing the subject visits with missing post-baseline assessments.

Replace missing values with the imputed baseline-like values (SAS Code Fragment 7.16).

Figure 7.9 shows the mean values for each treatment group and time point under the MAR assumption, and when it is assumed that for the experimental arm, withdrawals revert to a baseline-distributed value. As with the other plots in this chapter, the means are calculated from both the imputed and observed data. We have noted earlier that a joint modeling assumption such as "copy increment from reference"

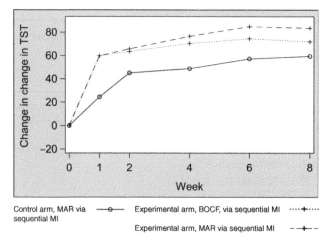

Figure 7.9   Mean change from baseline in TST for all subjects, assuming MAR versus assuming missing values in experimental arm revert to baseline-like values.

```
* select subjects whose last observation was on visit 1, and
use their visit 1 data to model all their future visits;
DATA imputeLV2 rest2; SET strtimp2;
  * only include subjects for whom this visit is their first
missing visit:
    such subjects model their own LOCF values best;
  IF lastvis NE 1
  THEN
    OUTPUT rest2;
  ELSE
    OUTPUT imputeLV2;
RUN;
```

SAS Code Fragment 7.17   Select subjects with last observation at Visit 1 to impute LOCF values for Visits 2, 3, 4 and 5 for these subjects.

cannot easily be implemented via sequential modeling. BOCF-like imputation may be an example where sequential modeling is more flexible than joint modeling.

The LOCF assumption can be implemented in a rather similar way using regression MI. SAS Code Fragments 7.12, 7.13, 7.14, 7.15 and 7.16 can be used almost unchanged, but must be implemented separately for each visit in the trial. In addition, for LOCF, subjects whose last observation was at a certain visit, and only those subjects, are used to model the distribution of values at that visit in order to use this distribution to sample LOCF-like values for subsequent missing visits. Note that if there are not many subjects discontinuing at a given visit, this may be problematic, and this restriction may be dropped. Provision should be made for this contingency in the SAP. Please see Appendix 7.C for a macro that programs all the steps to implement LOCF for the insomnia dataset. As an example, SAS Code Fragment 7.17 shows how subjects whose last observation was at Visit 1 are selected to model-imputed values for subsequent visits.

SAS Code Fragment 7.18 shows how to create last-observation-like imputed values, in a manner analogous to that for creating baseline-like imputed values shown in SAS Code Fragment 7.13.

The imputation step (SAS Code Fragment 7.19) differs slightly, in that post-baseline data up to the last observed visit may be used, whereas only baseline values could be used when implementing BOCF. SAS Code Fragment 7.18 indicates how the imputation step would differ from BOCF SAS Code Fragment 7.14 above, implementing LOCF to impute missing values of subjects who discontinued after Visit 1. In SAS Code Fragment 7.18, we call the values that will be used for LOCF "*itst_1*" in place of the "*ibase_tst*" used in the BOCF code. Just as we estimated the distribution of baseline values from which to draw samples of imputed values for later (post-baseline) visits, here we will estimate the distribution of Visit 1 values (last observed visit for subjects who discontinued after Visit 1) and use this distribution to draw samples for imputation of the subsequent missed visits (2, 3, 4 and 5), in keeping with the general idea of LOCF.

```
* for each subject, create extra records with missing observations;
DATA imputeLV2;
    SET imputeLV2;
    LENGTH subjid_ $10;
    subjid_=subjid;

    * create the variable that will be the response in the model
      of the last observation that is to be carried forward;
    itst=tst_1;
    OUTPUT imputeLV&visit;

    * Create records with missing values, one for every missing tst
      for the subjects who withdrew early due to AE ;
    IF lastvis=1
    THEN
        DO;
            DO ivisit=2 TO 5;
                subjid_=TRIM(LEFT(subjid))|| "_" || PUT(ivisit,1.0);
                itst=.;
                OUTPUT imputeLV2;
            END;
        END;
RUN;
```

SAS Code Fragment 7.18   Create LOCF-like values for subjects whose last observation was at Visit 1.

The "*itst_1*" variables in the *imputelv2* dataset have Visit 1 values from those observed in the trial (from which the imputation model will be estimated), but we have also added some records with missing values of "*itst_1*" variables. The records with missing "*itst_1*" values will now be imputed for later use as last observation-distributed values for missing visits of those subjects who discontinued after Visit 1.

```
* Call PROC MI to impute missing data using dataset imputeLV2 as
input. Age, sex, MDD type, and baseline, as well as values prior to
the last visit are used as model effects;
PROC MI DATA=imputeLV2 OUT=imputedLV2 NIMPUTE=1 SEED=&seed;
      BY _imputation_;
      CLASS agegrp sex trt;
      VAR trt agegrp sex base_sqs base_mss tst_0 itst;

      MONOTONE REGRESSION(itst = trt agegrp sex base_sqs base_mss
tst_0 trt*tst_0);
RUN;
```

SAS Code Fragment 7.19   Imputing last observation-distributed values, adapting the code from SAS Code Fragment 7.14.

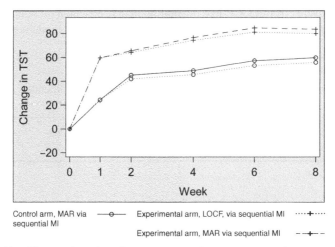

Figure 7.10   Change from baseline in mean TST, assuming MAR versus assuming LOCF-like values.

Figure 7.10 shows the mean imputed values for each treatment group and time point under the MAR assumption, and when it is assumed that, for both treatment groups, withdrawals are distributed as the last observed value for a similar subject in their treatment arm (similar based on baseline values and previous post-baseline assessments, and the fact they discontinued at the same time). As noted above, sequential modeling imputes LOCF values first for subjects who withdraw at Visit 1, then in a separate sequence of steps for those who withdraw at Visit 2 and so on.

In this case the assumption of LOCF produces poorer results for both treatment groups, compared to the MAR assumption.

The joint modeling macro package at www.missingdata.org.uk (Roger, 2012) implements LOCF using MI with joint modeling. The macro offers the choice of carrying forward observations drawn from a distribution whose mean is that of

- the withdrawer's at the last observed time point, – own last mean carried forward (OLMCF), or

- all subjects in the withdrawer's treatment group at the last observed time point for that subject – average last mean carried forward (ALMCF).

The SAS code for LOCF-like sequential modeling above (and in full in the appendix) models the subject's own mean at the last observed visit. The term "own mean" in this case represents a mean value adjusted for subject's covariables. The code uses baseline and previous post-baseline variables to do this. The above SAS code therefore implements an assumption similar to that of OLMCF. The standard error (SE) of the treatment difference is somewhat larger for the sequential method, probably because the models in sequential approach here are estimated on subsets of subjects (those that discontinued at a given visit), while the joint modeling approach uses all subjects to estimate parameters. As expected, the point estimates are similar – see Table 7.5.

Table 7.5   Results from LOCF-like imputation using sequential modeling approach for total sleep time (*tst*) as in Appendix 7.C, and from the joint modeling approach of Roger.

MI method	Treatment difference	SE of difference	*p*-value	Lower confidence limit	Upper confidence limit
Sequential modeling	19.7	7.5	0.0084	9.8	32.5
Joint modeling	19.9	6.4	0.002	7.3	37.2

SE, standard error.

7.4.5   The general principle of using selected subsets of observed data as the basis to implement "what if" stress tests

The approach illustrated in Sections 7.4.3 and 7.4.4 above can be modified and extended to implement other assumptions. Thus instead of baseline values (SAS Code Fragment 7.14) or last observed values (SAS Code Fragment 7.19), values from any chosen visit and/or subject subgroup may be modeled, and then imputations from this estimated model may be used in place of missing values for any other chosen visit, treatment group or otherwise defined subgroup of missing data. In a similar way, the joint modeling approach allows one to create desired functions of model parameters from any selected visit and treatment group to impute the values for any selected group of withdrawals. As noted, Roger's macro (Roger, 2012) implements this by allowing the user to "write their own" imputation method, using functions of the model parameters associated with study visits.

7.4.6   Using a mixture of "what ifs," depending on reason for discontinuation

In SAS Code Fragments 7.15 and 7.16 we selected all subjects from the experimental treatment arm (*trt* = 2) who did not complete the study (*lastvis* < 5), and implemented BOCF-like imputation for these subjects. We could have selected a different subset of subjects to be imputed in this particular way, simply by having a different IF-clause in SAS Code Fragment 7.13. SAS Code Fragment 7.20 shows how SAS Code Fragment 7.13 of the code implementing BOCF-like MI could be amended for example, to impute baseline-distributed value only for subjects who withdrew due to an adverse event.

Regulators sometimes require that BOCF be applied for all missing values in the experimental arm, or to selected missing values only. Code such as that in SAS Code Fragment 7.20 can be used to apply BOCF-like values to any subset of subjects, and has the advantage that the MI can reflect the uncertainty inherent in the missing data, thus avoiding the usual underestimation of variance associated with single-imputation BOCF. Sometimes it is judged clinically reasonable to apply BOCF to all treatment groups (control and experimental arms), and this is also straightforward to implement,

```
* Create new variables with baseline values that will be used on
  the left-hand side of the imputation model specification in
  PROC MI;
* Create records with non-missing baseline values to be used for
  estimation of the imputation model;
ibase_tst=base_tst;
OUTPUT;

* Create records with missing values of the newly created
  variables corresponding to each time point that has
  missing value for discontinued subjects. They will be
  imputed by PROC MI. On these records, subject number is
  transformed with a concatenation of a number
  representing a time point that needs to be imputed.;
* for testing, make it BOC for all trt=2;
 IF trt = 2 & reasond = "AE" AND lastvis < 5
   THEN
   DO;
     DO I=(lastvis+1) TO 5;
        subjid_=TRIM(LEFT(subjid))|| "_" || PUT(I,1.0);
        ibase_tst=.;
        OUTPUT;
     END;
  END;
RUN;
```

SAS Code Fragment 7.20 Imputing baseline-like values for subjects with reason for discontinuation = "AE."

by selecting all subjects with *lastvis* < 5 in SAS Code Fragment 7.13. BOCF may of course be judged as unlikely to favor the experimental treatment arm when, for example, it is expected that a higher proportion of subjects will withdraw early from the experimental arm, compared to the control arm.

More generally, clinicians and patients, as well as regulators, may find it plausible to assume different efficacy trajectories for withdrawals, depending on the reason for withdrawal with, for example, worse trajectory assumed for those who withdrew due to AE or due to lack of efficacy. We discussed in Chapter 4 that the approach of having a mixture of assumptions, depending on reason for discontinuation, seemed attractive for all three of our example trials. The code fragments above may be used in combination with little alteration to allow a variety of assumptions, depending on a subject's reason for discontinuation. We adopt this approach later for our illustrative PD dataset and provide code to implement that analysis in Appendix 7.F. A "by reason" approach can also be implemented using the joint modeling macro due to Roger (2012) – the assumption about missing values may be indicated at the level of subject using a special input variable *MethodV*.

The particular assumptions adopted for each type of discontinuation – BOCF, control-based values, LOCF and others, should be decided in advance in consultation with clinicians and in the light of historic data. The next section describes a final example – delta adjustment – of how MI can be used flexibly to impose assumptions about withdrawals. This delta-adjusting kind of assumption could also be applied selectively to certain types of withdrawal, if desired.

7.4.7   Assuming trajectory of withdrawals is worse by some δ: Delta adjustment and tipping point analysis

This section and Section 7.4.9 below are adapted from Ratitch *et al.* (2013).

Another sensitivity analysis that is quite broadly applicable imposes the assumption that subjects from the experimental treatment arm who discontinue at a given time point would, on average, have their unobserved efficacy score worse by some amount δ compared to the observed efficacy score of subjects that continue to the next time point, or indeed compared to any other supposed trajectory. Delta adjustment may form part of the assumption for all treatment groups, or may be used to "penalize" the experimental arm(s) only.

The NRC report on missing data (National Research Council, 2010) recommended delta adjustment as an informative sensitivity analysis. We note that the delta adjustment sensitivity analysis is a particularly useful approach when a trial has no control arm (and therefore control-based imputation is not an option), such as single-arm phase II oncology trials. More generally, delta adjustment can be useful when the primary alternative hypothesis is not superiority of the experimental arm. For example, in non-inferiority trials, assuming that withdrawals from both arms are similar (as is the case in the control-based method) would create bias in favor of demonstrating equivalence of the two treatments and would not be conservative. If the control arm can be reasonably expected to be at least as good as the experimental arm, then imputation based on the control arm could actually favor the experimental arm. It is clear that control-based imputation, which can often provide a plausible stress test of the conclusions of the trial, cannot do so in such a case. Delta adjustment can then usually provide a useful stress test.

We shall see that a series of delta adjustments of increasing severity can give information that helps the reader of the study report to assess the credibility of the result. But delta adjustment can also be used as a stand-alone analysis method if a specific δ of interest can be identified in advance based on some clinical justification.

Three variants are currently used to apply the delta adjustment. In the first, as described in the NRC report (National Research Council, 2010) and as clarified by Roderick Little in a private communication, the δ is applied just once, at the first visit that has missing data for each subject. An imputed δ-adjusted value at time point j is then used to calculate the subject's residual for the imputation of subsequent time points along with other variables (e.g., baseline) that might explain future values. This method matches the single event of dropping out with a single worsening (delta adjustment); the worsening imposed at this time point affects subsequent time points only via the correlations between visits that are estimated in the imputation model. Since the imputation model is estimated from the data of subjects who remained on study, the assumption of this analysis is that the future values of the discontinued subject (after the one-time delta adjustment) would resemble the outcomes of study completers who had a similar trajectory prior to the subject's discontinuation visit and a similar one-time worsening in the course of the study.

A second variation applies δ at each visit, from withdrawal up to the end of the trial, in addition to using previously delta-adjusted values to calculate a subject's residual as described in the previous paragraph. It explicitly enforces an assumption that the discontinuation is associated with worsening that persists throughout subsequent time points (and that the outcomes of withdrawals are persistently different from those of study completers) and does not rely exclusively on the estimated correlation between time points embedded in the imputation model in order to propagate the effect of δ through time.

Note that the effect on future missing values of these single or repeated impositions of worsening will depend on the imputation model used: if the model includes only one previous visit as predictor, the effect of any δ may be stronger, modeling worse values in the future, but if all previous visits are included as predictors, the effect may be weaker, if the subject had good scores prior to discontinuation. In all cases where δ-adjusted values are used in calculating a subject's residual for the imputation of later missing values, the strength of the effect of δ will depend in part on the correlations between time points.

The above two approaches are implemented by the macro due to Ratitch (2012b) that implements sequential modeling with delta adjustment, available at www.missingdata.org.uk.

A third approach imputes all values (all time points) using an MAR-based method and only then applies delta adjustments. In this case, the value of δ can, if clinically appropriate, be increased at each time point after withdrawal to impose a steady worsening as described in the second variation above. This method does not use delta-adjusted values at earlier visits as explanatory variables in the imputation model of the subsequent visits. This third method can be useful if it is desired to impose a fixed and definite set of quantities to encapsulate the change in efficacy associated with withdrawal. For example, a fixed delta adjustment could be used to impose a mean worsening over time that was observed in withdrawals in particular historic data. This variation is described in Carpenter and Kenward (2007, pp. 174–7) and Carpenter *et al.* (2013). This is the approach implemented by Roger's macro at www.missingdata.org.uk (Roger, 2012).

In practice, for delta adjustment via sequential MI, one first imputes a given visit under a "base" assumption then applies the delta adjustment to the imputed value at that visit prior to proceeding with the imputation of the subsequent visit. The base assumption is often MAR, and the delta adjustment is therefore applied to imputations after MAR imputation. Note that a control-based, LOCF-like or other assumption may be judged clinically plausible, rather than MAR. After a "base" assumption has been imputed, the imputed values are then worsened by a planned value δ. The direction of worsening (addition or subtraction of δ) would be determined by the nature of the efficacy endpoint. This would reflect the assumption that the experimental arm dropouts are doing worse than is assumed by the "base" assumption.

Often a satisfactory single fixed δ cannot be identified a priori, and a succession of δ adjustments may be applied. This so-called "tipping point" strategy has been suggested in the literature (Yan *et al.*, 2009) for analysis of both continuous and categorical outcomes with missing data. Tipping point analysis is a means of exploring the influence of missingness on the overall conclusion from statistical inference by positing a wide range of assumptions regarding the missingness mechanism (from less conservative to more conservative). The analysis finds a (tipping) point in this spectrum of assumptions, at which conclusions change from being favorable to the experimental treatment to being unfavorable or inconclusive. After such a tipping point is determined, clinical judgment can be applied as to the plausibility of the assumptions underlying this tipping point (in particular, concerning the plausibility of the δ value corresponding to the tipping point). This methodology would provide the regulators with a good picture of what it would take to overturn trial conclusions based on varying assumptions about missing data.

In the following example we apply delta adjustment to the dataset illustrative of a trial in mania.

7.4.7.1   Illustrative dataset for a clinical trial in mania

Data in this section have been patterned after typical clinical trials studying mania. Section 1.10.3 has a full description of the dataset, including definitions of the variables in the dataset. The dataset represents a large randomized, double-blind trial with 550 subjects in each of the two arms – the experimental treatment and a control treatment of lithium. Time points included in our example dataset represent study visits scheduled to occur prior to the commencement of the study treatment (referred to as baseline or Day 0), and then at post-baseline Days 4, 7, 14, 21 and 28. We have posited that the experimental arm in our illustrative trial is a treatment similar to valproate, with efficacy that is hoped to be somewhat better than lithium. The objective is to show superiority to the control treatment. In this case, the planned primary efficacy parameter is a binary responder variable derived from the Young Mania Rating Scale (YMRS). For the YMRS scale, lower scores are better. The primary test of the null hypothesis of no treatment difference in proportion of responders is at the Day 28 visit. For convenience, Tables 7.6 and 7.7 present summaries of discontinuation by reason and last observed visit.

Table 7.6   Reasons for discontinuation by treatment group for the mania dataset.

Reason for discontinuation	Experimental arm (%)	Control arm (%)
AE	3	1
Consent withdrawn	9	11
Decision of investigator	7	7
Lost to follow up	1	0
Other	4	11
Sponsor's request	1	0
Completed study	75	70

Table 7.7   Percentage of subjects remaining in the study after each visit.

Visit	Experimental arm (%)	Control arm (%)
Baseline	99	99
1	96	95
2	91	92
3	82	79
4	75	70

More subjects from the control arm discontinued early from the study, and the difference is mainly due to a markedly larger number of discontinuations with reason = "other" in that treatment group.

7.4.7.2   Implementing a delta adjustment

We show here examples of SAS code to indicate how delta adjustment can be implemented using sequential regression-based MI with selected trial data. Although the primary efficacy parameter for the mania trial was a binary response, we will first demonstrate delta adjustment on that trial's continuous YMRS score.

If the object is to stress test the MAR assumption, we might assume that the trajectory of withdrawals is close to that of apparent treatment failures in Figures 4.7 and 4.8 in Chapter 4. From Figure 4.7 we can calculate that in subjects who relapsed the mean increase (worsening) per week in YMRS from the time of relapse to the end of the fourth week (Lipkovich *et al.*, 2008) is about 2.8. Of the two non-responders in Figure 4.8 (Post *et al.*, 2005) one had an increase of about 1.2 per week and one of 4 per week in the YMRS scale. On the basis of these examples from the literature, given that it is unlikely that all withdrawals relapsed, a δ of 2.5 might be justified as a reasonable deviation from MAR that could stress test the MAR assumption. We apply $\delta = 2.5$ to each imputed visit after discontinuation here, in the experimental arm only.

SAS macro code to apply delta adjustment on a continuous outcome is available at the web page of the DIA SWG for missing data, on the www.missingdata.org.uk website as macro *delta_pmm* (Ratitch, 2012b). We will show template code here to demonstrate how delta adjustment may be applied straightforwardly in SAS.

As with other examples, we assume that the dataset has been rendered monotone missing, has one record per subject and is called *strtimp1*.

We first impute missing values for Visit 1 with a "base" assumption. As noted, this "base" assumption could be that withdrawals are modeled on similar subjects in the control arm. For simplicity we will assume MAR as the "base" assumption. This is implemented for Visit 1 in SAS Code Fragment 7.21.

The second step for the visit is to impose the delta adjustment as shown in SAS Code Fragment 7.22.

```
* Impute Visit 1 assuming MAR using regression-based MI;
PROC MI DATA=strtimp1 OUT=imputedmar1 NIMPUTE=1 SEED=34535499;
   BY _imputation_;
   VAR trt base_ymrs ymrs_1;
   MONOTONE REG(ymrs_1=trt base_ymrs);
RUN;
```

SAS Code Fragment 7.21 Imputing a base imputation before imposing a delta adjustment.

```
DATA strtimp2;
   SET imputedmar1;
   delta=0.56;
   IF lastvis = 0 AND trt=2
   THEN
      DO;
         ymrs_1 = ymrs_1 + delta;
      END;
RUN;
```

SAS Code Fragment 7.22 Adjust imputed value by an amount δ.

If it is desired to impose an unfavorable effect on the experimental treatment group for every visit after withdrawal, the above two steps are repeated for each subsequent visit, using values imputed and delta adjusted at one visit in calculating the residual of withdrawals so that the δ amount is reflected in the imputation of the next visit, via the between-visit correlation.

Figure 7.11 shows the difference in trend of the mean efficacy scores when an increase (worsening) in YMRS score of 2.5 is imposed at every visit after withdrawal. Under this, rather pessimistic, assumption that all withdrawals have a trajectory typical of treatment failures (relapsed subjects), the mean YMRS score for the experimental treatment group is considerably worsened and is much closer to the control group. Post-withdrawal outcomes were assumed to be MAR in the control arm. The treatment difference is now estimated as 1.6 (SE = 0.69, p = 0.0188), compared to 2.6 (SE = 6.8, p = 0.0001) under MAR.

We noted in Section 7.4.7 that Roger (2012) provides an implementation of the delta-adjustment method that imposes a δ after imputation at all visits is accomplished under MAR, and that this version could be useful if it were desired to impose a fixed worsening on imputed data. Roger's implementation could be useful here, where we have evidence of particular rates of worsening in relapsed subjects. SAS Code Fragment 7.23 shows how this can be done with the macro that implements MI with joint modeling (Roger, 2012). This code fragment uses *strtimp1* (dataset with a monotone missing pattern), as the previous fragment does.

Macro %Part1A checks parameters and sets up a master file for the job. Macro %Part1B uses PROC MCMC to in effect estimate the posterior distribution of MMRM

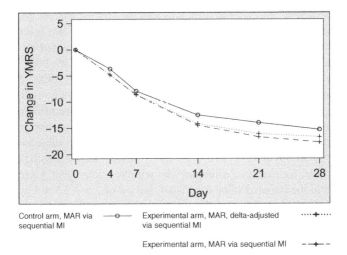

Control arm, MAR via sequential MI   —o—
Experimental arm, MAR, delta-adjusted via sequential MI   ····+····
Experimental arm, MAR via sequential MI   – –+– –

Figure 7.11   Change in mean YMRS, assuming MAR versus assuming an extra 2.5 worsening in YMRS at each visit for the experimental arm.

```
DATA strtimp1;
   SET strtimp1;
   * impose a delta for all subjects in treatment group 2;
   * do_delta is true (=1) when trt=2, false (zero) otherwise;
   do_delta=(trt=2);
run;

%part1A(Jobname=mania_GSK_delta, Data=strtimp1, Subject=subjid,
Response=ymrs, Time=visit, Treat=trt, cov=, catcov=,
covbytime=base_ymrs, catcovbytime=,
PEwhere=, ID=do_delta, covgroup=trt, debug=0);
%part1B(Jobname=mania_GSK_MAR, Ndraws=1000, thin=50, seed=34535499,
debug=0);
%part2A(Jobname=mania_GSK_MAR, Method=MAR, ref=1, debug=0)
%part2b(Jobname=mania_GSK_MAR, debug=0);

* then apply a delta to the MAR imputations;
%part3(Jobname=mania_GSK_delta, InName=mania_GSK_MAR, delta=2.5 2.5
2.5 2.5 2.5, DGroupsV=do_delta, debug=0);
PROC PRINT data=mania_GSK_delta_out;
   TITLE "Applying delta after all imputations ";
RUN;
```

SAS Code Fragment 7.23   Imposing a delta adjustment after all subjects have been imputed based on MAR assumption via MI with joint modeling as implemented by Roger.

regression coefficients and sample from it as specified by the analyst. Macro Part2A calculates the mean for each subject, once for each draw of the estimates of the regression coefficients. The calculation of the mean will be guided by the method specified in macro argument "method=" (the special variable *MethodV* can also be used). Macro Part2B calculates the imputations for the missing values. Macro Part3 performs a univariate analysis of imputed data by time point, applying Rubin's rules to provide an overall estimate of SAS LSMEANS estimates of the primary parameter scores for each treatment group, and the difference between treatment groups.

The macro argument DGroupsV allows the analyst to select subjects to whom to apply the δ. The default in this macro, used here, is to increase the δ with the time from withdrawal. Thus, for example, a subject who withdrew after Visit 3 would have a δ of 2.5 applied to the imputed value for Visit 4, but a δ of 2.5 + 2.5 = 5 applied to the imputed value for Visit 5. As noted, Roger's macro imposes the δ after the process of imputing all the missing data (at all study visits) is completed. This contrasts with the previous SAS Code Fragment 7.22, which imposes the δ after each individual visit is imputed, and does not increase the δ by time from withdrawal, but allows the δs imposed at successive visit to be "pulled through" and at least partially accumulated via the correlations between visits. The method implemented by Roger is "clean" in that the analyst can control the exact δ imposed at each visit. On the other hand, the method of SAS Code Fragment 7.22 can reflect the natural history of the indication by preserving the effect of previous δ adjustments, or allowing that effect to diminish over time, depending on the strength of the correlations found in the study. Generally, for a given δ (here 2.5) specified for each visit, Roger's implementation will impose a larger quantitative change than the method shown in SAS Code Fragment 7.22. Here, the method implemented by Roger results in an estimate of treatment difference at the final Visit 5 of -1.2 (SE 0.70, p = 0.0710), compared with an estimate from the *delta_pmm* macro of -1.6 (SE 0.69, p = 0.0188). The analyst should work closely with the clinician in deciding which of the approaches to delta adjustment makes sense for the indication, given the historic data available and given what is known about disease progression in the indication.

It is easy to implement a similar delta adjustment on a binary response. If a binary variable can be calculated from continuous variables, we recommend imputing the continuous variables and re-calculating the binary response from the imputed variables – Bunouf *et al.* (2012) give a nice example of this using pain data. This calculation of the binary response from imputed source variables is relatively straightforward to implement. However we want to show here how to deal with the more challenging case where the primary efficacy parameter is a binary one, with no direct source in a continuous variable or variables. For the purposes of the following example, therefore, and in the final section of this chapter also, we will assume that the responder (Y/N) variable is entered on the case report form (CRF) and cannot be calculated directly from other variables. For this somewhat artificial example, we will however assume that there is a related continuous baseline variable. Kenward and Carpenter (2013) note that, because of the invertible nature of the log odds, where explanatory variables are all observed and the model is correct, an estimate based on a binary response using only observed data are unbiased. Despite this, however, it may often be desired to improve the power of the analysis, by imputing based on partially observed binary responses, plus ancillary variables.

We note in passing a practical hurdle when imputing binary outcomes. When using logistic regression for imputation, as we do here, the analyst should be aware of a potential problem of perfect prediction. This does not happen with the following example, but can often be encountered in this setting. It may occur if the strata formed by the covariates included in the model form cells in which all available values of a dependent categorical variable are the same (e.g., available binary outcomes are all 0s or all 1s within a cell). This may result in the imputation model generating imputed values that are very different from observed ones (see Carpenter and Kenward (2013) for more details on this issue). In clinical trials, this may be more likely with the imputation of a binary responder status at earlier time points if achievement of response is not likely at the beginning of the study. Also, this may happen if covariates such as investigator site are included in the model, and there are sites with a relatively small number of subjects, all having the same response at a given time point. To deal with this potential problem, it is advisable to carry out a preliminary exploratory step by fitting logistic regression models to available data at each time point, for example, using PROC LOGISTIC, and carefully examining the resulting model parameters. PROC LOGISTIC will produce a warning of a "quasi-complete separation" in this case, and the analyst can subsequently modify the model by excluding or changing certain covariates to avoid this problem. Once the models have been appropriately selected for each time point, they can be specified in PROC MI by using a separate MONOTONE LOGISTIC statement with a distinct model for each variable.

For a binary response, the δ adjustment could consist of imposing an unfavorable or "non-responder" status on withdrawals with an extra pre-planned probability over and above that modeled by the MAR assumption. This is the assumption we implement here, imposing a 10% extra chance of being a treatment failure or "non-responder" over and above that assumed by MAR. Thus, for every 10 subjects imputed as responders under the MAR assumption, the delta adjustment randomly re-imputes about 1 subject to be a non-responder. (Note, of course, that some subjects may well be imputed as non-responders directly under MAR.)

We will illustrate the implementation of this approach using the mania example dataset. SAS code for the two steps for Visit 1 in the case of a binary response variable *resp_1* is given in SAS Code Fragment 7.24.

An example SAS macro to implement delta adjustment for this dataset is given in Appendix 7.D. The same procedure would be repeated for each visit where, as with the continuous outcome, responder status imputed and delta adjusted at one visit will be used in calculating a withdrawal's residual when imputing the next visit, and this will in turn influence that imputation via the between-visit correlations. Other ancillary variables can be added to the logistic model, and also delta adjusted if this is deemed clinically reasonable. The resulting proportions of responders imputed in the above case for all visits are shown in Figure 7.12.

As with the delta adjustment of the continuous efficacy score for this trial shown in Figure 7.7, this moderately conservative assumption makes a small but discernible impact on the results for the experimental arm.

```
* impute Visit 1 assuming MAR using logistic regression-based MI;
PROC MI DATA=strtimp1 OUT=imputedmar1 NIMPUTE=1 SEED=883960001;
   BY _imputation_;
   VAR trt base_ymrs resp_1;
   CLASS TRT resp_1;
   MONOTONE LOGISTIC(resp_1=trt base_ymrs);
RUN;


* Delta adjustment of a binary variable;
DATA strtimp2;
   SET imputedmar1;
   * Delta represents a probability of resetting imputed responder
     status to non-responder;
   delta=0.10;
   IF lastvis = 0 AND trt=2
   THEN DO;
      if ranuni(783)<delta
      then
         resp_1 = 0;
   END;
RUN;
```

SAS Code Fragment 7.24   Imposing an adjustment to imputed binary response with a probability δ.

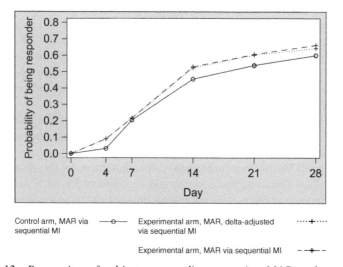

Figure 7.12   Proportion of subjects responding assuming MAR and assuming an extra 10% chance of treatment failure over and above MAR for withdrawals in the experimental arm.

Table 7.8   Mean number and percentage of responders calculated across 1000 imputed datasets after MAR imputation for the illustrative mania dataset, and with an assumption of an extra 10% chance of treatment failure over and above MAR for withdrawals in the experimental arm.

	Visit 1	Visit 2	Visit 3	Visit 4	Visit 5
Experimental arm, MAR	49 (9)	120 (21.8)	292 (53)	333 (60.6)	364 (66.2)
Experimental arm, with $\delta = 0.1$	49 (9)	119 (21.7)	289 (52.5)	331 (60.2)	354 (64.3)
Control arm, MAR	17 (3.1)	113 (20.5)	250 (45.5)	296 (54)	330 (60)

When withdrawals from the experimental arm are imputed to non-responders with 10% probability over and above that imputed by MAR, this results in 10 additional non-responders imputed for that arm (Table 7.8).

The effect of delta adjustment in this trial reflects the relatively high proportion of subjects who discontinued from the trial. We have noted in Section 4.2.3.3 that for indications where such a high proportion of discontinuations is expected, even a mild δ may lack clinical plausibility when applied to the entire experimental treatment group. For such indications, it may be more clinically plausible to impose a delta adjustment on a suitable subset of subjects, such as those who discontinued for reasons that suggest a poor outcome (e.g., "lack of efficacy," "AE," "subject's choice").

7.4.7.3   Implementing a "tipping point" sensitivity analysis

We have described in Section 7.4.7 how a "tipping point" analysis can stress test a result by imposing a succession of δ adjustments, each one more severe, until a positive trial conclusion is overturned. In this final "toolkit" example, we perform a "tipping point" analysis on the binary response. This is straightforward to implement. The SAS Code Fragment 7.25 simply runs the delta-adjustment macro given in Appendix 7.D for a succession of increasing amounts of worsening δ:

```
%MACRO run_tip(delta=, tipstep=, tipmaxiter=);
%let thisdelta=&delta;
%do tipiter=1 %to &tipmaxiter;
    %run_tdelta(delta=&&thisdelta);
    %let thisdelta=&&thisdelta + &tipstep;
%end;
%mend run_tip;

%run_tip(delta=0,tipstep=%left(0.05), tipmaxiter=4)
```

SAS Code Fragment 7.25   Call the *run_tdelta* macro repeatedly to implement a tipping point analysis.

The code in SAS Code Fragment 7.25 first performs an MAR analysis ($\delta = 0$), then implements successively harsher delta adjustments ($\delta = 0.05, 0.10, 0.15$). In practice, the progressively harsher delta adjustment will usually be continued until the p-value of the primary analysis (if significant) is rendered non-significant, where the level of significance is pre-defined.

For our example mania dataset, the proportions of responders resulting from δ values greater than 0 are plotted in Figure 7.13.

We can see that the imposition of an extra 15% chance of non-responder status for withdrawals, over and above that assumed by MAR, brings the result of the experimental arm quite close to that of the control arm.

In the later section on the mania dataset in this chapter, we shall see an example that illustrates the degree to which the results of statistical tests change as δ is increased to a "tipping point."

Code very similar to that of SAS Code Fragment 7.21 can be used to implement a "tipping point" analysis for a continuous variable, if used in conjunction with a macro similar to that in Appendix 7.D, applied to a continuous outcome.

SAS macros available at the DIA page of www.missingdata.org.uk (Ratitch, 2012b), implement both the delta adjustment and "tipping point" approaches for continuous outcomes and allows the user to specify the significance level stopping criterion or the maximum number of "tipping" iterations. If it is desired to use ancillary variables in the context of delta-adjustment and "tipping point" analyses, then we believe that it makes sense to make adjustments to all the post-baseline variables in the model that are consistent with the δ chosen. The Ratitch macros offer, in addition to the simple delta adjustment we show here, additional matching delta adjustment that could be applied to ancillary variables, both continuous and categorical.

Recall (Section 7.4.7) that one variant of delta adjustment imposes a δ visit-by-visit, using the adjusted imputed visit values as input to the model for future imputations at each visit after discontinuation; a second variant imposes a δ at a single visit (the first visit after discontinuation), and again uses the adjusted imputed values as input to the next visit, and through that visit to subsequent visits via model correlations. The Ratitch macros can be used to implement both of these variants of delta adjustment. If it is desired to implement the third variant of delta adjustment, which imposes δ after all imputation is completed under MAR, the macros by Roger at www.missingdata.co.uk can implement this variant (Roger, 2012).

For binary responses, another tipping point approach assesses scenarios where a given *number* of withdrawals are non-responders, rather than a proportion in excess of the MAR proportion. We have described this in Section 4.2.3.3 under the heading *Other MNAR approaches*. In practice, generally for this approach, every possible combination of response and non-response is considered for the missing values, and the primary null hypothesis is tested, for each of the many scenarios (Yan *et al.*, 2008). We have called this approach, *tipping point analysis via exhaustive scenarios*. It can be implemented by relatively simple SAS code. In Appendix 7.E, we include example code to implement it for the illustrative mania dataset. In Section 4.2.3.3 we suggested a variant of Yan *et al.*'s approach, which we call *tipping point analysis via deviation from imputed success*, where rather than an exhaustive set of scenarios for

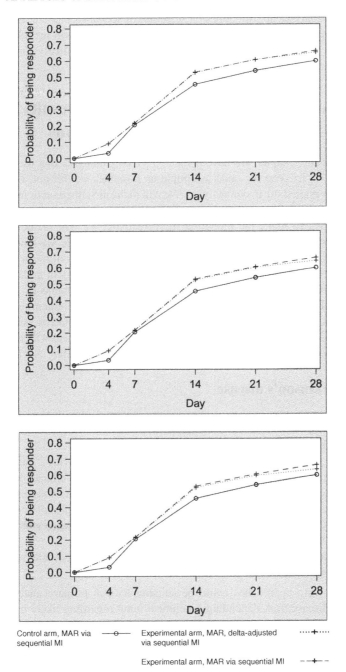

Figure 7.13 Proportion of subjects responding assuming MAR and assuming an extra 5%, 10% and 15% chance of treatment failure over and above MAR for withdrawals in the experimental arm.

withdrawals, analyses are run only of a selection of scenarios that are less favorable to the experimental arm than that of the primary analysis. We will include SAS code to implement this variant when we discuss below the strategy finally chosen for this illustrative mania dataset.

7.5 Examples of realistic strategies and results for illustrative datasets of three indications

Up to now in this chapter, we have presented MNAR analyses that used relatively simple models. To keep the code as simple as possible, we did not, for example, include site or pooled site in our analyses. We will in the next three sections implement for each of our three datasets approaches that might constitute a missing data strategy of a real study. To make the modeling more realistic, we will include covariates such as investigator/pooled site/country in the analyses. While we have presented the results of sensitivity analyses so far in the chapter via plots of mean values after imputations, we will now present the results almost completely in tables of means, confidence intervals and *p*-values. Rather than presenting fragments of "open" SAS code, we will in the upcoming sections refer to appendices containing SAS code, much of which consists of calls of sequential MI modeling macros available from www.missingdata.org.uk. These sequential modeling macros have, at their heart, code similar to the SAS code fragments presented up to now as building blocks.

7.5.1 Parkinson's disease

As a first illustration of how the principles of Chapter 4 may work out in practice using the methods of Chapters 5–7, we implement a sample strategy for the illustrative Parkinson's disease data.

As noted in the description of the PD dataset (Section 1.10.1), our illustrative trial has nine visits including a baseline visit, and its primary efficacy variable is a UPDRS sub-score represented by the variable *upd* when the dataset has one record per subject/visit or variables *base_upd* and *upd_1* . . . *upd_8* when the dataset is arranged with values for all visits in a single record per subject. The primary statistical test is at Visit 8.

Recall that in Section 4.2.3.1, we summarized potentially suitable strategies for our illustrative trial as follows:

The following approaches could be suitable for the primary analysis for the Parkinson's disease trial, depending on clinical input regarding likely outcomes for withdrawals:

- MAR approach implementable either via MI or MMRM;
- Control-based imputation for the experimental arm.

The following could be useful sensitivity analyses in this case:

- Control-based imputation for the experimental arm (if not used as primary);

- Assume a variety of outcomes for missing values, depending on reason for discontinuation;

- Tipping point analysis, using delta adjustment for subjects on experimental arm, increasing δ until primary conclusion is rejected.

If the experimental arm has notably more discontinuations than the control arm due to side effects, then the following analysis could be considered:

- Responder analysis imputing treatment failure for subjects with missing data.

From among these possibilities, we will implement the following strategy:

Primary analysis:

- MAR approach via MI with region and baseline as explanatory variables.

Sensitivity analyses, all using the same explanatory variables as the primary analysis, and implemented via sequential modeling:

- Control-based imputation for the experimental arm: assume that the experimental arm has visits correlated as for the control arm (i.e., has a trajectory similar to that of the control arm);

- Assume a variety of outcomes for missing values, depending on reason for discontinuation. In this analysis, for subjects in the experimental arm who withdraw due to AE, we will impose a δ (worsening) of 2 on the UPDRS sub-score to each MAR-imputed value at each visit. Other missing values will be imputed assuming MAR for both treatment groups;

- Tipping point analysis, using delta adjustment for all subjects on experimental arm, increasing δ until primary conclusion is nullified. Here, we will impose successively harsher δs on imputed values in the experimental arm, starting with a δ (worsening) of 1 on the UPDRS sub-score, and incrementing δ by 1 for four iterations or until the statistical significance of the hypothesis test is nullified (i.e., if $\delta > 4$ is needed for that);

- For reference purposes, an available cases analysis.

Appendix 4.A contains a sample protocol that describes and justifies the above strategy as it could be applied to our illustrative dataset, in particular the values of δ. All analyses will allow for separate estimation by treatment group of the between-visit correlation.

All the sensitivity analyses above can be implemented via macros available from the DIA page of www.missingdata.org.uk. SAS code to provide the planned sensitivity analyses, mostly consisting of calls to the www.missingdata.org.uk macros, is given in Appendix 7.F.

We will confine ourselves to hypothesis testing for the primary endpoint (change from baseline at Visit 8). Table 7.9 presents the results from the primary and sensitivity analyses. We also present the result from MMRM from Chapter 5 for reference.

Table 7.9   Results for PD example dataset, planned primary analysis and sensitivity analyses: least-squares means (LSMEANS) estimate of difference between treatments in change from baseline in UPDRS sub-score at Visit 8.

Analysis	Treatment difference, LSMEANS estimate	Standard error	95% CI, lower	upper	p-value
MAR (MI)	−5.1	2.5	−10	−0.4	0.0314
MAR (MMRM)	−4.9	2.3	−9.5	−0.2	0.0427
Trajectory like control	−4.8	2.7	−10.1	0.5	0.0774
Imputation varies by reason	−3.2	2.6	−8.2	1.9	0.2208
Tipping point, $\delta = 1$	−4.1	2.5	−9	0.9	0.1102
Tipping point, $\delta = 2$	−2.9	2.6	−8	2.2	0.2596
Tipping point, $\delta = 3$	−1	2.7	−5.8	3.8	0.6811
Tipping point, $\delta = 4$	0.3	2.6	−7.1	3.5	0.5023
Available cases	−4.3	2.3	−0.4	9	0.0724

CI: confidence interval; Imputation varies by reason: $\delta = 2$ applied to MAR imputations for subjects in the experimental arm who withdrew due to AE; Tipping point: δ was applied to all subjects in the experimental arm.

Recall from Section 1.10 that, as often with new treatments of PD, there was a higher proportion of withdrawals in the experimental arm than in the control arm, and that a higher proportion of the withdrawals in the experimental arm than in the control arm were due to AEs.

The analysis assuming MAR gives a p-value significant at the 5% level. Because of the rather high proportion of discontinuations in the experimental arm, this seems a case where the reader of the trial report (regulators, clinicians and subjects) would wish to explore the potential impact of missing data very thoroughly, and will value the sensitivity analyses above as an aid to assessing the robustness of the primary result. Given that the p-value from the primary analysis is rather close to 0.05, it is not surprising that the analysis assuming the trajectory of control arm subjects for withdrawals from the experimental arm gives a non-significant result (p = 0.0774). Not all sensitivity analyses should be required to be statistically significant. However, a variety of these analyses will provide a rounded picture, and the results of one analysis could help to put in perspective the conclusions from the others. The analysis that applied a penalty $\delta = 2$ to MAR imputations of UPDRS sub-score for subjects who withdrew from the experimental arm due to AE ("Imputation varies by reason" in Table 7.9) further undermines the credibility of the primary analysis, in this case. Again, given the patterns of missingness, this is not surprising.

A worsening of 1 point on the UPDRS scale is less than half a clinically important difference (CID) as estimated in the literature (see e.g., Shulman et al. (2010), which suggests 2.3–2.7 as a minimally CID in a UPDRS sub-score, and other references in

Appendix 4.A). We have noted (Section 4.2.3.3) that when the proportion of withdrawals is high, even a mild δ, when applied to the entire set of withdrawals in the experimental arm, may represent quite an extreme scenario clinically, and will often overturn a significant primary result. Here, δ is imposed on all experimental arm subjects, so the sensitivity analysis assumes that subjects with PD who discontinue treatment are likely to start deteriorating sooner than subjects who are still on treatment, and the rate of this additional worsening is likely to be 1 point on the UPDRS scale per visit. The tipping point analysis shows that even a δ of 1 on the UPDRS scale, applied to MAR imputations for all withdrawals from the experimental arm, changes the result of the primary analysis from significant to non-significant. Based on the interpretation of the CID in the available literature, this value of δ can be considered clinically plausible and the result of this analysis important to take into consideration. Thus all the sensitivity analyses tend to undermine the primary result in this case.

Were there no sensitivity analyses planned, the regulator, if he/she follows the recent guidance documents on missing data, would likely question the credibility of the result, even though the estimate of the efficacy of the experimental treatment in the primary analysis is positive. If the proportion of missing values was smaller, and/or the estimate of the treatment effect greater, the sensitivity analyses could have served as a defense of the credibility of the primary result. But the sensitivity analyses in this case do not support the credibility of the study result. The argument for the efficacy of the treatment would need to be made on the basis of the primary analysis alone. In this case it will be difficult to consider the trial as having a credible overall result in favor of the experimental arm. Indeed, many readers of the trial report would likely feel that for this trial, the missing data and some of the reasons for it (more AEs in the experimental arm than in the control arm), would lead them to question the interpretability of the primary result – the rejection of the null hypothesis by the primary statistical analysis would need to be qualified in some way to take account of the missingness in the study.

7.5.2   Insomnia

Next, we implement the sample strategy envisaged in Chapter 4 for the illustrative insomnia dataset. As noted in the description of the insomnia dataset (Section 1.10.2), our example trial has six visits including a baseline visit. Its primary efficacy variable is total sleep time (*tst*), and there are two related secondary efficacy variables, *sqs* and morning sleepiness score (*mss*). The proportions of withdrawals in the two treatment arms were similar (18% and 20% in the placebo and experimental arm, respectively). Reasons for discontinuation that could be entered on the CRF were: AE; consent withdrawn; lack of efficacy; lost to follow up; other and protocol violated.

In Chapter 4, suitable strategies for the illustrative insomnia dataset were summarized as follows:

Primary analyses could be any of the following:

- MAR approach implementable either via MI or MMRM;

- Control-based imputation for the experimental arm;

- Delta adjustment of MAR outcome for subjects in the experimental arm who discontinued for lack of efficacy, AEs, or through personal choice (reason = "lack of efficacy," "AE" or "consent withdrawn").

Potential sensitivity analyses in this case:

- Control-based imputation for the experimental arm (if not used as primary);

- Responder analysis imputing treatment failure for subjects with missing data;

- LOCF-like assumption for experimental arm with MAR assumption for control arm;

- Assume a variety of outcomes for missing values, depending on reason for discontinuation, perhaps as in the third option for primary analysis above;

- Tipping point analysis, using delta adjustment for subjects on experimental arm, increasing δ until the primary conclusion is nullified.

Before we finalize a strategy for the insomnia dataset, it will be useful in choosing delta adjustment and helpful in judging credibility of tipping point scenarios to identify a clinically significant change in the main efficacy measures. For TST, Mayer *et al.* (2009) suggest 30 min "could be considered clinically meaningful." Jungquist *et al.* (2012) call 23 min a "clinically significant improvement in total sleep time," where by improvement they mean improvement over baseline. Here we are using the CID to justify a criterion for an implausible or fairly extreme scenario for the change in score. The larger we define a CID to be, the greater the number of "plausible" scenarios that could potentially overturn the primary result. Therefore, in the context of judging a tipping point or imposing a δ, larger values are conservative. We might reasonably take 30 min as a clinically significant decrease in TST. The standard deviation (SD) of TST in our illustrative dataset is 87.9. The CID of 30 for TST is therefore one-third of its SD. The two other efficacy scores, SQS and MSS, range from 1–10 and better values are higher and lower, respectively. For these two scores the literature is not clear as to a clinically significant change, but for purposes of determining δs and of evaluating a tipping point we follow the approximate percentage of TST (about 6–8% of one night's sleep, or 20–26 min in terms of the mean sleep time at baseline) and posit a change of -1 in SQS as a clinically significant worsening. Similarly, we posit a change of 1 in MSS as a clinically significant worsening. The SD of SQS and MSS is 1.9 and 1.8, respectively, so the CID for these two parameters is a little more than one-half the SD. A δ of more than twice the clinically significant change might be regarded as lacking credibility as a clinical scenario for withdrawals.

From among the possibilities listed above, we will implement the following strategy:

Primary analysis:

- Control-based imputation for the experimental arm implemented via sequential modeling: assume that the experimental arm has visits correlated as for the control arm (i.e., has a trajectory similar to that of the control arm after discontinuation).

Sensitivity analyses:

- Delta adjustment of outcome as imputed for the primary analysis (i.e., control-based imputation) for subjects in the experimental arm who discontinued due to AEs or due to personal choice. Note that since we have chosen control-based imputation for the primary analysis, we have specified that the delta-adjusted analysis use control-based imputation rather than MAR imputation as a basis. Further, we have assumed that lack of efficacy would be adequately modeled by the control-based imputation, so will apply the planned δ, $\delta=30$, to each post-baseline visit for those who discontinued due to AEs or "consent withdrawn," but will not apply it to those who discontinued due to lack of efficacy;

- LOCF-like assumption for experimental arm with MAR assumption for control arm;

- Tipping point analysis, using delta adjustment for subjects on experimental arm who discontinued with reason = "AE" or "consent withdrawn," increasing δ for imputed TST from 15 min to 90 min in increments of 15 min, or until the primary statistical test has p-value > 0.20. As noted, SQS and MSS will be adjusted proportionately, with a step of 0.5;

- For reference purposes, an available cases analysis;

- Also for reference purposes, an MAR analysis implemented via MI;

- We will also present the results of Chapter 6, to facilitate comparison (but note the differences in the model of Chapter 6 discussed below).

The primary and LOCF-like analyses can be implemented directly via macros available from the DIA page of www.missingdata.org.uk. SAS code to provide the planned sensitivity analyses, including calls to the www.missingdata.org.uk macros, is given in Appendix 7.G. All analyses allow for separate estimation by treatment group of the between-visit correlations.

As with the PD example, we will confine our discussion to the hypothesis test for the primary endpoint (change from baseline at Visit 5 (Week 8) in TST) and will not present results from earlier visits. We will assume that for the sensitivity analyses, we have planned to use all three efficacy variables (*tst, sqs* and *mss*), and demographic variable *sexn* (a numeric version of *sex*). This is a slightly different model from that used in Chapter 6: the model in Chapter 6 included neither *mss* nor *sexn* (sex) as an explanatory variable. We present the results in Table 7.10.

As noted, for the sensitivity analyses we have used some additional explanatory covariates, compared to the MI analysis of Chapter 6. Also, we have estimated the between-visit correlations separately here for each treatment group, whereas these were estimated across treatment groups in Chapter 6. The LSMEANS estimate for the treatment difference under MAR using MI in Table 7.10 is nevertheless close to those of the three variants of MAR in Chapter 6, Table 6.2, which were 18.7, 17.3

Table 7.10   Results for insomnia example dataset, planned primary analysis and sensitivity analyses: least-squares means (LSMEANS) estimate of difference between treatments in change from baseline in total sleep time (min) at Visit 5.

Analysis	Treatment difference, LSMEANS estimate	Standard error	95% CI, lower	upper	p-value
Trajectory like control	18.4	6.3	6	30.8	0.0035
Imputation varies by reason	13.1	6.4	0.6	25.7	0.0399
OLMCF	19.1	6.5	6.4	31.8	0.0032
Tipping point, $\delta = 15$ min	15.8	6.3	3.4	28.3	0.0128
Tipping point, $\delta = 30$ min	13.1	6.4	0.6	25.7	0.0399
Tipping point, $\delta = 45$ min	10.5	6.5	−2.2	23.3	0.1059
Tipping point, $\delta = 60$ min	7.9	6.7	−5.1	20.9	0.2354
Available cases	16.3	6.4	3.6	28.9	0.0119
MAR (MI)	18.1	6.4	5.6	30.5	0.0045

"Trajectory like control": withdrawals from experimental arm are assumed to have correlations of control arm, and thus approximately similar trajectory with some drift towards the mean of the control arm; "Imputation varies by reason": for subjects in the experimental arm who withdrew due to "AE" or "Consent withdrawn," $\delta = 30$ (min sleep) applied to the control-based imputations ("Trajectory like control"); OLMCF: own last mean carried forward, a version of LOCF implemented via MI with joint modeling that takes account of the variability in the data – MAR is assumed for the control arm; "Tipping point . . . ": analysis as for "Imputation varies by reason, for a range of δs; "Available cases": include only subjects with data at Visit 8; "MAR (MI)": MAR implemented via MI. All analyses use baseline *tst, sqs* and *mss*, as well as *sexn* in the imputation and analysis model.

and 19.3, compared with 18.1 in Table 7.10; the SEs and the p-values are similarly close.

If the experimental arm has any benign effect, we expect the efficacy score for subjects in the experimental arm to have a better trajectory than subjects in the control arm. As noted in Chapter 4, it is a shortcoming of MAR that it normally assumes that withdrawals have the trajectory of their own treatment group, whereas one would expect withdrawals from the experimental arm to have a worse trajectory compared to similar completers in their arm. Hence the attractiveness of control-based imputation, where withdrawals from the experimental arm are assumed to have a trajectory similar to completers in the control arm that have similar post-baseline outcomes.

It would therefore be expected that the planned primary analysis, which uses control-based imputation, would give a less favorable estimate of treatment effect than MAR. However, we see in Table 7.10 that the primary analysis actually leads to a point estimate of treatment effect that is marginally more favorable to the study drug than does MAR. (This is found also when the same assumptions are implemented via the joint modeling macro. This macro's "copy reference" (CR) assumption is very

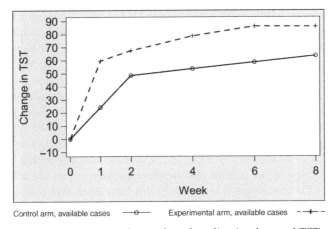

Control arm, available cases —⊖— Experimental arm, available cases --+--

Figure 7.14   Mean change from baseline in observed TST.

similar to the sequential modeling implementation of the "trajectory like control" assumption, with a slightly different model (see Section 7.3.6.2). In Roger's implementation, the estimate of treatment effect under CR is likewise more favorable to the experimental treatment group than that under MAR, at 19 versus 19.2 for MAR and CR, respectively.) In our experience it is very unusual for the CR result to be more favorable to the experimental arm than the MAR result. To see why it could be so with this dataset, recall that "trajectory like control" assumes that, after withdrawal, the values of a subject from the experimental arm would have control-group-like correlations with their previous values. In practice, this means that, starting from the value last observed, withdrawal's values will take on a trajectory similar to that of the control group, with some drift towards the mean of the control group.

The plots of mean change in TST in Figure 7.14 (observed values only) may help to explain why it could be more favorable to the experimental arm to assume that its trajectory is that of the control arm, for this particular illustrative dataset. The plot shows that the trajectory of the control arm observed values is better (steeper) than that of the experimental arm in the period from Visit 1 to Visit 2 (Week 1 to Week 2), and from Visit 4 (Week 6) to the final visit. Consider a subject from the experimental arm whose last observed value was at Visit 1 (Week 1). Other things being equal, that subject would under MAR be assumed to have a slope like that of the red dashed line in Figure 7.14. Under the "trajectory like control" assumption, the subject's slope would be like that of the black solid line, overall a slightly steeper, (more rapidly improving) slope – the plot shows that from Week 1 to the end of the study the mean improvement in the placebo arm is about 30 min, while the mean improvement in the experimental treatment arm in the same period is just over 20 min. Thus, for a subject from the experimental arm last observed at Week 1 with a typical (high) value last observed, the "trajectory like control" assumption is actually more favorable than MAR. The same is true for an experimental arm subject last observed at Week 6 – the placebo arm had a mean increase in TST of about three minutes from Week 6 to Week 8, while in the experimental treatment group the mean TST actually decreased slightly in the same period. On the other hand, subjects from the experimental arm with last observed values at Week 1 or 2 are likely to have a slightly *better* outcome under MAR than under "trajectory like control." All discontinuations in this dataset happened after Week 1, that is, after there was the most separation between the treatments. As a result, withdrawals from the experimental arm are very likely to start their post-discontinuation trajectory from a better value compared to control subjects, and to continue on a trajectory with a better slope compared to their fellow experimental subjects. Overall, it seems from Table 7.10, the "trajectory like control" assumption is marginally more favorable to the experimental treatment group than the MAR assumption. Thus, in this case the assumption that withdrawals have the trajectory of the control arm happens actually to provide a (very small) advantage for the experimental arm. Could this have been anticipated in advance for this indication? The trajectories for placebo versus experimental treatment from historic data in Figures 4.4 and 4.5 are ambiguous. Figure 4.4 is actually quite similar to that in Figure 7.14, with the placebo slope indicating marginally more rapid improvement than the experimental arm, except for the first post-baseline visit, and could suggest that the trajectory of control might favor the experimental arm; but the slope of the placebo group in Figure 4.5 is uniformly and substantially worse than that of the experimental arm – relying on Figure 4.5 alone one would infer that the trajectory of control would strongly disadvantage the experimental arm. This example demonstrates that it is important to consider the likely timing of discontinuations with respect to the anticipated trajectory of disease symptoms, the likely timing of the treatment effect onset, and the likely trajectory of the control arm at all time points.

Be that as it may, the planned primary analysis provides evidence ($p = 0.0035$) to reject the primary hypothesis of no difference between treatment groups.

In this illustrative dataset, withdrawal rates are moderate (18% and 20% in the control and experimental arms, respectively). Withdrawal rates are similar across treatment groups, and the treatment groups do not differ greatly with respect to reason for withdrawal as collected on the CRF.

In the first sensitivity analysis ("imputation varies by reason") we use the planned primary analysis as a basis, (i.e., withdrawals in the experimental arm have trajectory close to that of the control arm) but apply a δ of 30 min less sleep time at each visit for subjects in the experimental arm who discontinue with reason "AE" or "consent withdrawn." As expected, the change in assumption with regard to missing data moderates the clinical and statistical significance of the result of the primary analysis. However, this sensitivity analysis does not substantially undermine the conclusion of superiority of the experimental arm. The estimate and confidence interval of treatment difference in change from baseline in TST still strongly favors the experimental arm.

Note that in the method used for delta adjustment here, the δ applied to a visit influences the value of the next visit via the correlation between visits. This means that the cumulative δ at the final visit will be less than or equal to the sum of all the δs applied. The idea here is to model a clinically reasonable worsening, modulated via all the other factors that are associated with a subject's changes in TST. Thus if, for example, it happens that baseline values have a very strong association with the result at the final visit, and is included in the MI model, then this association with baseline values may dwarf any effect of δs from previous visits. This way of implementing the delta adjustment can be argued to reflect a clinically realistic scenario. However, it may be desired to implement a delta adjustment after all imputation is done, giving a known and definite change in trajectory to the experimental arm for selected cases or for all cases. As noted earlier, this approach is available in Roger's macro, available on the DIA page of the www.missingdata.org.uk website.

The next sensitivity analysis is based on an LOCF-like assumption ("OLMCF") for the experimental arm, and MAR assumption for the control arm. The assumption that a subject's outcomes remain "as is" after discontinuation is not particularly clinically plausible, so we would recommend this approach only as a sensitivity analysis; but use of an LOCF-like approach may be considered by some to be attractively "conservative" here because, given expected natural improvement over time with no treatment in this indication and similar rates of withdrawal in the two treatment arms, earlier withdrawals should, on average, have lower (worse) TST. Thus, assuming that these worse early values would persist in subjects discontinued from the experimental arm, while allowing withdrawals from the control arm to continue on the trajectory of natural improvement would provide a stress test which is not favorable to the experimental arm. We have noted in Section 4.2.2.3 how MI can be used to implement LOCF-like analyses that reasonably account for variability (as opposed to conventional single-imputation LOCF, which can often underestimate variance). We implement this LOCF-like analysis using joint modeling with MI, via the macro due to Roger (2012). The OLMCF analysis performs a version of LOCF that does reflect the variability of the data. The variance under the assumption of OLMCF is close to that for the primary analysis and the MAR analysis, and the estimate of treatment effect is marginally less favorable to the experimental arm than the planned primary analysis.

The final sensitivity analysis applies successively harsher δs to selected subjects until the p-value of the primary analysis becomes >0.2. As planned, the δ was applied to the primary analysis's control-based imputations. We had set a change of 30 min as clinically significant, and a change of more than 60 min as bordering on lack of plausibility as a clinical scenario for withdrawals. Here, the "tipping point" is reached at a δ of 60 min ($p = 0.2354$).

The estimate of treatment effect from the available cases analysis, provided for reference only, is in this case somewhat less favorable to the experimental arm than the planned primary analysis.

The sensitivity analyses here suggest that the rejection of the null hypothesis by the primary analysis is fairly robust to the missing data. The three sensitivity analyses give quite strong evidence of the robustness of the primary result. The "tipping point" analysis nullifies the conclusion of the primary analysis only when it is assumed that discontinuations due to AE or subject choice had 60 min less improvement in TST than was imputed from the model based on control arm subjects. Given the criteria set, such a scenario may be regarded as clinically implausible, and regulators, subjects and clinicians may well be able to conclude that the study conclusions are credible despite the missing data.

In this kind of case, a full discussion of the results should of course be included in the study report, and it may be that additional *post hoc* analyses, such as are discussed in the European Medicines Agency Guidance (European Medicines Agency, 2010), could be justified to further stress test the primary analysis. For example, we have seen that the sensitivity analysis that assumed that withdrawals from the experimental arm had *trajectory* like that of the control arm was somewhat favorable to the experimental arm. Therefore, one might add an analysis that assumes that withdrawals from the experimental arm were *distributed* (i.e., had mean and correlations) similar to the control arm. This assumption is a variant of Roger's "J2R" (or "jump to reference") (Roger, 2012). It may sometimes be difficult to justify J2R's assumption of abrupt worsening of post-withdrawal outcomes clinically, but perhaps in this case it could mimic potential withdrawal effects that could be associated with treatment for insomnia (see the discussion in Section 4.2.3.2).

7.5.3   Mania

The illustrative dataset for a clinical trial in mania had six visits including a baseline visit. Its primary efficacy parameter was a binary responder variable (responder status Yes or No).

Recall that, as noted earlier in this chapter, for this illustrative dataset we wish to explore the more challenging scenario where the binary responder variable is entered directly on the CRF, similarly to the Clinical Global Impression of Improvement measure. We are therefore assuming for this section that the mania responder variable has no direct source in a continuous variable, although we will allow it to be associated with the continuous baseline variable *base_ymrs*. Recall from Section 1.10.3 that reason for discontinuation can take values "AE," "consent withdrawn," "decision of investigator" or "other."

The sample strategy for the illustrative study in mania in Chapter 4 allowed for the following options:

Primary analyses could be either

- MAR approach using MI; or

- worst-case imputation, that is, a subject with missing response is assumed to be a treatment failure (responder status equals No).

Whichever of the options above that was not selected for the primary analysis should be included as a sensitivity analysis.

Other potential sensitivity analyses in this case:

- Assume a variety of outcomes for missing values, depending on reason for discontinuation;

- Tipping point analyses, using successively more extreme scenarios until the primary conclusion is nullified, for subjects with a reason for discontinuation that suggests the possibility of relapse, side effect or treatment failure (note that this sensitivity analysis is a development of the previous one):

o tipping point analysis via deviation from imputed probability of success (i.e., from assumed probability of being a responder);

o tipping point analysis via deviation from imputed success.

In Chapter 4, we noted that subjects with mania can have sudden shifts in symptoms. It is also acknowledged that discontinuation of treatment in mania can result in relapse (Cavanagh *et al.*, 2004). These characteristics of the outcome make it plausible to impose some worsening on subjects who withdraw, on the supposition that at least some will be without treatment for a period (even if they revert to their pre-study treatment later). We have seen that delta adjustment of an imputed binary response can be accomplished by rendering the MAR-imputed binary response a "failure" (responder = No) with a probability δ ("deviation from imputed probability of success," Section 4.2.3.3). For this indication and outcome, the historic data are such that it is difficult to identify a reasonable range for δ on clinical grounds. To identify reasonable values for δ we would need to identify a (presumably) increased probability that withdrawals turn out to be "relapsers" rather than "responders." We can then implement successively harsher δs for the tipping point analysis, starting at some relatively small value, and continuing until a statistically significant primary result is rendered non-significant. Cavanagh *et al.* (2004) found that a statistically significantly higher proportion of subjects who discontinued treatment relapsed, compared to those who continued to be treated. The rates of relapse reported, for example, for depressive episodes for subjects after discontinuation of treatment (Altshuler *et al.*, 2003, Table 3) are almost twice that of subjects continuing treatment. These rates are similar to those found in the example studies in Table 4.4, which all report relapse rates of around 50%. Thus, since a rather high absolute rate of relapse is expected by the end of study, perhaps an approximately 25% extra chance of failure to respond would constitute a reasonable value for δ. For a tipping point analysis, δ could be planned to start at 10% and increase by 5% increments until any significant result is rendered non-significant. We have already seen in Figure 7.13 that δs of this magnitude have a considerable effect on the overall probability of being a responder – here we will examine associated estimates and test statistics. We will also perform a tipping point analysis using "deviation from imputed success" (as opposed to deviation from imputed *probability* of success, see Section 4.2.3.3), plotting p-values of results where an increasing *number* of successes imputed under the MAR assumption are posited as failures. Collectively, these analyses may help the reader of the clinical study report to make their own judgment about the credibility of the study result, given the deviation from MAR needed to nullify the primary statistical test.

Given the binary response and the data on relapse, then, from among the possible analyses listed above we will implement the following strategy:

Primary analysis:

• MAR approach using MI.

Sensitivity analyses:

- Worst-case imputation, with withdrawals counted as non-responders for both arms;

- Worst-case imputation, with withdrawals counted as non-responders for the experimental arm and assuming MAR for control arm;

- Assume MAR; for discontinuations due to AE or consent withdrawn in the experimental arm, impose a "failure" (responder = N) outcome with an additional 25% probability (i.e., $\delta = 0.25$);

- Tipping point analysis, changing successes imputed under MAR to be failures with a probability of δ, where δ is (0.1, 0.15, 0.20, 0.25, 0.30), or until the primary conclusion is nullified, for subjects in the experimental arm with a reason for discontinuation that suggests the possibility of relapse, side effect or treatment failure ("tipping point via deviation from imputed probability of success");

- Tipping point analysis as above, but changing increasing *numbers* of successes imputed under MAR to be failures, for subjects with a reason for discontinuation that suggests the possibility of relapse, side effect or treatment failure ("tipping point via deviation from imputed success");

- For reference purposes, an available cases analysis.

Of the reasons for discontinuation available in the illustrative dataset, the following are judged to suggest the possibility of relapse, side effect or treatment failure: "adverse event," "consent withdrawn" and "decision of investigator." See Section 1.10.3 for a discussion of efficacy profiles for withdrawals by reason for discontinuation. (We note that for this illustrative dataset the only other reason available is "other.")

We will assume that pooling of sites was envisaged in the SAP, and that a pooling based on country was included in the primary model. We note that the sensitivity analyses will involve visit-by-visit imputation, and so will force a country-by-visit interaction to be included, even though differences between visits in the effect of country may not be envisaged.

We have noted elsewhere that MMRM and MI that assumes MAR should give very similar results. Recall that the generalized linear mixed model (GLMM) featured in Chapter 5 can give results close MAR but is not an MAR model. Nevertheless, to assess the similarity of its results to those of MI, we will include not only the Chapter 5 GLMM result for that dataset, but also include the result from a GLMM whose model matches the primary MI analysis exactly in including a country-by-visit interaction. All analyses except that from Chapter 5 allow for separate estimation by treatment group of the between-visit correlations.

SAS code to provide the planned sensitivity analyses is given in Appendix 7.H.

Table 7.11 shows that, although the GLMM analysis in Chapter 5 was borderline significant ($p = 0.05$), the planned primary analysis using MI fails to reject the null

Table 7.11   Results for mania dataset, planned primary analysis and sensitivity analyses: least-squares means (LSMEANS) estimate of difference between treatments in the logit of the probability of response at Visit 5.

Analysis	Treatment difference, LSMEANS estimate	Standard error	Odds ratio	95% CI, lower	95% CI, upper	p-value
MAR (MI)	0.26	0.15	1.30	0.96	1.75	0.0847
Impute worst case	0.27	0.12	1.31	1.03	1.67	0.0254
Impute worst case, experimental arm	−0.36	0.14	0.70	0.54	0.91	0.0106
Imputation varies by reason	0.12	0.15	1.13	0.84	1.50	0.418
Tipping point, $\delta = 0.1$	0.19	0.15	1.21	0.90	1.62	0.2084
For reference						
GLMM (Chapter 5)	0.28	0.14	1.32	1	1.75	0.05
GLMM (matching MAR MI)	0.26	0.14	1.30	0.98	1.72	0.0666
Available cases	0.18	0.15	1.20	0.89	1.61	0.2439

MAR(MI): MI analysis assuming MAR, imputed using a model that includes previous post-baseline outcomes, treatment group*visit, country*visit and baseline YRMS score*visit; "Impute worst case": assume that subjects with missing response were non-responders; "Impute worst case, experimental arm": assume that subjects from the experimental arm with missing response were non-responders, assume that subjects from the control arm were MAR; "Imputation varies by reason": assumes MAR using model as for MAR (MI), but subjects in the experimental arm who discontinued with reason "AE," "Consent withdrawn" or "Decision of investigator" and imputed as responders by MAR changed to non-responders with extra probability of 0.25 "Tipping point, $\delta = 0.1$": as previous analysis, but use probability 0.1; "Available cases" uses only non-missing response data; logistic regression GLMM (Chapter 5): analysis from Table 5.11, row 7, including treatment group*visit, country, baseline and baseline*visit as explanatory variables; logistic regression GLMM (matching MAR MI): as previous analysis, but including country*visit interaction as explanatory variable and estimating visit correlations separately for each treatment group.

hypothesis ($p = 0.0847$). The MI analysis, being visit-by-visit, included a country-by-visit interaction absent from the GLMM analysis; the MI analysis also estimated the between-visit correlations separately for each treatment, while the GLMM in Chapter 5 estimated these across treatment groups. When the GLMM analysis is performed with the additional *country*visit* factors and by-treatment estimation of correlations that matches the primary MI analysis, the p-value is somewhat closer to that of the primary analysis (0.0666 and 0.0847 for the GLMM and MI analyses, respectively). As the primary analysis does not give a significant p-value, sensitivity analyses in this case have less urgency in terms of approval or non-approval of the treatment. Even if certain sensitivity analyses result in a p-value of less than 0.05 (as here), it is not envisaged by the regulatory guidance that this could make a "success" out of a failed or a borderline trial.

The MI-based sensitivity analyses "imputation varies by reason" and "tipping point, $\delta = 0.1$" are implemented as deviations from this base "MAR (MI)" analysis.

The sensitivity analyses provide some interesting results. Recall that there was a fairly high dropout rate in the trial, and there were more withdrawals from the control arm than from the experimental arm (32% and 22%, respectively). In the planning stage, this imbalance in rate of withdrawal was not predicted, based on historic data. As it turns out, the imbalance in withdrawals means that the "worst-case" assumption, when applied to both arms, favors the experimental treatment group (by penalizing the control treatment group to a greater extent). As a result, this sensitivity analysis provides the only result that favors the experimental arm at the 5% significance level ($p = 0.0254$). The next sensitivity analysis assumes the worst case (i.e., assumes treatment failure) only for the experimental arm. The clinical plausibility of this stress test may be questionable because there is no reason to believe that the experimental treatment will act in such a way as to cause a relapse in *all* of the subjects after discontinuation, and that the controls would follow a more moderate natural course of disease. In this sensitivity analysis, the experimental arm is actually estimated to be significantly worse than the control group. Perhaps the most clinically plausible of the stress tests is that where for subjects in the experimental arm who discontinued due to reason "AE," "consent withdrawn" or "decision of investigator," MAR-imputed responders were changed to be non-responders with a probability of 0.25. This assumption draws from historic data which shows that in some cases subjects who discontinue treatment for mania relapse quite rapidly. Not all subjects who discontinued this study would be expected to discontinue all treatment, of course, but the assumption of extra probability of worsening, compared to subjects remaining in the study, could reflect a reasonable clinical scenario. This stress test provides no evidence supporting the rejection of the primary hypothesis ($p = 0.4180$). This is not surprising with this example, because the conclusion under a milder MAR assumption is also that of no statistical significance. The "tipping point" analysis in Table 7.11 likewise does not support the study objective even on its first (least harsh) iteration, again failing to provide supportive evidence regarding the rejection of the primary hypothesis. That "tipping point" analysis is of the kind that we have denominated "deviation from imputed probability of success" – withdrawals imputed to be successes are changed to be failures *with a certain probability* δ. Figure 7.15 shows the result of the final sensitivity analysis, (results not shown in Table 7.11), a second version of the tipping point analysis, of the kind that we have denominated "deviation from imputed success," where in successive analyses a growing *number* of withdrawals that were imputed successes are changed to be failures.

Figure 7.15 shows how rapidly the p-value increases from that of the primary MAR analysis, as more MAR-imputed responders are changed to be non-responders from the group of subjects discontinuing for a reason that could be associated with relapse. When about 33 subjects in the experimental arm are changed to non-responders, the estimate of the odds ratio for response begins to favor the control group.

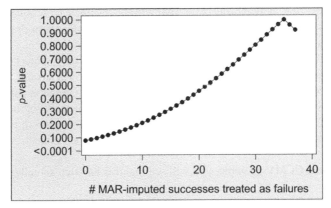

Figure 7.15 P-values from tipping point analysis using deviation from imputed success. *Primary analysis is run with increasing numbers of MAR-imputed responders in the experimental arm who discontinued with reason "AE," "consent withdrawn" or "decision of investigator" changed to be non-responders. One hundred imputations were used for each of the analyses. In the 100 imputed datasets, the range of experimental arm withdrawals imputed as responders under MAR was [45, 69] out of 123 with missing outcomes. The x-axis denotes the absolute number of imputed responders changed to be non-responders. The same number of imputed responders was changed to be non-responders for each set of imputed datasets.*

We note that the "available cases" analysis, which is often viewed as potentially biased because it includes only subjects who were capable of completing the study, does not favor the experimental arm here.

In the case of this illustrative trial, all but one of the sensitivity analyses would have failed to support the rejection of the null hypothesis, which the primary statistical test itself failed to overturn. In this case, it is clear that overall the trial has failed to overturn the null hypothesis. If it had been planned to use the GLMM analysis from Chapter 5 as the primary analysis, whose p-value was 0.05, the sensitivity analyses above would have provided strong evidence that this GLMM result was not robust to missing data, and the trial would still likely be judged not to have conclusively rejected the primary null hypothesis, given the missing data.

Appendix 7.A How one could implement the neighboring case missing value assumption using visit-by-visit multiple imputation

One could implement NCMV for the trial described in Section 7.3.1 via sequential MI as follows. Recall that the fictitious trial had two post-baseline visits, Visit 1 and Visit 2.

Step 1: Perform MI for subjects with missing Visit 1 by including in the input dataset only subjects with missing Visit 1 and subjects with non-missing Visit 1 but missing Visit 2 – the "neighboring cases." MI will now estimate regression parameters for Visit 1 using only subjects who withdrew after Visit 1. Posterior draws of those regression parameters will then be used to impute Visit 1.

Step 2: To impute Visit 2, include in the input dataset only subjects with missing Visit 2 and completers – completers are the "neighboring cases" for subjects who withdrew after the second-last visit. MI will estimate regression parameters for Visit 2, and will be able to use completers only, because they are the only subjects who have information about likely values at Visit 2. Posterior draws of those regression parameters will then be used to impute Visit 2, for all subjects with Visit 2 missing.

As with the CCMV example, you will see that this last step actually includes all subjects.

Appendix 7.B SAS code to model withdrawals from the experimental arm, using observed data from the control arm

SAS macro based on the code in Section 7.3

The following macro for the Parkinson's disease dataset assumes that withdrawals have the correlations found in the control arm. This will result in missing values being imputed to have approximately the trajectory of the control arm, with some drift towards the mean of the control arm (because correlations are not exactly unity). This assumption is that of the "copy reference" reference assumption discussed in Section 7.3.5 and sketched in Figure 7.2.

```
* perform reference-based CR-type imputation for a succession
of visits using sequential regression-based MI;

%MACRO imp_vis(SEED=-1, var=, visit=);
* step 1. Select observations to be imputed (LASTVIS<&visit), plus
the observations to be used to model the imputation (trt=1);
DATA impute&visit rest&visit;
  SET strtimp&visit;
  * Put to one side subjects from experimental arm (trt=2)
that have data at time-point &visit;
  IF trt = 2 AND lastvis >=&visit
  THEN
    OUTPUT rest&visit;
  * Select all other subjects for the time-point &visit
imputation step;
  ELSE
    OUTPUT impute&visit;
run;

* only perform imputation for this visit if there are some missings;
```

```
PROC SQL NOPRINT;
SELECT count(*) INTO :anymiss
     FROM impute&visit(WHERE=(&var._&visit IS MISSING));
QUIT;
%IF &anymiss>0
%THEN
  %DO;

* Step 2. Call PROC MI to impute missing data at time-point &visit
using dataset IMPUTE&visit;
ODS LISTING CLOSE;
PROC MI DATA=impute&visit OUT=imputed&VISIT NIMPUTE=1 SEED=&seed;
    BY _imputation_;
    VAR base_&var &var._1-&var._&visit;
    MONOTONE REGRESSION(&var._&visit = base_&var %do _iv=1 %to
%eval(&visit-1); &var._&_iv %end;);
RUN;
ODS LISTING;

   %END; * of &anymiss>0;

%IF &anymiss=0
%THEN
   %DO;
DATA imputed&visit;
   SET impute&visit;
RUN;
   %END;

* Step 3.  Re-assemble the dataset, now with time-point &visit
imputed;
DATA strtimp%EVAL(&visit+1);
    SET rest&visit imputed&visit;
RUN;
PROC SORT DATA=strtimp%EVAL(&visit+1);
    BY _imputation_;
RUN;
%MEND imp_vis;

* name dataset appropriately as input for visit 1;
DATA strtimp1;
    SET updrsh;
RUN;
* impute non-monotone missing values as in SAS Code Fragment 7.3
[not included here];

* perform the visit-by-visit MI, for the 8 post-baseline visits;
%MACRO run_RBI();
%DO I=1 %TO 8;
```

```
        %imp_vis(seed=34535499, var=UPD, visit=&i);
%END;
%MEND run_RBI;
%run_RBI();


* convert dataset from horizontal format (all time points on one
record for a subject) to vertical format (one time point per record
for a subject), ready to be analyzed with a by _imputation_
statement;
DATA PD_RBI;
     SET strtimp9;
     %MACRO makevert();
        %DO i=1 %TO 8;
           UPD=UPD_&i;
           CFG_UPD=UPD-BASE_UPD;
           visit=&i;
           OUTPUT;
        %END;
     %MEND makevert;
     %makevert();
run;
```

Identical implementation via an SAS macro by the authors, available from DIA pages at missingdata.org.uk

```
%include "cbi_pmm.sas";
%include "PMMUtilityMacros.sas';
%cbi_pmm(datain=UPDRS, trtname=trt, subjname=subjid,
visname=visit, poolsite=, basecont=%str(base_upd),
baseclass=%str(), postcont=%str(upd), postclass=%str(),
seed=34535499, nimp=1000, primaryname=upd,
analcovarcont=%str(base_upd), analcovarclass=%str(), trtref=1,
analmethod=ancova, repstr=, dataout=PD_RBI_Q_MACRO_DATAFULL,
resout=PD_RBI_results);
```

Note: as for all implementation of control-based imputation, for non-monotone missing data this call to the macro assumes MAR.

Implementation of similar analysis using five-part SAS macro by James Roger and GlaxoSmithKline, available from DIA pages at missingdata.org.uk

```
* impose trajectory of control via Roger option CR = Copy
Reference;
* note that the Roger macro offers variants on this approach
including CIR = Copy Increment from Reference (method=CIR);
%include "part1a_28.sas";
%include "part1b_40.sas";
```

```
%include "part2a_35.sas";
%include "part2b_40.sas";
%include "part3_45.sas";
data UPDRS(drop=subjid rename=(lsubjid=subjid));
  set dd.UPDRSmono(where=(visit ne 0));
  * numeric subjid seems to be required by GSK macro;
  length lsubjid 8;
  lsubjid=left(trim(subjid))+0;
run;
%part1A(Jobname=PD_RBI_GSK_CR, Data=UPDRS, Subject=subjid,
Response=upd, Time=visit, Treat=trt, cov=, covbytime=base_upd,
PEwhere=, ID=, covgroup=trt);
%part1B(Jobname=PD_RBI_GSK_CR, Ndraws=1000, thin=50, debug=0,
seed=34535499);
%part2A(Jobname=PD_RBI_GSK_CR, Method=CR, ref=1)
%part2b(Jobname=PD_RBI_GSK_CR);
%part3(Jobname=PD_RBI_GSK_CR);
```

Implementation of the "jump to reference" (J2R) assumption using five-part SAS macro by James Roger and GlaxoSmithKline, available from DIA pages at missingdata.org.uk

To implement the "jump to reference" assumption, use the call in the previous section, with a new Jobname, say, PD_RBI_GSK_J2R (any Jobname can be chosen), and for the call to the PART2A macro, substitute the following:

```
%part2A(Jobname=PD_RBI_GSK_J2R, Method=J2R, ref=1);
```

Example call of Roger/GlaxoSmithKline macro to plot the imputations made by the above five-part macro, also available at the DIA page of missingdata.org.uk

To plot the imputations with the "copy reference" assumption generated by the jobname PD_RBI_GSK_J2R, use the following call of the plotter macro:

```
%include "plotter3.sas";
%plotter(jobname=PD_RBI_GSK_CR,where=,file=PD_RBI_GSK_CR,
Xlabel=Visit,YLabel=UPDRS, Title=PD_RBI_GSK_CR);
```

To plot the imputations with the "jump to reference" assumption, use the following call:

```
%plotter(jobname=PD_RBI_GSK_J2R,where=,file=PD_RBI_GSK_J2R,
Xlabel=Visit,YLabel=UPDRS, Title=PD_RBI_GSK_J2R);
```

The outputs from these plotting macros are available in the cgm format, which can be imported easily into Word documents.

SAS macro to implement the "jump to reference" assumption via sequential modeling based on the code in Section 7.3

The following macro for the Parkinson's disease dataset follows the logic exemplified in SAS Code Fragment 7.11. That is, it assumes that withdrawals have the mean of the control group at each visit, conditional only on the withdrawal's baseline covariables. No account is taken, therefore, of a withdrawal's post-baseline outcomes. Whether a withdrawal had relatively good or relatively poor post-baseline outcomes, the mean of that withdrawal's imputed missing values, as imputed by this macro, will be very close to that of the control arm for each visit. (If baseline has a strong correlation with outcomes, a withdrawal's baseline will influence that withdrawal's imputed values, of course, but, due to randomization, the expectation is that baseline will be similar for all treatment groups.) This contrasts with the first macro in this Appendix, which also uses sequential modeling, but which included a withdrawal's post-baseline outcomes in the imputation model and reflected a withdrawal's post-baseline outcomes in imputations via between-visit correlations. See Section 7.3.5 for a discussion of how J2R can be implemented either taking account of post-baseline outcomes (using the joint modeling implementation of MI as in the SAS code immediately above) or omitting post-baseline outcomes from the imputation model (using either the sequential modeling macro or the joint modeling implementation).

The macro here assumes that as a first step we have created dataset *strtimp1*, in which the control arm is already imputed assuming MAR as in the first part of SAS Code Fragment 7.10.

```
* Impute visit using only information from control (trt=1);
%MACRO imp_J2R(seed=-1, var=, visit=);
* select observations to be imputed (LASTVIS<&visit), plus the
observations to be used to model the imputation (trt=0);
DATA impute&visit rest&visit;
  SET strtimp&visit;
  * Put to one side subjects from experimental arm (trt=2) that
have data at time-point &visit;
  IF trt = 2 AND lastvis >=&visit
  THEN
     OUTPUT rest&visit;
  * Select all other subjects for the time-point &visit
imputation step;
  ELSE
     OUTPUT impute&visit;
RUN;
```

```
* only perform imputation for this visit if there are some missings;
PROC SQL NOPRINT;
SELECT Count(*) INTO :Anymiss
     FROM impute&visit(WHERE=(&var._&visit IS MISSING));
QUIT;
%IF &Anymiss>0
%THEN
    %DO;

* Step 2. Call PROC MI to impute missing data at time-point &visit
using dataset IMPUTE&visit;
ODS LISTING CLOSE;
PROC MI DATA=IMPUTE&visit OUT=IMPUTED&visit NIMPUTE=1 SEED=34535499;
    BY _Imputation_;
    VAR base_&var &var._&visit;
    MONOTONE REGRESSION(&var._&visit = base_&var);
RUN;
ODS LISTING;

    %END; * of &Anymiss>0;

%IF &Anymiss=0
%THEN
    %DO;
DATA imputed&visit;
    SET impute&visit;
RUN;
    %END;

* Step 3.  Re-assemble the dataset, now with time-point &visit
imputed;
DATA strtimp%eval(&visit+1);
    SET rest&visit imputed&visit;
run;
PROC SORT DATA=strtimp%eval(&visit+1);
    BY _Imputation_;
RUN;
%MEND imp_J2R;

* perform the visit-by-visit MI, for the 8 post-baseline visits;
%MACRO run_J2R();
%DO i=1 %TO 8;
    %imp_J2R(seed=34535499, var=UPD, visit=&i);
%END;
%MEND run_J2R;
%run_J2R();
```

Appendix 7.C SAS code to model early withdrawals from the experimental arm, using the last-observation-carried-forward-like values

SAS macro for the insomnia dataset based on SAS Code Fragments 7.12 and 7.13

```
* perform LOCF via reference-based imputation for a succession
of visits using visit-by-visit regression-based MI;
%MACRO impLOCFv(seed=883960001, var=, visit=);
* only perform imputation for this visit if there are dropouts
in the previous visit;
PROC SQL NOPRINT;
SELECT count(*) INTO :anymiss
     FROM strtimp&visit(WHERE=(lastvis=&visit-1));
QUIT;
%IF &anymiss>0
%THEN
  %DO;
* step 1. select subjects whose last observation was on visit
&visit-1, and use their data for this visit to model all their
future visits;
DATA imputeLV&visit rest&visit; SET strtimp&visit;
  * subjects for whom this visit is their first missing visit
model their own LOCF values best;
  IF lastvis NE &visit-1
  THEN
    OUTPUT rest&visit;
  ELSE
    OUTPUT imputeLV&visit;
RUN;
* step 2. for each subject, create extra records with missing
observations,
  as many records as there are visits to impute;
DATA imputeLV&visit;
  SET imputeLV&visit;
  LENGTH subjid_ $10;
  subjid_=subjid;

  * create the variable that will be the outcome in the model
    of the last observation that is to be carried forward;
  i&var=&var._%eval(&visit-1);
  OUTPUT imputeLV&visit;

  * Create records with missing values, one for every missing
&var
```

```
       for the subjects who withdrew;
    IF lastvis=&visit-1
    THEN
       DO;
          DO ivisit=&visit TO 5;
             subjid_=TRIM(LEFT(subjid))|| "_" ||
PUT(ivisit,1.0);
             i&var=.;
             OUTPUT imputeLV&visit;
          END;
       END;
RUN;
* step 3. impute likely LOCF values for those who withdraw at
visit &visit-1;
PROC SORT DATA=imputeLV&visit;
   BY _imputation_ subjid;
RUN;
ODS LISTING CLOSE;
PROC MI DATA=imputeLV&visit OUT=imputedLV&visit NIMPUTE=1
SEED=&seed;
     BY _imputation_;
     CLASS agegrp sex trt;
     VAR trt agegrp sex base_sqs base_mss
     %DO j=0 %TO &visit-2;
     &var._&j
     %END;
     i&var;
     MONOTONE REGRESSION(i&var = trt agegrp sex base_sqs
base_mss
   %DO j=0 %TO %EVAL(&visit-2);
   &var._&j trt*&var._&j
   %END;
   );

RUN;
ODS LISTING;

* step 4. store the imputed values
   in the variables representing post-baseline assessments;
PROC TRANSPOSE
DATA=imputedLV&visit(WHERE=(INDEX(subjid_,"_")>0))
OUT=imputedLV&visit.&var PREFIX=&var;
          BY _imputation_ subjid;
          * imputed &var;
          VAR i&var;
          ID ivisit;
RUN;
* Step 5. Merge LOCF-imputed efficacy scores with the original
dataset;
```

```
DATA strtimp%EVAL(&visit+1);
  MERGE imputELV&visit(WHERE=(INDEX(subjid_,"_")=0))
        imputedLV&visit&var
        ;
     BY _imputation_ subjid;

        ARRAY &var.o(5) &var._1 - &var._5;
        ARRAY &var(5) &var.1 - &var.5;

        DO j=1 TO 5;

             IF &var.o [j]=. THEN &var.o[j]=&var[j];
        END;
RUN;
DATA strtimp%eval(&visit+1);
     SET strtimp%eval(&visit+1) rest&visit;
RUN;
  %END; * of test for any dropouts in Visit &visit-1;

* if there were no dropouts in Visit &visit-1,
  move all data to the dataset for the next visit;
%IF &anymiss=0
%THEN
  %DO;
DATA strtimp%eval(&visit+1);
  SET strtimp&visit;
RUN;
  %END;

%MEND impLOCFV;

DATA strtimp1;
  SET monotone;
RUN;

PROC SORT DATA=strtimp1;
  BY _imputation_ subjid;
RUN;

* perform the visit-by-visit MI, for the 5 post-baseline
visits;
%MACRO run_LOCF();
%DO v=1 %TO 5;
   %impLOCFV(seed=883960001, var=TST, visit=&v);
%END;
%MEND run_LOCF;

%run_LOCF();
```

Appendix 7.D SAS macro to impose delta adjustment on a responder variable in the mania dataset

```
%macro delta(seed1=-1, seed2=-1, var=, visit=,  delta=0,
condn=);
* only perform imputation for this visit if there are some
missings;
PROC SQL NOPRINT;
SELECT count(*) INTO :anymiss
   FROM strtimp&visit(WHERE=(&var._&visit IS MISSING));
QUIT;
%IF &Anymiss>0
%THEN
   %DO;
ODS LISTING CLOSE;
PROC MI DATA=strtimp&visit OUT=imputedmar&visit NIMPUTE=1
SEED=&seed1;
   BY _imputation_;
   VAR trt base_ymrs
   %if &visit=2 %then %do;
      resp_1
                   %end;
   %if &visit>2 %then %do;
      resp_1-resp_%eval(&visit-1)
                   %end;
   resp_&visit;
   CLASS TRT resp_1-resp_&visit;
   MONOTONE LOGISTIC(
      resp_&visit=trt base_ymrs
   %DO _iv=1 %TO %EVAL(&visit-1);
      resp_&_iv trt*resp_&_iv
   %END;
   );
RUN;
ODS LISTING;
   %END; * of there being any missing values to impute;
* impute failure with probability δ over and above MAR-imputed
failure
DATA strtimp%eval(&visit+1);
   SET imputedmar&visit;
   IF lastvis<&visit AND trt=2 &condn
   THEN DO;
      IF ranuni(&seed2)<&delta
      THEN
         resp_&visit = 0;
   END;
RUN;
```

```
%MEND delta;
* perform the visit-by-visit MI, for the post-baseline visits;
%MACRO run_tdelta(delta=);
%DO I=1 %TO 5;
   %delta(seed1=34535499, seed2=34535500, var=resp, visit=&i,
delta=&delta);
%END;
%MEND run_tdelta;
%run_tdelta(delta=0.1);
```

Appendix 7.E SAS code to implement tipping point via exhaustive scenarios for withdrawals in the mania dataset

```
* FDA-defined (Yan, 2008) tipping point analysis: assign
failure to all possible combinations of the missing values in both
treatment groups;
* do analysis just for final visit;
* find number of missings by treatment group;
DATA resptip;
   SET resp(where=(visit=5));
   randnum=ranuni(883960001);
   merger=1;
RUN;
* count missing values;
PROC SQL NOPRINT;
CREATE TABLE missing AS
SELECT trt, count(*) AS missing
     FROM resptip(WHERE=(resp IS MISSING))
     GROUP BY trt
     ORDER BY trt;
QUIT;
PROC TRANSPOSE DATA=missing OUT=missings PREFIX=miss_;
   VAR missing;
   ID trt;
RUN;
DATA missings;
   SET missings;
   merger=1;
RUN;

DATA resptip;
   MERGE resptip
         missings;
   BY merger;
RUN;
```

```
* if miss_1 and miss_2 are the number of withdrawals in each
treatment group,
  create miss_1 * miss_2 datasets containing all possible
combinations of numbers of successes and failures for the
withdrawals;

* sort by random number allows cumulative imputation of
failure/success to subjects in random order;
PROC SORT DATA=resptip;
   BY randnum;
RUN;
DATA resptip;
   SET resptip;
   ARRAY randcount(2);
   ARRAY t(2);
   RETAIN randcount 0;
   newresp=resp;
   IF resp=.
   THEN
      randcount(trt)+1;
   * output miss_1 * miss_2 scenarios, i.e., all possible
combinations of results for missings for the two treatment
groups;
   * when t1 is x, x subjects with missing data will be
imputed as failures;
   do t1=1 TO miss_1;
     DO t2=1 TO miss_2;
      IF resp=.
      THEN
         DO;
             IF randcount(trt)<=t(trt)
             THEN
                newresp=0;
             ELSE
                newresp=1;
             OUTPUT;
         END;
      ELSE
         OUTPUT;
    END;
   END;
RUN;
proc sort data=resptip;
   by t1 t2 trt country;
run;
TITLE;
ODS LISTING CLOSE;
```

```
ODS RESULTS OFF;
PROC GENMOD DATA=resptip;
  CLASS trt country;
  MODEL newresp/denom = trt country base_ymrs/DIST=BIN;
  LSMEANS trt/DIFF=control("1") EXP CL;
  BY t1 t2;
  ODS OUTPUT diffs=diffs;
RUN;
ODS LISTING;
ODS RESULTS ON;
* standard output from this tipping point analysis is a plot
of the p-values in diffs by T1 and T2;
```

Appendix 7.F SAS code to perform sensitivity analyses for the Parkinson's disease dataset

The following code assumes that a monotone-missing dataset *updrs* is available, with one record per subject visit, and that the macros *cbi_pmm.sas, delta_pmm.sas, delta_and_tip.sas* and *PMMutilityMacros.sas* have been %INCLUDEd in the program.

- We implement control-based imputation using Ratitch's macro *cbi_pmm*. Note that for the *cbi_pmm* and *delta_pmm* and *delta_and_tip* macros, the variable entered for the parameter *poolsite* will not be used in the preliminary step which imputes non-monotone missings, due to limitations with handling classification variables in PROC MI's MCMC method. However, the *poolsite* parameter variable is used in the imputation model for monotone missing data and in the analysis model. In the following call, *region* is the *poolsite* parameter variable.

```
%cbi_pmm(datain=updrs, trtname=trt, subjname=subjid,
visname=visit, poolsite=region,
basecont=%str(base_upd), baseclass=%str(), postcont=%str(upd),
postclass=%str(),
seed=34535499, nimp=1000,
primaryname=upd, analcovarcont=%str(base_upd),
analcovarclass=%str(region), trtref=1, analmethod=ancova,
repstr=,
dataout=ddw.PD_RBI_Q_macro_study_datafull,
resout=ddw.PD_RBI_study_results, imptrtbytime=Y
);
```

- We implement MAR imputation with delta adjustment (worsening) for subjects from the experimental arm who withdrew due to AE, using Ratitch's macro *delta_pmm*. Note that if a δ of zero is specified for the *delta_pmm* macro, a simple MAR analysis is performed. Here we call *delta_pmm* twice: once to impute missings assuming MAR, and once to impose $\delta = 2$. We then combine the two imputed datasets, selecting from the $\delta = 2$ imputation only subjects from the experimental arm who withdrew due to AE.

```
* perform MAR via delta=0;
%delta_pmm(
datain=updrs, trtname=trt, subjname=subjid, visname=visit,
poolsite=region,
basecont=%str(base_upd), baseclass=%str(), postcont=%str(upd),
postclass=%str(),
seed=34535499, nimp=1000,
deltavis=all,
deltacont=%str(0), deltacontarm=%str(2),
deltacontmethod=%str(meanabs), favorcont=%str(low),
primaryname=upd, analcovarcont=%str(base_upd),
analcovarclass=%str(region), trtref=1, analmethod=ancova,
repstr=, dataout=PD_MAR_study_datafull,
resout=PD_MAR_study_results,
imptrtbytime=Y
);
data ddw.PD_MAR_study_datafull;
   set PD_MAR_study_datafull;
run;
data ddw.PD_MAR_study_results;
   set PD_MAR_study_results;
run;

* impute imposing a delta of 2;
%delta_pmm(
datain=updrs, trtname=trt, subjname=subjid, visname=visit,
poolsite=region,
basecont=%str(base_upd), baseclass=%str(), postcont=%str(upd),
postclass=%str(),
seed=883960001, nimp=1000,
deltavis=all,
deltacont=%str(2), deltacontarm=%str(2),
deltacontmethod=%str(meanabs), favorcont=%str(low),
primaryname=upd, analcovarcont=%str(base_upd),
analcovarclass=%str(region), trtref=1, analmethod=ancova,
repstr=,
dataout=PD_delta_study_datafull,
resout=ddw.PD_delta_study_results, imptrtbytime=Y
);
data ddw.PD_delta_study_datafull;
   set PD_delta_study_datafull;
run;

* add reason for discontinuation to both imputed datasets;
proc sort data=updrs(keep=subjid reasond) out=reasond
nodupkey
```

```
    by subjid;
run;
proc sort data=PD_delta_study_datafull;
    by subjid;
run;
proc sort data=PD_MAR_study_datafull;
    by subjid;
run;
data PD_MAR_study_datafull;
    merge PD_MAR_study_datafull
          reasond;
    by subjid;
run;
data PD_delta_study_datafull;
    merge PD_delta_study_datafull
          reasond;
    by subjid;
run;

data PD_by_reason_study_datafull;
    set PD_MAR_study_datafull(where=(trt=1 or reasond^="AE"))
      PD_delta_study_datafull(where=(trt=2 and
reasond="AE"));
run;
data ddw.PD_by_reason_study_datafull;
    set PD_by_reason_study_datafull;
run;
proc sort data=upd;
  by visit _imputation_;
run;

* use analyze macro from PMMutilityMacro.sas, also available
from www.missingdata.org.uk, to analyze and call PROC
MIANALYZE;
title2 "Allow imputation to differ by reason for withdrawal";
title3 "continuous endpoint (upd)";
%analyze(datain=upd, dataout=PD_by_reason_study_results,
trtname=trt, trtref=1, subjname=subjid, visname=visit,
primaryname=upd, analcovarcont=upd,
          analcovarclass=region, analmethod=ANCOVA);
title2;
title3;
```

- We implement a tipping point analysis using Ratitch's *delta_and_tip.sas* macro. We first apply a $\delta = 1$ (*deltacont = 1*) to MAR-imputed values from the experimental arm; then increase δ by 1 (*tipstepcont = %str(1)*) for four iterations (*tipmaxiter = 4*). We could choose to iterate until a non-significant *p*-value is reached (e.g., until $p > 0.1$, *tipalpha = 0.1*), but we choose here to look at four iterations irrespective of the significance of the result, by specifying *tipalpha = 0.99*.

```
%delta_and_tip(
datain=updrs, trtname=trt, subjname=subjid, visname=visit,
poolsite=region,
basecont=%str(base upd), baseclass=%str(), postcont=%str(upd),
seed=34535499, nimp=1000,
deltavis=all,
deltacont=%str(1), deltacontarm=%str(2),
deltacontmethod=%str(meanabs), favorcont=%str(low),
primaryname=upd, analcovarcont=%str(base_upd),
analcovarclass=%str(region), trtref=1,
analmethod=ancova,
dataout=PD_tip_study_datafull, resout=PD_tip_study_results,
tipstepcont=%str(1.0), tiparm=2, tipalpha=0.99, tipmaxiter=4,
imptrtbytime=Y
);
```

Appendix 7.G SAS code to perform sensitivity analyses for the insomnia dataset

```
* primary analysis: assume experimental arm has correlations
similar to control: should have trajectory close to control,
with some drift towards the mean of the control group;
%cbi_pmm(
datain=tst, trtname=trt, subjname=subjid, visname=visit,
poolsite=,
basecont=%str(base_tst base_sqs base_mss),
baseclass=%str(sexn), postcont=%str(tst sqs mss),
postclass=%str(),
seed=883960001, nimp=1000,
primaryname=tst, analcovarcont=%str(base_tst base_sqs
base_mss), analcovarclass=%str(sexn), trtref=1,
analmethod=ancova, repstr=,
dataout=ddw.sleep_RBI_Q_macro_study_datafull,
resout=ddw.sleep_RBI_Q_macro_study_results, imptrtbytime=Y
);

* 1st sensitivity analysis: delta-adjust those discontinuing
due to AE or personal choice, using control based imputation
as a basis;
* no ready-made sequential-modeling macro for this, so use
handmade macro for RBI with addition of delta;
```

```
* perform reference-based imputation for a succession of
visits using visit-by-visit regression-based MI;
%MACRO imp_vis(SEED=-1, var=, visit=, delta=);
* select observations to be imputed (lastvis<&visit) ;
DATA impute&visit rest&visit;
     SET strtimp&visit;
* Put to one side subjects from experimental arm (trt=2) that
have data at time point &visit;
     IF trt = 2 AND lastvis >=&visit
  THEN
    OUTPUT rest&visit;
  * Select all other subjects for the time point &visit
imputation step;
  ELSE
    OUTPUT impute&visit;
run;


* only perform imputation for this visit if there are some
missings;
PROC SQL NOPRINT;
SELECT count(*) INTO :anymiss
     FROM impute&visit(WHERE=(&var._&visit IS MISSING));
QUIT;
%IF &anymiss>0
%THEN
  %DO;


* Step 2. Call PROC MI to impute missing data at time point
&visit using dataset IMPUTE&visit;
ODS LISTING CLOSE;
PROC MI DATA=impute&visit OUT=imputed&visit NIMPUTE=1
SEED=883960001;
     BY _imputation_;
     VAR base_mss base_sqs base_tst sexn %DO i=1 %TO &visit;
tst_&i sqs_&i mss_&i %END;;
     %if &visit=1
     %then
        %do;
     MONOTONE REGRESSION(mss_&visit=sexn base_tst base_sqs
base_mss);
     MONOTONE REGRESSION(sqs_&visit=sexn base_tst base_sqs
base_mss);
     MONOTONE REGRESSION(tst_&visit=sexn base_tst base_sqs
base_mss);
     %end;
     %if &visit>1
     %then
        %do;
     MONOTONE REGRESSION(MSS_&visit =sexn base_tst base_sqs
```

```
base_mss %DO i=1 %TO %eval(&visit-1); trt*tst_&i sqs_&i
trt*tst_&I mss_&i trt*mss_&i %END;);
      MONOTONE REGRESSION(sqs_&visit =sexn base_tst base_sqs
base_mss %DO i=1 %TO %eval(&visit-1); trt*tst_&i sqs_&i
  trt*tst_&I mss_&i trt*mss_&i %END;);
      MONOTONE REGRESSION(tst_&visit =sexn base_tst base_sqs
base_mss %DO i=1 %TO %eval(&visit 1); trt*tst_&i sqs_&i
trt*tst_&I mss_&i trt*mss_&i %END;);
       %end;
RUN;
ODS LISTING;
* apply delta;
DATA imputed&visit;
      SET imputed&visit;
      IF  lastvis<&visit AND trt=2 AND reasond in ("AE,"
"Consent withdrawn")
      THEN DO;
          tst_&visit  = tst_&visit + &delta;
          * apply delta to other efficacy variables
proportionately: for every 30 minutes, a score of 1 on the (1-
10) SQS and MSS scores;
          sqs_&visit  = sqs_&visit + (&delta/30);
          * for MSS (morning sleepiness score), higher is
worse: reverse the sign for the delta;
          mss_&visit  = mss_&visit - (&delta/30);
   END;
RUN;
  %END; * of &anymiss>0;

%IF &anymiss=0
%THEN
  %DO;
DATA imputed&visit;
  SET impute&visit;
RUN;
  %END;

* Step 3.  Re-assemble the dataset, now with time point &visit
imputed;
DATA strtimp%EVAL(&visit+1);
      SET rest&visit imputed&visit;
RUN;
PROC SORT DATA=strtimp%EVAL(&visit+1);
  BY _imputation_;
RUN;
%MEND imp_vis;

* call the macro once for each visit;
* dataset monotone is in vertical format (one record per
```

```
subject) and contains the original mania dataset with non-
monotone missings imputed using MCMC;
DATA strtimpl;
  SET monotone;
RUN;
%MACRO run_RBI(delta=);
%DO I=1 %TO 5;
  %imp_vis(seed=883960001, var=tst, visit=&i, delta=&delta);
%END;
%MEND run_RBI;
%run_RBI(delta=-30);


* third sensitivity analysis: assume LOCF-like outcomes for
the experimental arm and MAR for control arm, via GSK-
sponsored joint modeling macro;
options missing=.;
* dataset monotonv is as monotone above, but has one record
per subject and visit;
DATA tstGSK(DROP=subjid RENAME=(lsubjid=subjid));
  SET monotonv(WHERE=(visit NE 0));
  * numeric subjid works with GSK macro;
  LENGTH lsubjid 8;
  lsubjid=LEFT(TRIM(subjid))+0;
run;


* checks parameters and sets up a master file for the job;
%part1A(Jobname=sleep_GSK_OLMCF, Data=tstGSK, Subject=subjid,
Response=tst, Time=visit, Treat=trt,
cov=, catcov=, covbytime=base_tst base_sqs base_mss,
catcovbytime=sexn, PEwhere=, ID=, covgroup=trt,
debug=0);
* estimate the MMRM-like model parameters;
%part1B(Jobname=sleep_GSK_OLMCF, Ndraws=1000, thin=2, debug=0,
seed=883960001);


* estimate means for each subject, one per draw, assuming MAR;
%part2A(Jobname=sleep_GSK_MAR, Inname=sleep_GSK_OLMCF,
Method=MAR, ref=1, debug=0);
* calculate the imputed values;
* the multiply imputed datasets are in <jobname>_datafull;
%part2b(Jobname=sleep_GSK_MAR, debug=0);


* estimate means for each subject, one per draw, but assuming
LOCF-like values;
%part2A(Jobname=sleep_GSK_OLMCF, Method=OLMCF, ref=1, debug=0)
* calculate the imputed values;
* the multiply imputed datasets are in <jobname>_datafull;
%part2b(Jobname=sleep_GSK_OLMCF, debug=0);
```

```
* amalgamate MAR and OLMCF imputations (for control and
experimental arm, respectively);
DATA sleep_GSK_OLMCF_datafull;
   SET sleep_GSK_OLMCF_datafull(WHERE=(trt=2))
       sleep_GSK_MAR_datafull(WHERE=(trt=1));
RUN;


* perform univariate analysis by time point;
%part3(Jobname=sleep_GSK_OLMCF, debug=0);


* fourth sensitivity analysis: tipping point analysis, using
the run_RBI macro given in Appendix 7.B;
%MACRO sleep_tip(delta=, iter=);
%run_RBI(delta=&delta);
* convert dataset from horizontal format (all time points on
one record for a subject) to vertical format (one time point
per record for a subject);
DATA sleep_reason_study&iter;
  SET strtimp6;
  %MACRO makevert();
    %DO i=1 %TO 5;
      tst=tst_&i;
      visit=&i;
      OUTPUT;
    %END;
  %MEND makevert;
  %makevert();
RUN;


* write permanent file;
DATA ddw.sleep_reason_study&iter;
  SET sleep_reason_study&iter;
RUN;


* use macro from PMMutilityMacro.sas to analyze the imputed
data;
TITLE2 "Insomnia data by reason: RBI, delta=&delta for
experimental arm when reason=AE or subject choice, iteration
&iter";
TITLE3 "continuous endpoint (TST)";
%analyze(datain=sleep_reason_study&iter,
dataout=ddw.sleep_reason_study_results&iter,
trtname=trt, trtref=1, subjname=subjid, visname=visit,
primaryname=tst,
analcovarcont=base_tst base_sqs base_mss,
          analcovarclass=sexn, analmethod=ANCOVA);
TITLE2;
TITLE3;
%MEND sleep_tip;
```

```
%sleep_tip(delta=-15, iter=1);
%sleep_tip(delta=-30, iter=2);
%sleep_tip(delta=-45, iter=3);
%sleep_tip(delta=-60, iter=4);
```

Appendix 7.H SAS code to perform sensitivity analyses for the mania dataset

The following code assumes that (1) a monotone-missing dataset *resp* is available, with one record per subject visit; (2) dataset *strtimp1*, like *resp* but with one record per subject, is available; (3) the macros *cbi_pmm.sas, delta_pmm.sas, delta_and_tip.sas* and *PMMutilityMacros.sas* have been %INCLUDEd in the program.

```
* primary analysis: MAR MI;
ODS LISTING CLOSE;
PROC MI DATA=strtimp1 OUT=imputedMAR NIMPUTE=1
SEED=883960001;
   BY _imputation_;
   VAR trt country base_YMRS resp_1-resp_5;
   CLASS TRT country resp_1-resp_5;
   MONOTONE logistic(resp_1=trt country base_YMRS);
   MONOTONE logistic(resp_2=trt country base_YMRS
                         resp_1 trt*resp_1);
   MONOTONE logistic(resp_3=trt country base_YMRS
                         resp_1 trt*resp_1
                         resp_2 trt*resp_2);
   MONOTONE logistic(resp_4=trt country base_YMRS
                         resp_1 trt*resp_1
                         resp_2 trt*resp_2
                         resp_3 trt*resp_3);
   MONOTONE logistic(resp_5=trt country base_YMRS
                         resp_1 trt*resp_1
                         resp_2 trt*resp_2
                         resp_3 trt*resp_3
                         resp_4 trt*resp_4);
RUN;
ODS LISTING;


* 1st sensitivity analysis, worst-case analysis: count all
withdrawals as non-responders;
DATA respwors;
   SET resp;
   IF resp=.
   THEN
      resp=0;
RUN;
```

```
ODS LISTING CLOSE;
ODS RESULTS OFF;
PROC GENMOD DATA=respwors;
  CLASS trt country;
  MODEL resp/denom = trt country base_ymrs/DIST=BIN;
  LSMEANS trt/DIFF=control("1") EXP CL;
  BY visit;
  ODS OUTPUT LSMEANS=lsm DIFFS=diffs;
RUN;
ODS LISTING;
ODS RESULTS ON;

* 2nd sensitivity analysis, worst-case analysis, but only
count withdrawals from experimental treatment arm as non-
responders, assume withdrawals from control arm are MAR;
* use MI output from primary analysis, which assumes MAR;
data Mania_binary_sdy_MAR_datafull;
  set imputedMAR;
  resp=0;
  visit=0;
  output Mania_binary_sdy_MAR_datafull;
  %macro makevert();
    %do i=1 %to 5;
      resp=resp_&i;
      visit=&I;
      output Mania_binary_sdy_MAR_datafull;
    %END;
  %mend makevert;
%makevert();
DATA Mania_binary_worse2_datafull;
   SET Mania_binary_sdy_MAR_datafull(DROP=resp_0-resp_5);
   IF lastvis<visit AND trt=2
   THEN
    resp=0;
RUN;

proc genmod data=Mania_binary_worse2_datafull;
  class trt country;
  model resp = trt country base_ymrs/dist=bin;
  lsmeans trt /diff;
  by visit _imputation_;
  ods output lsmeans=lsm diffs=diffs;
run;

proc mianalyze data=diffs;
modeleffects Estimate;
stderr stderr;
ods output parameterestimates=diff2  VarianceInfo=diffs_V;
run;
```

```
* 3rd sensitivity analysis, imputation varies by reason;
* for experimental arm subjects discontinuing with reason AE,
Consent withdrawn or Decision of investigator,
* change MAR-imputed responder to non-responder with
probability 0.25;
* use the %delta macro from appendix 7.D;
* perform the visit-by-visit MI, for the post-baseline visits;
%MACRO run_delta();
%DO I=1 %TO 5;
  %delta(seed1=883960001, seed2=883960002,
      var=resp, visit=&i, delta=0.25,
      condn=%str(AND reasond IN ("AE," "Consent withdrawn,"
      "Decision of investigator")));
%END;
%MEND run_delta;
%run_delta();
* 4th sensitivity analysis, tipping point version of previous
analysis, using run_tdelta macro from Appendix 7.D;
%MACRO run_tip(deltacont=, tipstepcont=, tipmaxiter=);
%LET thisdelta=&deltacont;
%DO tipiter=1 %TO &tipmaxiter;
    %run_tdelta(delta=&&thisdelta);
    %let thisdelta=&&thisdelta + &tipstepcont;
%END; *of do loop for &tipiter
%MEND run_tip;
%run_tip(deltacont=0.10, tipstepcont=%left(0.05),
tipmaxiter=2);
```

Appendix 7.I Selection models

Theory

In Section 7.2.2, we noted that PMMs decompose the joint probability of outcome and missingness, conditional on observed covariates, in the following way:

$$p(Y_{obs}, Y_{mis}, R|X) = p(R|X)p(Y_{obs}, Y_{mis}|R, X)$$

Selection models decompose the joint probability of outcome and missingness as follows:

$$p(Y_{obs}, Y_{mis}, R|X) = p(Y_{obs}, Y_{mis}|X)p(R|X, Y_{obs}, Y_{mis})$$

A selection model approach presupposes that one can model the complete outcome (missing and observed) jointly with the missingness, and the two models can be linked not only by common explanatory covariates X, but also because the missing outcomes Y_{mis} can form part of the expression defining the likelihood of the binary missingness variable, R.

Regression coefficients for Y_{mis} in the model for R can allow the model to test for dependence on unobserved data. However, importantly, as noted in Chapter 4, this test itself relies on untestable assumptions about the distribution of the data, and so is not a useful test of dependence – it cannot be used to "prove" that the data are or are not MAR, for instance. However, some experts view such estimated regression coefficients as interesting and informative. Further, scenarios of greater or lesser dependence (again, given the untestable assumptions about the distribution of the data) can be played out by assigning larger or smaller values to the coefficient for Y_{mis} in the model, and assessing the resulting estimates of treatment effect. As noted in Section 4.2.4.2, we add a caveat that these estimates can be difficult to interpret in a clinically meaningful way.

Implementation

Hedeker and Gibbons (2006) describe selection models, and Hedeker (2012) shows an example implementation of a selection model in the mixed effects setting for a binary response with a linear time effect, using SAS's PROC NLMIXED. Zheng and Lin (2012) have made available at www.missingdata.org.uk a SAS macro to implement a selection model for a continuous outcome with missing data assuming a linear time effect. The user can specify the model for Y, and can choose from a set of scenarios via a user-selected choice of dependency on unobserved outcomes. The macro uses PROC IML to do the integration necessary to estimate the regression parameters across the two probability models (i.e., the full data model and the missingness model). Finally, Chen (2013) provides an implementation of selection models by means of PROC MCMC, which uses a very compact piece of code that clarifies how selection modeling links the probability of the missingness with the probability of the full data.

Example

We use the DIA macro to implement a selection model for the semi-continuous YMRS efficacy score in the illustrative mania dataset. We note that, at least in the DIA implementation, similar issues arise with selection models as with MMRM and GLMM approaches, with regard to convergence. The DIA macro allows the user to specify the following variance–covariance structures (codenames in parentheses):

- unstructured (UN);
- autoregressive (AR[H]);
- Toeplitz (TOEP[H]);
- compound symmetry (CS[H]);

with the [H] indicating that heterogeneity of variance is allowed for. Our application of the selection model to the mania dataset would converge only for the compound symmetry structure. We allowed for heterogeneity of variance. We first implement an MAR analysis, where the model does not include a dependence on unobserved outcomes. A second call specifies macro parameter *mech* = "MNAR" to allow the modeling of a dependence of *R* on the unobserved outcome through regression parameters *psi5* and *psi6* for the control and active treatment groups, respectively. SAS code to call the macro for the mania dataset assumes that the dataset *maniah* has one record per subject visit, and is as follows:

```
* rename variables as required by macro;
DATA ymrs(rename=(subjid=patient visit=seq));
  SET maniah(where=(visit>0));

  * create character treatment code;
  LENGTH therapy $10;
  IF trt=1
  THEN
   therapy="Control";
  ELSE
   therapy="Experiml";

  * center the YMRS score approximately ;
  ymrs=(ymrs-30)/7;
  base_ymrs=(base_ymrs-30)/7;
  change=ymrs-base_ymrs;
RUN;

PROC SORT DATA=ymrs;
   BY patient seq;
RUN;

* first, perform an MAR analysis, with missingness modeled as
not depending on unobserved values of YMRS;
%Selection_Model2(
     inputds = ymrs,
     covtype = CSH,
     response = change,
     modl = base_ymrs therapy seq therapy*seq base_YMRS*seq,
     clasvar = therapy seq,
     mech = MAR,
     const = 4,
     derivative = 1,
     method = %str(QN),
     out1 = Ch_7_SM1_mania_estimates,
     out2 = Ch_7_SM1_mania_diffs,
     out3 = _Ch_7_SM1_mania_lsmeans,
     debug = 1
);
```

```
* now perform a MNAR analysis, allowing dependency between
unobserved outcome and missingness to be modeled via
coefficients psi5 and psi6 for dependency between missingness
and the unobserved outcome (dependency for control
and active treatment groups, respectively);
%Selection_Model2(
     inputds = ymrs,
     covtype = CSH,
     response = change,
     modl = base_ymrs therapy seq therapy*seq base_YMRS*seq,
     clasvar = therapy seq,
     mech = MNAR,
     const = 4,
     derivative = 1,
     method = %str(QN),
     out1 = Ch_7_SM2_mania_estimates,
     out2 = Ch_7_SM2_mania_diffs,
     out3 = Ch_7_SM2_mania_lsmeans,
     debug = 1
);
```

The coefficient for treatment effect at the final visit assuming MAR and its SE are estimated at 0.22 (SE 0.092, p-value $= 0.0161$). We note that the contrast here subtracts the mean for the experimental treatment group from that of control; lower YMRS is better, so the result is in favor of the experimental treatment group. When we assume MNAR and allow a dependence to be estimated between missingness and the unobserved Y, the regression coefficients for this dependence are large relative to their SEs (-1.33 (SE 0.151) and 1.58 (SE 0.348) for the control and experimental treatment groups, respectively). It is notable that the direction of the regression coefficients differs between treatment groups. Recall that lower YMRS scores are better. It seems that the higher (worse) the unobserved YMRS score for the control group, the lower the probability of missingness is estimated; while for the experimental treatment group, the higher the YMRS the higher the estimated risk of missingness. Given these large values for *psi5* and *psi6*, as one might expect, the estimate of treatment effect under the MNAR assumption differs from that under MAR: it is perhaps surprising that the coefficient for treatment effect at the final visit is now estimated to be in favor of the control treatment group, at -0.18 (SE 0.100, p-value $= 0.0689$).

To explore the MNAR assumption, we force the values of the regression coefficients for dependence on unobserved values to be stronger, by specifying values for psi5 and psi6 that are larger in magnitude than estimated in the above step:

```
* MNAR analysis estimated psi5 and psi6 as -1.33 and 1.59,
respectively - posit values more extreme than this to see if
result changes under the more extreme assumption about MNAR);
```

```
%Selection_Model2(
     inputds = ymrs,
     covtype = CSH,
     response = change,
     modl = base_ymrs therapy seq therapy*seq base_YMRS*seq,
     clasvar = therapy seq,
     mech = MNARS,
     psi5 = -2.00,
     psi6 = 2.00,
     const = 4,
     derivative = 1,
     method = %str(QN),
     out1 = Ch_7_SM3_mania_estimates,
     out2 = Ch_7_SM3_mania_diffs,
     out3 = _Ch_7_SM3_mania_lsmeans,
     debug = 1
);
```

The results are even more clearly in favor of the control treatment group: treatment effect is estimated as −0.26 (SE 0.073, p-value = 0.0063). If we posit values for *psi5* and *psi6* that are approximately half of those estimated (−0.7 and 0.8, respectively), the estimate is non-significant ($p = 0.8478$) but still favors the control group, at −0.018 (SE 0.093).

It would be difficult to draw conclusions with regard to a primary MAR analysis of YMRS from the above selection model analyses, because the implementation required a rather simple compound-symmetric structure for the variance–covariance matrix, which makes strong assumptions compared to the unstructured variance–covariance matrix that is the ideal one to use in this context. Nevertheless, the differences in results under different scenarios is striking, and could prompt further analyses.

Appendix 7.J Shared parameter models

Theory

Shared parameter models decompose the joint probability of outcome and missingness as follows:

$$p\left(Y_{obs}, Y_{mis}, R|X\right) = p(Y_{obs}, Y_{mis}|X, B)p(R|X, B)$$

The first part of the decomposition on the right-hand side is the same as that for the selection model in Appendix 7.I, except for the addition of a (latent) random variable B. The second part on the right-hand side is linked to the outcome data not by conditioning on the Y as in selection models, but by likewise including B.

Implementation

Hedeker (2012) gives an implementation in the mixed effects setting for a binary response with a linear time effect, using SAS's PROC NLMIXED.

As with the selection model, members of the DIA SWG for missing data have made available on www.missingdata.org.uk a SAS macro to implement shared parameter models that, like Hedeker's code, uses PROC NLMIXED (Lin and Xu, 2012; Xu and Lin, 2012). The Lin and Xu macro allows for up to three (latent) random variables. As with Hedeker's implementation, trial visit or time point is treated as a continuous variable. For the probability of Y, in addition to the usual model effects the user may request that the model include:

- a random intercept;

- a random intercept and a random slope over time; or

- a random intercept, a random slope over time and a random slope over time squared.

These requests are made by giving the value "none," "linear" and "quad," respectively, for macro parameter RANDOM_SLOPE.

If g here is the variable indicating visit or time point, b is used to represent random variables and ε the residual variance, the three models for the Y corresponding to the three requests above could, for example, look like this:

- $Y_{ik} = \beta_0 + \beta_1 g_{ik} + \dots + b_{i0} + \varepsilon_{ik}$

- $Y_{ik} = \beta_0 + \beta_1 g_{ik} + \dots + b_{i0} + b_{i1} g_{ik} + \varepsilon_{ik}$

- $Y_{ik} = \beta_0 + \beta_1 g_{ik} + \beta_2 g_{ik} g_{ik} + \dots + b_{i0} + b_{i1} g_{ik} + b_{i2} g_{ik} g_{ik} + \varepsilon_{ik}$

The macro estimates parameters by maximizing the joint likelihood of the requested model for Y and the model for the missingness variables R. For any of the above three requests, the macro does the estimation in three different ways, allowing for progressively more complex "sharing" of the (latent) random variables between the models for Y and R by modifying the model for R:

- no sharing – no random variables included in the model for R;

- sharing ignoring treatment group – random variables are included in the model for R;

- sharing allowing different regression coefficients for the random variables for each treatment group in the model for R.

Thus for any dataset and β, a total of nine variants of the selection model are available (if we count "no sharing" as a variant).

Note that the model for Y does not change in the above three variants.

Let Φ be some probability function for a binary variable and let f_{il} be the indicator for treatment group ($f_{il} = 0$, $1 \Rightarrow$ subject i is randomized to control, experimental treatment arm, respectively). Let Ψ be the regression coefficients in the model for R.

Then, for example, if the user requests a random intercept and a random slope over time, the three models for the R with progressively more complex sharing would look like this:

- $P(R_{ik} = 0 | R_{i.k-1} = 1) = \Phi\left(\psi_{i0} + \psi_{i1} f_{i1}\right)$
- $P(R_{ik} = 0 | R_{i.k-1} = 1) = \Phi\left(\psi_{i0} + \psi_{i1} f_{i1} + \psi_{i3} b_{i0} + \psi_{i4} b_{i1}\right)$
- $P(R_{ik} = 0 | R_{i.k-1} = 1) = \Phi(\psi_{i0} + \psi_{i1} f_{i1} + \psi_{i3} f_{i1} b_{i0} + \psi_{i4} f_{i1} b_{i1} + \psi_{i5}(f_{i1} - 1) b_{i0} + \psi_{i6}(f_{i1} - 1) b_{i1})$

Note that, apart from the (latent) random variables, in this implementation the model for missingness is constrained to be simple, consisting only of an intercept and a factor for treatment group ($\psi_{i0} + \psi_{i1} f_{i1}$).

Macro

We use the DIA macro to implement a shared parameter model for the continuous TST efficacy score in the illustrative insomnia dataset. It is assumed that the *tsth* dataset has the *tst* scores, with one record per subject visit. As before, TST at baseline is held in the variable *base_tst*. The joint likelihood would not converge when the full five post-baseline visits were included, but did converge when just the first and final visits were included. Accordingly, the following analysis includes only these two post-baseline visit records.

SAS code to call the macro for the insomnia dataset is as follows.

```
DATA tsth;
    SET tsth(WHERE=(visit>0 AND (visit=1 OR visit=5)));
    * treatment groups must be 0 (=control) and 1
(=experimental);
    trt=trt-1;
    change=tst-base_tst;

    * help convergance by standardising efficacy score;
    tst=(tst-339)/100;
    base_tst=(base_tst-339)/100;
    change=tst-base_tst;
RUN;


* works with slope=none, but not slope=linear or =quad;
options mprint;
%shared_parameter(
    INPUTDS=tsth,
    SUBJVAR=subjid,
    TRTVAR=trt,
    TIME=visit,
    quadtime=,
    Additional_Class=%STR( ),
    MODL=%STR(CHANGE= base_tst trt visit visit*trt
```

```
base_tst*visit),
   LINK=logit,
   RANDOM_SLOPE=%STR(none),
   DEBUG=0
);
```

The option RANDOM_SLOPE=%STR(none) requests that the model for Y and the model for R have a single random variable, an intercept, in common. The likelihood for the other options of RANDOM_SLOPE did not converge for the dataset, so we do not present results for these options here.

Whichever option the user chooses via RANDOM_SLOPE, the macro displays in three columns the estimates, SEs and p-values for regression coefficients, under each of the three assumptions for the linking of the models for Y and R. Coefficients for the Y model begin with the letter "b"; coefficients for the R model (including the coefficients for the random effects) begin with the letter "a." The coefficients for the random effects are labeled "aInt," "aSlp" and (if a quadratic random slope is modeled) "aSlp2." If separate regression coefficients are estimated for the random effects for the two treatment groups, the regression coefficients for the random effects for $f_{i1} = 0$ begin with "a" and the regression coefficients for the random effects for $f_{i1} = 1$ begin with "aD" – that is, they are labeled "aDint," "aDslp" and "aDslps."

In our case, for all estimates, the regression coefficients for the random variables were not significantly different from zero ($p = 1$). Given that the model failed to identify a latent-variable link between the missingness and the outcome models, one would in this case expect the results from the selection model to be close to those from an equivalent MAR analysis. The macro output includes results from a conventional MMRM analysis assuming MAR as well as the selection model results. Here, as expected, the results from the MAR and the selection model analyses are indeed identical.

References

Altshuler L, Suppes T, Black D, Nolen W, Keck P, Frye M, McElroy S, Kupka R, Grunze H, Walden J, Leverich G, Denicoff K, Luckenbaugh D, Post R (2003) Impact of anti-depressant discontinuation after acute bipolar depression remission on rates of depressive relapse at 1-year follow-up. *American Journal of Psychiatry* **160**: 1252–1262.

Bunouf P, Grouin J-M, Molenberghs G (2012) Analysis of an incomplete binary outcome derived from frequently recorded longitudinal continuous data: application to daily pain evaluation. *Statistics in Medicine* **31**: 1554–1571.

Carpenter JR, Kenward MG (2007) *Missing Data in Randomized Controlled Trials – A Practical Guide*. National Health Service Co-ordinating Centre for Research Methodology, Birmingham, available at www.hta.nhs.uk/nihrmethodology/reports/1589.pdf, accessed 18 June 2013.

Carpenter JR, Kenward MG (2013) *Multiple Imputation and its Application*. James Wiley and Sons, New York.

Carpenter JR, Roger JH, Kenward MG (2013) Analysis of longitudinal trials with protocol deviation: a framework for relevant, accessible assumptions and inference via multiple imputation. *Journal of Biopharmaceutical Statistics*, **23**(6): 1352–1371. DOI: 10.1080/10543406.2013.834911

Cavanagh J, Smyth R, Goodwin G (2004) Relapse into mania or depression following lithium discontinuation: a 7 year follow-up. *Acta Psychiatrica Scandinavica* **109**: 91–95.

Chen F (2011) *Missing no more: using the PROC MCMC procedure to model missing data.* SAS Global Forum 2013, available at http://support.sas.com/resources/papers/proceedings13/436-2013.pdf, accessed 29 November 2013.

European Medicines Agency (2010) Guideline on missing data in confirmatory clinical trials, EMA/CPMP/EWP/1776/99 Rev.1, available http://www.ema.europa.eu/docs/en_GB/document_library/Scientific_guideline/2009/09/WC500003460.pdf, accessed 22 March 2013.

Glynn R, Laird N, Rubin DB (1986) Selection modeling versus mixture modeling with nonignorable nonresponse. In: H. Wainer (ed.), *Drawing Inferences from Self-Selected Samples.* Springer-Verlag, New York.

Glynn R, Laird N, Rubin DB (1993) Multiple imputation in mixture models for nonignorable nonresponse with follow-ups. *Journal of the American Statistical Association* **88**: 984–993.

Hedeker D (2012) *Missing data in longitudinal studies,* available at http://www.uic.edu/classes/bstt/bstt513/missbLS.pdf, accessed 20 June 2013.

Hedeker D, Gibbons R (2006) *Longitudinal Data Analysis.* John Wiley and Sons, New York.

Jungquist C, Tra Y, Smith M, Pigeon W, Matteson-Rusby S, Xia Y, Perlis M (2012) The Durability of Cognitive Behavioral Therapy for Insomnia in Patients with Chronic Pain. *Sleep disorders,* available at http://www.hindawi.com/journals/sd/2012/679648/, accessed 20 June 2013.

Kenward M, Carpenter J (2009) Multiple imputation. In: M Davidian, G Fitzmaurice, G Molenberghs, G Verbeke (eds.), *Longitudinal Data analysis: A Handbook of Modern Statistical Methods.* Chapman and Hall, London, pp. 477–500.

Lin Q, Xu L for the Eli Lilly and Company Advanced Analytic Missing Data Hub (2012) *shared_parameter1.sas,* available at http://missingdata.lshtm.ac.uk/dia/Selection%20Model_20120726.zip, accessed 20 June 2013.

Lipkovich I, Houston J, Ahl J (2008) Identifying patterns in treatment response profiles in acute bipolar mania: a cluster analysis approach. *BMC Psychiatry* **8**: 65.

Little R (1993) Pattern-mixture models for multivariate incomplete data. *Journal of the American Statistical Association* **88**: 125–134.

Little R, Yau L (1996) Intention-to-treat analysis for longitudinal studies with drop-outs. *Biometrics* **52**: 1324–1333.

Mallinckrodt C (2013) *Preventing and Treating Missing Data in Longitudinal Clinical Trials.* Cambridge University Press, Cambridge.

Mayer G, Wang-Weigand S, Roth-Schechter B, Lehmann R, Staner C, Partinen M (2009) Efficacy and safety of 6-month nightly ramelteon administration in adults with chronic primary insomnia. *Sleep* **32**: 351–360.

National Research Council. Panel on Handling Missing Data in Clinical Trials. Committee on National Statistics, Division of Behavioral and Social Sciences and Education (2010) *The Prevention and Treatment of Missing Data in Clinical Trials.* The National Academies Press, Washington, DC.

Post R, Altshuler L, Frye M, Suppes T, McElroy S, Keck P, Leverich G, Kupka R, Nolen W, Luckenbaugh D, Walden J, Grunze H (2005) Preliminary observations on the effectiveness of levetiracetam in the open adjunctive treatment of refractory bipolar disorder. *Journal of Clinical Psychiatry* **66**: 370–374.

Ratitch B (2012a) *Fitting Control-Based Imputation (Using Monotone Sequential Regression) Macro Documentation.* available at http://missingdata.lshtm.ac uk/dia/PMM%20Delta%20Tipping%20Point%20and%20CBI_20120726.zip, accessed 20 June 2013.

Ratitch B (2012b) *Tipping Point Analysis with Delta-Adjusting Imputation (Using Monotone Sequential Regression) Macro Documentation.* http://missingdata.lshtm.ac.uk/dia/PMM%20Delta%20Tipping%20Point%20and%20CBI_20120726.zip, accessed 20 June 2013.

Ratitch B, O'Kelly M (2011) *Implementation of Pattern-Mixture Models Using Standard SAS/STAT Procedures.* PharmaSUG 2011, available at http://pharmasug.org/proceedings/2011/SP/PharmaSUG-2011-SP04.pdf, accessed 20 June 2013.

Ratitch B, O'Kelly M, Tosiello R (2013) Missing data in clinical trials: from clinical assumptions to statistical analysis using pattern mixture models. *Pharmaceutical Statistics*, **12**: 337–347, http://onlinelibrary.wiley.com/doi/10.1002/pst.1549/pdf, accessed 20 June 2013.

Roger J (2010) Discussion of Incomplete and Enriched Data Analysis and Sensitivity Analysis, presented by Geert Molenberghs. Drug Information Association (DIA) Meeting, Special Interest Area Communities (SIAC) – Statistics, January 2010.

Roger J (2012) *Fitting pattern-mixture models to longitudinal repeated-measures data,* available at http://missingdata.lshtm.ac.uk/dia/Five_Macros20120827.zip, accessed 20 June 2013.

Roger J, Ritchie S, Donovan C, Carpenter J (2008) *Sensitivity Analysis for Longitudinal Studies with Withdrawal.* PSI Conference, May 2008, available at http://www.psiweb.org/docs/2008finalprogramme.pdf, accessed 20 June 2013.

Rubin DB (1987) *Multiple Imputation for Nonresponse in Surveys.* John Wiley and Sons, New York.

Rubin DB (1996) Multiple imputation after 18+ years. *Journal of the American Statistical Association* **91**: 473–489.

Shulman L, Gruber-Baldini A, Anderson K, Fishman P, Reich S, Weiner W (2010) The clinically important difference on the unified Parkinson's disease rating scale. *Archives of Neurology* **67**: 64–70.

Xu L, Lin Q (2012) *Shared parameter model for informative missing data,* available at http://missingdata.lshtm.ac.uk/dia/Selection%20Model_20120726.zip, accessed 20 June 2013.

Yan X, Lee S, Li N (2009) Missing data handling methods in medical device clinical trials. *Journal of Biopharmaceutical Statistics* **19**: 1085–1098.

Yan X, Li H, Gao Y, Gray G (2008) *Case study: sensitivity analysis in clinical trials.* AdvaMed/FDA conference, http://www.amstat.org/sections/sigmedd/Advamed/advamed08/presentation/Yan_sherry.pdf, accessed 20 June 2013.

Zheng W, Lin Q, for the Eli Lilly and Company Advanced Analytic Missing Data Hub (2012) *Sensitivity Analysis on Incomplete Longitudinal Data with Selection Model.* http://missingdata.lshtm.ac.uk/dia/Selection%20Model_20120726.zip, accessed 20 June 2013.

Table of SAS Code Fragments

7.1   Simplified MI model to illustrate interaction by visit.
7.2   Simplified direct likelihood MMRM model to illustrate interaction by visit.
7.3   Use MCMC to impute non-monotone missing values.
7.4   Use regression imputation to complete the MAR imputation, to match an MMRM where covariances are estimated across all treatment groups.
7.5   Use regression imputation to complete the MAR imputation; the inclusion of interactions with treatment is consistent with an MMRM where covariances are estimated separately for each treatment group (as with the GROUP=*trt* option in PROC MIXED).
7.6   Select observations so as to impute Visit 1 using model based on control arm.
7.7   Impute Visit 1 using model based on control arm.
7.8   Re-assemble the dataset to impute missing values at the next visit.
7.9   Impute Visit 2 using model-based control arm.
7.10   Create dataset with missing values for reference treatment imputed assuming MAR, as preparation for J2R.
7.11   Impute distribution of control to Visit 2 value in experimental arm with baseline as the only covariable.
7.12   Perform the MI assuming MAR for the control arm.
7.13   Prepare to model the distribution of baseline values for BOCF-like imputation.
7.14   Impute baseline-like values for the subject visits with missing outcomes.
7.15   Transpose imputed values to obtain a dataset with one record per subject with all imputed values for a subject on the same record.
7.16   Use baseline-distributed values for imputing the subject visits with missing post-baseline assessments.
7.17   Select subjects with last observation at Visit 1 to impute LOCF values for Visits 2, 3, 4 and 5 for these subjects.
7.18   Create LOCF-like values for subjects whose last observation was at Visit 1.
7.19   Imputing last observation-distributed values, adapting the code from SAS Code Fragment 7.14.
7.20   Imputing baseline-like values for subjects with reason for discontinuation = "AE."
7.21   Imputing a base imputation before imposing a delta adjustment.
7.22   Adjust imputed value by an amount δ.
7.23   Imposing a delta adjustment after all subjects have been imputed based on MAR assumption via MI with joint modeling as implemented by Roger.
7.24   Imposing an adjustment to imputed binary response with a probability δ.
7.25   Call the *run_tdelta* macro repeatedly to implement a tipping point analysis.

See the Appendices to this chapter for additional SAS code examples.

8

Doubly robust estimation

Belinda Hernández, Ilya Lipkovich
and Michael O'Kelly

Key points

- Inverse probability weighting (IPW) weights subjects by the inverse probability of their being observed. In this way, subjects that are fully observed but have a small probability of being fully observed are treated as being representative of those with missing values. Such subjects are given a larger weight to compensate for missing data on subjects who would have similar outcome profiles, but whose data is not available because they dropped out.

- Doubly robust (DR) estimators augment the IPW estimator by making use not only of subjects with fully observed data but also the subjects with partially observed data which are used to predict (or impute) missing outcome values.

- DR estimators use three models: one, which models the probability of being observed (the missingness model), another which estimates missing values by modeling the relationship between the observed data and the response (the imputation model), and an analysis model which models the overall scientific question of interest.

- With DR estimators, if the imputation model or the missingness model are misspecified (but not both) the resulting estimates will still be unbiased. This

---

Clinical Trials with Missing Data: A Guide for Practitioners, First Edition. Michael O'Kelly and Bohdana Ratitch.
© 2014 John Wiley & Sons, Ltd. Published 2014 by John Wiley & Sons, Ltd.

provides the statistician with two opportunities to specify a correct model and obtain consistent unbiased estimates.

- Vansteelandt *et al.* (2010) propose a DR method for dealing with missingness in the response variable, which will be described in this chapter.

8.1   Introduction

Doubly robust (DR) estimators combine three models: an imputation model which models the response variables Y on the covariates X; a missingness model which calculates π_{ij}, the probability of being observed for each subject i at trial visit j; and a final analysis model which is the model that would have been used if there were no missing values in the dataset or, in other words, the model which answers the overall scientific question of interest. With DR methods, either the imputation model or the missingness model, but not both, can be misspecified and the trialist will still obtain unbiased estimates, thus giving the analyst two opportunities to correctly specify a model and get valid, consistent results. DR estimators augment the inverse probability weighted estimator by adding a term based on an imputation model that has an expected value of zero, if the inverse probability weighting (IPW) model is correctly specified. DR estimators can be more efficient than IPW estimators, which is not surprising because they make use of not only the fully observed subjects but also the information contained in partially observed subjects. We will first introduce the concept of IPW estimators before going on to describe DR estimation. We will also discuss the assumptions, advantages and limitations of each of these methods in turn.

The chapter will then focus on a particular implementation of DR estimation proposed by Vansteelandt *et al.* (2010) before finally providing example code showing how to implement this method in SAS. The code described here can also be implemented using a macro called "*Vansteelandt_method.sas*" which is available at the Drug Information Association (DIA) Special Working Group on Missing Data web page on the www.missingdata.org.uk site. As explained in Chapter 7, we feel that it is useful to provide sample code to show the reader how to implement this method using standard SAS procedures not only for ease of interpretation but also for use if an independent programmed quality control (QC) check is needed to support the validity of the analysis performed using the macro. Section 8.5 will provide SAS code fragments and results obtained from the analysis of two illustrative clinical trial datasets referred to throughout the book: the illustrative insomnia and mania datasets.

8.2   Inverse probability weighted estimation

Inverse probability weighted estimators are a form of complete case analysis that can give unbiased estimates when the missing at random (MAR) assumption holds. Here, π_{ij}, the probability of subject i being observed at the jth occurrence, is calculated separately for each visit j and the inverse of this probability is then applied to

Table 8.1   IPW example used in Carpenter and Kenward (2006).

x_i	A	A	A	B	B	B	C	C	C
y_i	1	1	1	2	2	2	3	3	3
r_i	1	0	0	1	1	1	1	1	0
π_i	1/3			1	1	1	2/3	2/3	
r_i/π_i	3	0	0	1	1	1	1.5	1.5	0

the outcome model for subject i. As often is the case, we are interested in estimating parameters which will be valid for the entire population of interest, extending inference not only for populations of subjects represented by those subjects fully observed, but also to those with missing data. Weighting subjects with the inverse of the probability of being observed results in constructing a "pseudo-population" in which subjects with certain covariate profiles who were under-represented in the observed data receive higher weights. Conversely, those kinds of subjects that were over-represented in the observed data receive lower weight. With IPW, then, patients who were actually observed, but had low probability of being observed, are treated as being representative of subjects with missing outcomes in the data, who would have similar outcome profiles, had they been observed, and as such receive a higher weight (Robins *et al.*, 1994).

The intuition behind IPW methods is very clearly explained in a simple example by Carpenter and Kenward (2006), which we will reiterate here. In this example, the target for the inference is the mean of the response, and the IPW estimator is defined in Equation 8.1.

$$\mu_{ipw} = \frac{\sum_{i=1}^{N} (r_i/\pi_i) y_i}{\sum_{i=1}^{N} r_i/\pi_i} \tag{8.1}$$

Here r_i is an indicator variable which is 1 when the ith subject is observed and 0 otherwise; y_i is the outcome or response for ith subject and π_i is the probability of being observed that is computed based on some fully observed covariate X with 3 possible levels (A, B and C). Example data is illustrated in Table 8.1.

Table 8.1 presents π_i, the probability of being observed for each level of the covariate x_i. As can be seen, the mean of the outcome variable y_i is 2 for the full data (including both complete and incomplete cases). This "full data mean" is an unbiased estimate of the true mean in the population. If complete cases only are used, the estimated mean would be 2 1/6, which probably overestimates the true mean. The bias is caused by the fact that subjects with $x_i =$ "A" (which has lower expected outcome) are represented in the observed sample by a single subject, whereas the category $x_i =$ "C" with higher expected outcome is represented by two subjects (over-represented compared with the group with $x_i =$ "A"). However, if for the observed cases, the outcome is weighted by r_i/π_i (the inverse probability of being observed), we see that the estimated mean is 2 ((3 + 2 + 2 + 2 + 4.5 + 4.5)/9), and the bias is removed.

Of course, the example above is a very simple one. However, we can still see how IPW estimators, by weighting the outcome by the inverse probability, put higher importance on the observations that have a low probability of being observed. In this way, we can estimate the true parameter of interest in the entire population of observed and missing observations.

8.2.1   Inverse probability weighting estimators for estimating equations

The objective of most clinical trials is not to estimate a simple population mean but rather to estimate some (functions of) model parameters, so as to quantify, for example, the effect of treatment versus control. We can show that for such functions the same logic applies with regard to IPW estimators.

In the following explanation we use a similar notation to Daniel and Kenward (2012). For a parametric or non-parametric model, the form of the IPW estimator is as shown in Equation 8.2.

$$\sum_{i=1}^{N} \frac{r_i}{\hat{\pi}_i} U_\theta \left(W_i, \theta^{ipw} \right) = 0 \tag{8.2}$$

where W_i is the complete data vector $W_i = (X_i^{T}, Y_i^{T})^{T}$; X_i are the fully observed baseline and post-baseline covariates; θ^{ipw} is the vector of parameters which we wish to estimate; r_i is an indicator variable which takes the value 1 when y_i is observed and 0 otherwise, $\hat{\pi}_i$ is the estimated probability of y_i being observed, and U_θ (.) is the score function. If we take the Gaussian case then the IPW estimation of the parameters β are the solution to the following normal estimating equations for β over the observed cases:

$$\sum_{i=1}^{N} \frac{r_i}{\hat{\pi}_i} X_i \left(y_i - X_i^{T} \hat{\beta} \right) = 0 \tag{8.3}$$

For Equation 8.3 we can see that the parameter estimates $\hat{\beta}$ are consistent as long as the estimates for π_i are consistent, that is, as long as the missingness model for π_i is correctly specified (Robins et al., 1994).

With repeated measures, such as a clinical trial with more than one post-baseline visit, π_{ij} (the probability for subject i being observed at visit j), is estimated by creating dichotomous variables R_{ij} which indicate patient i being observed at visit j and then performing a separate logistic regression for each visit j using R_{ij} as the response. These probabilities can then be transformed into the vertical format of one observation per subject/visit to give the overall weight $\frac{r_{ij}}{\hat{\pi}_{ij}}$ in the IPW model.

Of course, as mentioned above, the obvious limitation to this approach is that the model for the probability of being observed has to be correct in order for the resulting estimator to be unbiased. If the wrong model is used for estimating π_i, then the observations will be weighted incorrectly and so will not be able to properly represent the missing data. As, in practice, there is no way of knowing if the probability model is correct, this assumption may be rather strong, thus limiting the use of the IPW method. Also, if an observation has a very small estimated probability of being observed, the inverse weight on this observation will be extremely large and so could unduly dominate the analysis. This concept is slightly counterintuitive, as it means that the more accurately the IPW model predicts the probability of subjects who are the most representative of the missing observations, the more unstable the IPW solution becomes. However, it is hard to adjust for bias caused by missing subjects when there are only very few corresponding observed representatives in the sample, as it is hard to make inference based on small sample size in general, and it is impossible in the extreme case when there are no observed representatives corresponding to certain kinds of missing data. Note that probabilities estimated close to the boundaries (0 or 1) may simply reflect the non-probabilistic mechanism behind generation of missing values. This may happen if there is a provision in the protocol that investigators should discontinue a subject from the study once a certain criteria has been met as in this case, the logic of IPW does not apply. Because of these issues great care needs to be taken by the trialist when using IPW estimation to ensure that one or a small number of cases are not receiving extremely large weights or zero probability. Kang and Schafer (2007) suggest techniques such as the truncation of large weights to avoid a small subset of subjects dominating the analysis, or revision of the missingness model if either of these situations is encountered. They also advise against the removal of subjects which receive extreme weights, which is a warning we would like to reiterate here. Although removal of outliers may be a valid approach in other modeling methods, in the case of IPW estimation, the subjects who receive the highest weights are likely to be the subjects we are most interested in modeling, as they are the most representative of the missing subjects and so their removal could result in a biased model.

8.2.2   Summary of inverse probability weighting advantages

- IPW is designed to correct for the bias inherent in available cases or complete cases analysis by incorporating a missingness model, and weighting cases according to their probability of being observed.

- When the model for missingness is correctly specified and the missingness mechanism is MAR, this method will give unbiased estimates.

8.2.3   Inverse probability weighting disadvantages

- The model for missingness must be correctly specified. If this model is mis-specified then the resulting estimates may be biased. This is because if the model is incorrect then the resulting probabilities of being observed will also be misspecified, which will result in the incorrect weights being given to the observations.

- If the model is approximately correct but some observations have a very low probability of being observed, those observations will receive a very large weight which, while approximately correctly estimated, may inappropriately dominate the analysis.

- As with all missing data approaches, the analysis model (the model that would have been used in the event of no missingness) must also be correctly specified in order to give unbiased estimates.

8.3 Doubly robust estimation

We describe double robustness in the framework used by Robins *et al.* (1994) for estimating regression coefficients pertaining to the population from incomplete data. We also follow the framework of Vansteelandt *et al.* (2010).

DR methods require three models to be specified: one that explains the missingness in the data (π_i or missingness model), one which describes the population of responses (imputation model) and the model that would have been used if there were no missing values in the data (analysis model). As mentioned in the previous section, in order for the IPW estimator to be consistent, the model for the probability of being observed π_i has to be correctly specified. The final analysis model must also be correctly specified. Equally, for imputation methods such as multiple imputation, (MI, described in Chapter 6) both the model for imputing the missing values and the final analysis model must be correctly specified in order to obtain consistent estimators. DR methods build on the IPW estimator to include a model for the missing data given the observed (which could be, e.g., a linear regression, generalized estimating equations (GEEs) and so on or even MI) and are more robust to model misspecification than IPW or imputation methods alone.

Because the main section of this chapter describes the implementation of the method proposed in Section 4.2 of Vansteelandt *et al.* (2010), we will explain DR methods following Vansteelandt *et al.* (2010), where the assumption is that all baseline and post-baseline covariates are fully observed and so missingness is only permissible in the response variable Y. Their paper also describes an extension of this estimator where the covariates can contain missing values as long as the response is fully observed. Note that there are many possible ways of obtaining a DR estimator. For example, Teshome *et al.* (2011) suggested novel DR methods that combine MI with GEEs, Daniel and Kenward (2012) proposed a DR version of MI where missingness is confined to the response variable and Tchetgen (2009) implemented a likelihood-based approach to double robustness. We describe the implementation of Vansteelandt *et al.* as it can be implemented using standard SAS procedures and provides DR estimates which are calculated in a transparent manner and can be easily reproduced if a QC check is required.

8.3.1   Doubly robust methods explained

This section will explain how DR estimators offer greater protection against model misspecification than other methods. A formal description of the DR method can be seen in the formula below:

$$\sum_{i=1}^{n} \left[\overbrace{\frac{r_i}{\hat{\pi}_i} U_\theta \left(W_i, \theta^{DR} \right)}^{\text{first term}} - \overbrace{\left(\frac{r_i}{\hat{\pi}_i} - 1 \right) \Psi \left(r_i, W^{obs}, \theta^{DR} \right)}^{\text{second term}} \right] = 0 \qquad (8.4)$$

where W^{obs} refers to the observed part of the complete data W and θ^{DR} to the vector of parameter estimates estimated using this approach. Note that $U_\theta(\cdot)$ is the score function for the full data, not just the observed data. Only the observed cases are used because this function is multiplied by r_i, and $r_i = 1$ only when the data is observed.

Equation 8.4 above has two parts which we will hereafter refer to as the first term and the second term. The first term of this DR estimator is the IPW estimator described in Section 8.2, which inversely weights the observed responses in the dataset. $U_\theta(\cdot)$ is the final analysis model or in other words the model that would have been used if the data had been fully observed. In the second term, $\Psi(\cdot)$ represents the model for the missing data given the observed. We refer to $\Psi(\cdot)$ as the imputation model; in the literature this is also referred to as the probability of data (POD) model or the propensity model (Daniel and Kenward, 2012; Kang and Schafer, 2007). The model in the second term includes data from both fully observed subjects and those with missing values and thus has the potential to improve the efficiency of the IPW estimator. Because its expectation is zero (provided the model for missingness is correct) the overall estimator remains consistent (Molenberghs and Kenward, 2007, pp. 130–132).

8.3.1.1   Linear regression example

The general DR case described in Equation 8.4 can be re-written as in Equation 8.5 for the case of linear regression. To simplify notation, we omit the visit index j in the equations below for outcomes y_{ij} and missingness indicators r_{ij}, with the understanding that each specified model is a linear regression model for a particular visit. In Equation 8.5, X is an $N \times (S + 1)$ matrix which has N observations and S parameters where the first column of X is a column of 1s to allow for an intercept term. The 0 on the right-hand side of the equation is also a vector of zeros which has N elements. Note that Equation 8.5 can be evaluated using only observed data and each of the N observations contributes non-trivially to Equation 8.5: the missing cases contribute 0 to the first term because $r_i = 0$, but have non-zero contributions to the augmented part. Non-missing cases contribute to both terms.

$$\sum_{i=1}^{N} \left[\frac{r_i}{\hat{\pi}_i} X_i \left(y_i - X_i^T \beta \right) - \left(\frac{r_i}{\hat{\pi}_i} - 1 \right) \left\{ \hat{E} \left\{ X_i \left(y_i - X_i^T \beta \right) | X \right\} \right\} \right] = 0 \qquad (8.5)$$

If we assume that the missingness model is correctly specified, we can see that the expected value of the second term is zero because

$$E\left(\left(\frac{r_i}{\hat{\pi}_i} - 1\right)\hat{E}\left(X_i\left\{y_i - X_i^T\beta\right\}\right)\right) = E\left(E\left\{\left(\frac{r_i}{\hat{\pi}_i} - 1\right)\hat{E}\left(X_i(y_i - X_i^T\beta)\right)|y_i, X_i\right\}\right)$$

$$= E\left(\frac{r_i}{\hat{\pi}_i} - 1|X_i\right)E\left(\hat{E}\left(X_i(y_i - X_i^T\beta)\right)\right)$$

Note that we can separate the first expectation and drop its conditioning on y because of MAR. Under the weak law of large numbers $\hat{\pi}_i \overset{P}{\to} \pi_i$ and the first expectation tends to $E\left(\frac{r_i}{\pi_i} - 1|X_i\right) = \frac{Prob(r_i=1|X_i)-\pi_i}{\pi_i} = \frac{\pi_i-\pi_i}{\pi_i} = 0$ (Kang and Schafer, 2007). Because the second term of Equation 8.5 is zero in expectation, we are now just left with the first term which we already noted is the IPW estimator and provides consistent estimates as long as the missingness model is correctly specified. Thus we see from Equation 8.5 that when the missingness model is correctly specified we get unbiased estimates of the parameter estimates β regardless of the imputation model used.

Now, if we multiply out the second term of Equation 8.5, we can see that Equation 8.5 can be written as in Equation 8.6.

$$\sum_{i=1}^{N}\left[\frac{r_i}{\hat{\pi}_i(X)}X_i\left(y_i - \hat{E}\left\{y_i|X\right\}\right) + X_i\left\{\hat{E}\left\{y_i|X\right\} - X_i^T\beta\right\}\right] = 0 \qquad (8.6)$$

If we now assume that the imputation model $\hat{E}\left\{y_i|X\right\}$ is correctly specified we can see that the expected value of the residual term in the first term of Equation 8.6, which amounts to the residual of a linear regression, is zero and only the second term remains. Because the imputation model is correctly specified, the predicted values of y_i will be consistent and so the solution to the equation described by the second term of Equation 8.6 will provide consistent estimates regardless of the missingness model. Hence, DR estimators provide consistent estimates when either the missingness model or the imputation model or both are correctly specified.

8.3.2   Advantages of doubly robust methods

- DR methods provide consistent estimates, if either the missingness model or the imputation model (model of the observed data given the missingness) is correct. This offers more protection against model misspecification than other missing data approaches such as IPW, mixed models for repeated measures with categorical time effects (MMRM) or imputation alone.

8.3.3   Limitations of doubly robust methods

- As with all missing data methods, the final analysis model, that is, the model that would have been used if there were no missingness, must be correctly specified if the resulting estimates are to be unbiased.

- The missingness mechanism is assumed to be MAR.

- As DR methods incorporate the IPW estimator in their methodology they attract the limitations mentioned in Section 8.2, mainly that subjects with a very low probability of being observed will receive large weights which may dominate the analysis. Because of this, care must also be taken when implementing DR methods.

8.4   Vansteelandt *et al.* method for doubly robust estimation

Section 4.2 of Vansteelandt *et al.* (2010) describes a form of DR estimation that can easily be performed using standard statistical techniques such as logistic regression and GLM, and can be implemented in SAS using standard procedures such as PROC LOGISTIC and PROC MIXED. Vansteelandt *et al.* (2010) describe their DR method for the non-longitudinal case only. Hernández and O'Kelly have implemented an extension of this method for use on longitudinal data, available as the *Vansteelandt_method.sas* macro from the www.missingdata.org.uk site. We first describe the Vansteelandt *et al.* method. We then explain the extended method used to provide consistent estimates for longitudinal analysis.

As stated in Section 8.3, the Vansteelandt *et al.* method is valid when there is missingness in the response variable only. It is assumed that all covariates are fully observed and estimates will only be consistent if this is the case.

Vansteelandt *et al.* (2010) divide all the available covariates X into two sets. The first, which we will refer to as Z, are the covariates whose coefficients we wish to estimate (e.g., the measure of treatment effect); these variables are to be included in the final analysis model. The second group of covariates, F, explains the relationship between the response variable, Y, and the missingness in the data. We are not directly interested in evaluating the relationship between F and Y. Because F helps explain the missingness in the data, these variables should be included in the missingness and imputation models but not the final analysis model. In the description of the Vansteelandt *et al.* method below, we see that in computing the IPW estimator in step 1 both the covariates F and Z are used to model the missingness in Y and they are also used in the model which imputes the values of Y (the imputation model). However, only the covariates Z are used in the final model described in step 3 as these are the only covariates of primary interest. Note that some variables in which we are directly interested may also predict the missingness in Y. If this is the case, these variables should be included in the subset Z, so that they will be used in all the three models described below. Only variables whose relationship with Y we are not directly interested in calculating, but which predict the missingness in Y, should be included in F.

The procedure as laid out in Section 4.2 of Vansteelandt *et al.* (2010) for calculating a DR estimator is as follows:

1. Fit a logistic regression model for the probability of being observed as a function of F and Z. Let π_i denote the fitted probability for each subject i.

2. Fit a generalized linear model (GLM) to the response y_i using all covariates F and Z for the data where y_i is observed. This GLM should be a weighted regression using the weights π_i^{-1} as calculated in step 1. Let $m^*(F, Z)$ denote the fitted values of the response y_i for all subjects, that is, those which were fully observed and also those who had missing values for y_i.

3. Replace the values of the response y_i with the fitted values $m^*(F, Z)$ as calculated in step 2. Fit another GLM for all subjects (both fully observed and those that had a missing outcome) to the new response $m^*(F, Z)$ using only the covariates Z.

4. The resulting coefficient estimates will be consistent if either the model in step 1 or the model in step 2 is correctly specified, provided that the model in step 3 is correctly specified.

8.4.1   Theoretical justification for the Vansteelandt *et al.* method

Equation 8.7 is a reiteration of Equation 8.6 showing the covariate space spanned by X split into the two subspaces: Z (covariates whose relationship with response we are interested in evaluating) and F (covariates which further help to explain the relationship between the response Y and the missingness) described in the previous section.

$$\sum_{i=1}^{n} \left[\frac{r_i}{\hat{\pi}_i\,(F,Z)} Z_i \left(y_i - \hat{E}\left\{ y_i | F, Z \right\} \right) + Z_i \left\{ \hat{E}\left\{ y_i | F, Z \right\} - Z_i^T \beta \right\} \right] \qquad (8.7)$$

Here $\hat{\pi}_i(F, Z)$ refers to the model for the probability of being observed, and again $\hat{E}\left\{ y_i | F, Z \right\}$ refers to the imputation model, both of which may be estimated using all available covariates F and Z.

The Vansteelandt *et al.* method proposes a special case of Equation 8.7 and suggests the use of the IPW estimator to calculate $\hat{E}\left\{ y_i | F, Z \right\}$. This can be seen in Equation 8.8 where S describes the full covariate space enhanced by a column of 1s to allow for an intercept term in the models $(1, F, Z)$. In this case we can see that when $\hat{E}\left\{ Y_i | F, Z \right\} \equiv \hat{E}^{IPW}\left\{ y_i | F, Z \right\}$, the first term in Equation 8.8 is zero. This is because $\hat{E}^{IPW}\left\{ y_i | F, Z \right\} = \mu^{IPW}$, therefore the first sum in Equation 8.8 comprises estimating equations for the IPW model evaluated at its solution μ^{IPW}, which of course is 0; therefore the first term of Equation 8.8 vanishes.

$$\sum_{i=1}^{N} \left[\frac{r_i}{\hat{\pi}_i\,(S)} S_i \left(y_i - \mu_i^{ipw}(S) \right) \right] + \sum_{i=1}^{N} \left[Z_i \left\{ \mu_i^{ipw}(S) - Z_i^T \beta \right\} \right] = 0 \qquad (8.8)$$

Because of the above, Equation 8.8 can then be simplified to the unweighted equations described in Equation 8.9 where both the fully observed subjects and subjects with missing outcomes whose values have been predicted through $\mu_i^{ipw}(S)$ all contribute to the overall coefficient estimates.

$$\sum_{i=1}^{N} \left[Z_i \left\{ \mu_i^{ipw}(S) - Z_i^T \beta \right\} \right] = 0 \qquad (8.9)$$

As we can see, Equation 8.9 is exactly the estimating procedure in Vansteelandt *et al.* whereby the IPW estimator is calculated for the full covariate space $S = (1, F, Z)$. The fitted values from this are then used as the response for an unweighted regression on all the observations for the covariates of interest Z. This last model is the one that must also be correct if the estimate is to be DR.

As noted in Vansteelandt *et al.* (2010), this method will also work in a more general framework of GEEs where $E\{y_i\} = g(Z_i^T \beta)$ and $g(\cdot)$ is an inverse link function.

8.4.2   Implementation of the Vansteelandt *et al.* method for doubly robust estimation

The macro to implement the Vansteelandt *et al.* method was written with the aim of facilitating DR estimation in longitudinal clinical trials. Missingness for a visit is estimated given baseline and available post-baseline data. In addition, the overall results from the macro provide the trialist with a report showing the estimated change from baseline by treatment group for each visit, as well as the difference between treatment and control effects for each visit. This report indicates the mean, standard error and the upper and lower 95% confidence limits of each estimate as well as the *p*-value for the significance of the difference between treatment levels at each visit compared to baseline. In the case of a binary response, the macro will report both the log odds and the odds for treatment effects for each visit as well as the difference in log odds and the odds ratio for each visit.

Thus the SAS macro extends the DR method outlined in Vansteelandt *et al.* (2010) to allow for longitudinal analysis; it also provides bootstrap estimates of the standard errors of estimated treatment effects.

8.4.2.1   Bootstrap estimates of the variance

It is clear that the standard SAS output for the variance of the estimators using the Vansteelandt *et al.* method will underestimate the true variance, as the response values for the final analysis GLM (step 3, Section 8.4) are the predicted values from a previous, often very similar, weighted GLM (step 2, Section 8.4). Because of this, the estimate of the standard error from the standard output could not be used. The standard errors of the estimated treatment effect are obtained using non-parametric bootstrap procedure: the procedure is run on multiple datasets, each dataset consisting of a sample with replacement from the original set of subjects. The mean of the parameter estimates denoted $\hat{\theta}^*(.)$ is then calculated as: $\hat{\theta}^*(.) = \frac{1}{B} \sum_{b=1}^{B} \hat{\theta}^*(b)$ where $\hat{\theta}^*(b)$ refers to the parameter estimate for the bootstrap sample b. Note that this estimate is produced by applying the entire four-step DR procedure as described earlier in this section, including re-estimation of IP weights, to each bootstrap sample. The standard error of the parameter estimate is calculated as $\left\{ \sum_{b=1}^{B} \left[\hat{\theta}^* (b) - \hat{\theta}^* (.) \right]^2 / (B-1) \right\}^{\frac{1}{2}}$ where B denotes the total number of bootstrap samples. In addition to capturing all the sources of variability in the estimated parameters, the bootstrap estimate of the standard error has the advantage that no assumptions about the distribution of the data are made. The procedure is non-parametric and it mimics the true sampling distribution of the test statistic with the distribution of the estimates from multiple bootstrap (re)samples. The confidence interval for $\hat{\theta}^* (.)$ is then calculated using a normal approximation based on the bootstrap estimate of the standard error. The random seed used to generate the bootstrapped datasets and also the number of bootstrap samples required can be specified by the trialist in the macro call to ensure fully reproducible results.

Bootstrap theory states that the estimates of the standard error are asymptotically unbiased, meaning that estimates are valid under the assumption of infinite bootstrap samples. If too few samples are taken, the estimate of the standard error is not guaranteed to be unbiased. Efron and Tibshirani (1993, pp. 50–53) suggest that for the majority of examples between 50 and 200 bootstrap samples will provide satisfactory results. They also suggest that the number of bootstrap samples needed to obtain acceptable results can be effectively estimated by calculating the coefficient of variation (the ratio of the standard deviation to the expected value of the standard deviation). In this way the statistician can calculate the difference between the true standard error to its estimated value and can decide whether a larger number of bootstrap samples B are needed (the smaller the coefficient of variation the better). Because of this we recommend that care be taken when deciding the number of bootstrap samples used to calculate the standard error of estimates $\hat{\theta}^* (.)$ and in particular we caution against using too few samples.

8.4.2.2   Missingness model for longitudinal data

Recall that for each subject i at visit j, π_{ij} is the probability of being observed. In order to calculate π_{ij}, a separate logistic regression is run for each visit, j, where the response R_{ij} is an indicator variable with value 1 if the outcome is observed for subject i at visit j, and 0 otherwise. The default missingness model implemented by the macro for visit j includes baseline covariates plus, if available, post-baseline and response variables for visits 0 to $j - 1$. Monotone missingness, where data is missing for a subject after a given time point, is assumed. In other words, it is assumed that once data is missing for a subject at a particular visit, data for all subsequent visits are also missing. For each visit, the probability of being observed is conditional on being observed at previous visits and so any subject that is missing at visit j will not be included in the probability calculation in subsequent visits. To calculate the full unconditional probability of being observed at visit j, the product of the probabilities for the current and previous visits for each subject i are calculated: $\pi_{ij} = \prod_{a=1}^{j} \hat{\pi}_{ia}$. It is the inverse of this product that is used as the weights for the first GLM (described in step 2 of Section 8.4).

It is possible for the response variable for some bootstrap samples at a particular post-baseline visit to be either fully observed or contain only missing values. If this is the case then the response variable for that visit will only have one level (it will contain either 1 for every subject or 0 for every subject) and so PROC LOGISTIC will fail, as it will only have one group, not two, to model. The macro will automatically check if a visit is fully observed for the original or any bootstrap dataset. If it is, then the $\hat{\pi}_{ij}$ for visit j will be updated with the probability for the previous visit. As there was no change in subject dropout between the visits, there is thus no change in the estimate of the cumulative probability of being observed. If the response variable for a given bootstrap dataset contains only missing values, that bootstrap dataset will be deleted, as the weighted GLM (described in step 2 of Section 8.4) will not run for a dataset with no response values.

Another common issue addressed by the macro is non-convergence of PROC LOGISTIC due to quasi or complete separation of data points, which can result in unreliable predicted values for $\hat{\pi}_{ij}$. If this issue is encountered at a particular visit – and with the bootstrap sampling we find in practice that it does occur – the macro will continue to the next calculable visit and calculate the probability of being observed at the current visit conditional on all the previous fully observed/non-converging visits. The probability of being observed is then pooled across the current visit j and previous $q - 1$ fully observed/non-converging visits as $\sqrt[q]{\hat{\pi}_{ij}}$. The unconditional probability of being observed at each visit is then calculated by calculating the product of the $\hat{\pi}_{ij}$ over the j visits as before. More details on the calculation of these models can be found in the "Users Guidebook for Vansteelandt" also available on the www.missingdata.org.uk website.

8.4.2.3   Final analysis model

As discussed in Section 8.4 the final analysis model should only include covariates which are needed to gain the desired estimate, usually an estimate of treatment effect. The Vansteelandt *et al.* method macro calculates least-squares means for each treatment group effect at each visit, and the differences between these least-squared means. The statistician can specify other explanatory covariables for this analysis model, for example, baseline and demographic or medical history variables. We would, in general, advise against the addition of any post-baseline variables in this model as they may dilute the estimated treatment effect and render it difficult to interpret. For example, if a post-baseline variable were related to the response and also to treatment then its inclusion would lead to underestimating the effect of treatment (Vansteelandt *et al.*, 2010). Also, including too many coefficients in the final analysis model can lead to model over-specification which may inflate the variance of the estimates (Freund *et al.*, 2006, pp. 238–240).

8.4.2.4   Characteristics of Vansteelandt *et al.* method macro for calculating doubly robust estimates of treatment effects

Here we will summarize the main characteristics of the Vansteelandt *et al.* method macro.

Non-monotone missing data

1. This method assumes monotone missingness; if the trial data are non-monotone the macro cannot be used.

How regression parameters are estimated

2. All trial data are used to calculate the predicted values of the response described in step 2 of the Vansteelandt *et al.* method in Section 8.4. The statistician can also specify which covariates that are desired to be included in the final analysis model.

Restrictions on regression parameters

3. The statistician may specify which variables should be included in each of the imputation and final analysis models. They can also specify their own missingness models for any or all of the post-baseline visits if the default model is not desirable. An option is also included to revert to the default model if the user specified model does not converge.

Missing covariates

4. No covariates can contain missing values.

Binary covariates

5. The macro allows categorical or continuous covariates.

Binary responses

6. The macro allows binary or continuous outcomes. For the imputation and final analysis models, the macro will automatically use a sequential linear regression imputation if the response is continuous and a logistic regression if the response is binary.

Auxiliary variables

7. Auxiliary variables can be included in the missingness and imputation models in a straightforward manner.

8.5   Implementing the Vansteelandt *et al.* method via SAS

This section will provide code fragments showing how to calculate the Vansteelandt *et al.* method for two illustrative clinical trial datasets referred to throughout the book: mania (a binary outcome) and insomnia (a continuous outcome).

8.5.1   Mania dataset

As mentioned previously, the mania dataset is an illustrative dataset that is patterned after typical clinical data studying mania in an adult population with bipolar disorder (see Section 1.10.3). The response variable in this trial data is a binary variable derived from the Young Mania Rating Scale (YMRS). For the YMRS scale, lower scores are better. We suppose that the purpose of the trial in the case of this dataset is to compare the treatment effect of a mania treatment of a type similar to valproate to a control drug such as lithium.

As in Chapter 7, the code excerpts in this section will refer to the example data in both vertical (one observation per subject and visit) and horizontal formats (one observation per subject). See Section 1.10.3 for a description of variables included in the dataset.

8.5.1.1   Implementing the Vansteelandt *et al.* method for the illustrative mania dataset

The following section will show the equivalent analysis for a continuous response. A full implementation of the Vansteelandt *et al.* method for the mania trial data can be seen in Appendix 8.A. Appendix 8.A also gives code implementing the equivalent analysis using the macro described in Section 8.4 above. We assume that the data are monotone missing and the dataset in its horizontal format is called *maniah*.

As we estimate the variance of the DR estimates using the bootstrap, all calculations are done on a set of bootstrap samples of the original data. Bootstrap samples are drawn in SAS Code Fragment 8.1. One hundred bootstrap samples equal to the number of subjects in the original data (1100 subjects) are taken. As stated in Section 8.4 we would recommend that at least 100 samples be taken to ensure that the estimates of the standard error are consistent and unbiased.

```
ODS LISTING CLOSE;
PROC SURVEYSELECT DATA=maniah  METHOD = urs SAMPSIZE=1100
   REP=100 SEED=883960001 OUT=ymrs_boot_samples OUTHITS;
RUN;
ODS LISTING;
```

SAS Code Fragment 8.1   Take a bootstrap sample.

```
*Create missingness indicators for each visit Rij which
take the value 1 if the response is observed and 0 if not;

%MACRO create_missing_indicators();
DATA ymrs_boot_samples;
    SET ymrs_boot_samples;
    %DO i=1 %TO 5;
        IF resp_&i EQ . THEN r_&i = 0;ELSE r_&i = 1;
    %END;
    OUTPUT;
RUN;
%MEND create_missing_indicators;

%create_missing_indicators();
```

SAS Code Fragment 8.2   Simple macro to create missingness indicators.

We then create the missingness indicators R_{ij} which are 1 if the response (*resp_1,...,resp_5*) is observed for subject i at visit j and 0 if the response is missing (see SAS Code Fragment 8.2).

A logistic regression is then run for each visit separately. For each visit, only subjects who were observed at previous visits are included in the model. Hence the model for each visit calculates the conditional probability of being observed at the current visit given the subject was observed at previous visits.

When the logistic regression shown in SAS Code Fragment 8.3 was run on the original data (*maniah* dataset) for the first visit the following warning message was received.

```
WARNING: There is possibly a quasi-complete separation of data points.
The maximum likelihood estimate may not exist.
```

```
*Run logistic regression for being observed at visits 1;
ODS LISTING CLOSE;
PROC LOGISTIC DATA=maniah DESCENDING;
    CLASS trt resp_0 country;
    MODEL r_1=base_ymrs resp_0 trt country;
    BY replicate;
    OUTPUT OUT=p_1 P=prob_1;
    ODS OUTPUT CONVERGENCESTATUS =convstat;
RUN;
QUIT;
ODS LISTING;
```

SAS Code Fragment 8.3   Code to calculate the probability of being observed at the first visit.

```
*Run logistic regression for being observed at visits 1 or 2;
ODS LISTING CLOSE;
PROC LOGISTIC DATA=ymrs_boot_samples DESCENDING;
    CLASS trt resp_0 country;
    MODEL r_2=base_ymrs resp_0 trt country;
    BY replicate;
    OUTPUT OUT=p_2 P=prob_2;
    ODS OUTPUT CONVERGENCESTATUS =convstat;
RUN;
QUIT;
ODS LISTING;
```

SAS Code Fragment 8.4   Code to calculate the probability of being observed at the first or the second visit.

This warning can occur because a linear combination of covariates exists that can perfectly predict the response and so PROC LOGISTIC will not give reliable estimates, as the maximum likelihood cannot be calculated if there is no overlap in the distribution of the two groups. Thus, the predicted probabilities from an analysis with this warning message cannot be used. In the case of non-convergence, such as this, we continue to the next visit which did converge for the original dataset (*maniah*), which in our example is Visit 2. The code to implement the logistic regression on the bootstrapped datasets for Visit 2 can be seen in SAS Code Fragment 8.4.

The analysis performed in SAS Code Fragment 8.4 calculates the probability of a subject being observed at either Visit 1 or Visit 2. Since some subjects will have missing values for Visit 1, no covariates relating to Visit 1 were included in the model. To approximate the probability of being observed at Visit 1, we apportion the predicted probability of being observed at Visits 1 or 2 by estimating each visit's probability as $\sqrt[q]{\hat{\pi}_{ij}}$, where q is the number of visits we are pooling across (two in this case). The unconditional probability of being observed at Visit 2 is then $\hat{\pi}_{i1} * \hat{\pi}_{i2}$. The probabilities for Visits 3, 4 and 5 are calculated similarly to those for Visits 1 and 2. SAS Code Fragment 8.5 describes how to calculate the overall probability of being observed at Visits 1, 2 and 3.

Once the probability of being observed at each visit has been calculated, the inverse of this probability needs to be obtained (SAS Code Fragment 8.6). The inverse probability weight each subject will receive at each visit has now been calculated, and it is these weights which will be used in the GLM referred to in step 2 of the description of the Vansteelandt *et al.* method in Section 8.4.

Before the GLM can be performed the data must first be converted to vertical format, one record per visit per subject. SAS Code Fragment 8.7 shows how to do this for our example. Once the data are in vertical format, a weighted logistic regression is performed using PROC GLIMMIX (although the model does not include a random effect). This step models the binary response, *resp*, on all available covariates: *base_ymrs, country* and *trt*. Note that the IPW is included in this model by use of the "WEIGHT *inverse_prob*"; statement.

```
*Calculate the product of the probabilities of being observed from
visits 1 to j-1;

*PROC LOGISTIC for visit 1 didn't converge so pooled probability is
sqrt(prob_2);
DATA p_2;
    SET p_2;
    prob_2=SQRT(prob_2);
RUN;

*The unconditional probability of being observed at visit 2 is
prob(observed at visit 1) * prob(observed at visit 2),since the data
are monotone missing;

DATA overall_probability;
    SET p_2;
    prob_1=prob_2;
    prob_2 = prob_1*prob_2;
RUN;

*Likewise for visit 3 the overall probability of being observed
at visit 3 is the probability of being observed at visit 1*visit
2*visit3 as the data are monotone missing;

DATA overall_probability;
    MERGE overall_probability p_3;
    BY replicate subjid trt;
    *prob 2 is now prob_1*prob2;
    prob_3 = prob_2*prob_3;
RUN;
```

SAS Code Fragment 8.5   Code to calculate the unconditional probability of being observed at each visit.

```
*Get the inverse probability of being observed at each visit;
    %MACRO get_inverse_prob();
    DATA overall_probability;
    SET overall_probability;
        %DO i = 1 %TO 5;
            inverse_prob_&i = 1/prob_&i;
        %END;
    RUN;
    %MEND get_inverse_prob;
    %get_inverse_prob();
```

SAS Code Fragment 8.6   Calculate the inverse probability of being observed.

```
*Convert the data back to vertical format;

DATA ymrs_boot_vert;
  SET ymrs_boot_samples;
  %MACRO makevert();
    %DO i=1 %TO 5;
      resp=resp_&i;
      r=r_&i;
      inverse_prob=inverse_prob_&i;
      visit=&i;
      OUTPUT;
      DROP resp_&i r_&i inverse_prob_&i;
    %END;
  %MEND makevert;
  %makevert();
RUN;


*Sort the data appropriately;
PROC SORT DATA=ymrs_boot_vert;
    BY replicate DESCENDING trt DESCENDING visit;
RUN;


*Run a weighted GLM (to get the IPW predictions). This model can
make use of both baseline and post-baseline variables;

ODS LISTING CLOSE;
PROC GLIMMIX DATA=ymrs_boot_vert;
    CLASS trt visit country;
    MODEL resp=base_ymrs country trt trt*visit/DIST=binomial
    LINK=logit;
    BY replicate;
    WEIGHT inverse_prob;
    OUTPUT OUT=first_glm_out PRED(ILINK)=pred;
RUN;
ODS LISTING;
```

SAS Code Fragment 8.7   Convert the dataset to vertical format and run the weighted imputation model.

The predicted probability obtained from the logistic regression shown in SAS Code Fragment 8.7 is then used as the new response for a second logistic regression (the final analysis model) as described in Section 8.4. Because the mania dataset has a binary response, the final analysis model uses the equivalent binominal notation where the response is written in the form of $\frac{number\ of\ successes}{number\ of\ trials}$, where the number of successes is the probability of being a responder on the mania scale (the response from the model in SAS Code Fragment 8.7) and the number of trials for each subject/visit is one. SAS Code Fragment 8.8 runs the final analysis model. Note that

```
*set new response to be the predicted response from the previous GLM;
DATA ymrs_boot_vert;
    MERGE ymrs_boot_vert first_glm_out(KEEP=pred replicate subjid
    visit);
    BY replicate visit subjid;
    resp=pred;
    DROP pred;
RUN;


PROC SORT DATA= ymrs_boot_vert;
    BY replicate DESCENDING trt DESCENDING visit;
RUN;


*Run the second logistic regression using the predicted probability
of being observed obtained from the first logistic regression. To do
this, need to use the binomial notation where the probability is the
number of successes and 1 is the number of trials;
DATA ymrs_boot_vert;
    SET ymrs_boot_vert;
    denom=1;
RUN;


*Run final analysis model using only the covariates for which
coefficient are required(in this case treatment effects are each
visit);

ODS LISTING CLOSE;
PROC GLIMMIX DATA= ymrs_boot_vert;
    CLASS trt visit;
    MODEL resp/denom=trt visit trt*visit/DIST=binomial LINK=logit;
    BY replicate;
    LSMEANS trt*visit /odds ODDSRATIO cl DIFF=control("1" "5");
    OUTPUT OUT=YMRS_Final_Analysis_out PRED(ILINK)=pred;
    ODS OUTPUT DIFFS=diffs LSMEANS=lsms;
RUN;
QUIT;
ODS LISTING;
```

SAS Code Fragment 8.8   Set the predicted outcome from the imputation model as the new response and run the final analysis model.

the covariates in this model are only those for which we are directly interested in calculating coefficients, in this case *trt* and *visit*. The LSMEANS statement with the DIFFS qualifier provides estimates of the expected log odds of response for each treatment group, and of the difference between two groups at each visit for each bootstrap dataset. The "/ODDS ODDSRATIO" in the LSMEANS statement provides these results on the odds scale as well as the log odds scale.

```
*Get overall estimates of mean and standard error of treatment effect
at final visit;
*Dataset "lsms" contains the estimates of the treatment effect for
each visit over the 100 bootstrap samples
Here, we are interested in the final visit.;

DATA lsms;
    SET lsms;
    IF visit NE 5 THEN DELETE;
RUN;

PROC SORT DATA=lsms;
    BY trt;
RUN;

*Get the mean and standard error of estimates over the bootstrap
samples to get the overall bootstrapped estimate;

PROC MEANS DATA=lsms;
    VAR estimate;
    BY trt;
    *stddev gives the bootstrap standard error of the overall
    estimate(arithmetically identical to that specified in
    section 8.4);
    OUTPUT OUT=lsm_estimates MEAN=lsm STDDEV=se;
RUN;
```

SAS Code Fragment 8.9   Use LSMEANS to get the treatment effect at the final visit for each bootstrap sample and PROC MEANS to get the overall estimate of treatment effect.

The DR estimate of the mean and standard error of the effect of valproate over lithium for the mania dataset is calculated as the mean and standard deviation of the estimates over all the bootstrap datasets. SAS Code Fragment 8.9 shows how to obtain the overall DR estimates of the mean and standard error of the effects of valproate and lithium at the final visit, which are easily calculated using PROC MEANS (see Appendix 8.B for SAS code which shows that this is equivalent to calculating the formula described in Section 8.4).

The DR estimates for the effect of experimental and control treatment groups, as well as the difference between these at the final visit, can be seen in Table 8.2. The code to perform the equivalent analysis using the Vansteelandt *et al.* method macro can also be seen in Appendix 8.A. From Table 8.2 we can see that the results of this analysis are in line with the MI analysis on this dataset shown in Table 6.5 which reports a treatment difference in the LSMEANS estimate of 0.1 and also shows no evidence of a significant difference between treatments at the final visit (p-value = 0.0849).

Table 8.2 Results for Vansteelandt *et al.* method for mania dataset: least-squares means (LSMEANS) estimate of treatment (TRT) effects and the difference between treatments in the logit of the probability of response at Visit 5.

TRT level	LSMEANS TRT estimate (log odds)	Std. error TRT	Odds	TRT difference, LSMEANS estimate	Std. error	Odds ratio	*p*-value
1	0.5	0.1	1.7				
2	0.7	0.1	2.1	0.2	0.1	1.2	0.1454

The results of the DR approach are reasonably consistent with those of MI in Table 6.5 ($p = 0.0849$), given that a different model was used for Table 6.5.

8.5.2 Insomnia dataset

This section will show the equivalent DR analysis for data with a continuous response and will use the insomnia trial data described as an illustrative example in Section 1.10.2. The primary efficacy variable for the insomnia data is the total sleep time (TST). The insomnia trial contains data for six visits in total, one baseline and five post-baseline visits. Two secondary efficacy variables: sleep quality score (SQS) and morning sleepiness score (MSS) were also measured as part of this trial. However, because the values for SQS and MSS contain missing values they cannot be used in the Vansteelandt *et al.* analysis, as it is an assumption of this method that all covariates are fully observed. Because of this, analysis for this data will model the primary efficacy TST based on the baseline MSS score and the treatment by visit effect only. Section 1.10.2 includes a description of all variables in the dataset.

Again, the following is given as an illustrative example only. It should be noted that if a dataset has a high number of explanatory variables with missing values, this implementation of the Vansteelandt *et al.* method will be at a disadvantage compared to, for example, MI. This is because MI can, for example, make use of post-baseline data from incompletely observed subjects to give potentially less biased or more precise estimates of the response.

Since this implementation uses the bootstrap to estimate variance, the procedure is repeated for a number of bootstrap samples. As a first step, therefore, a number of bootstrap samples of the dataset should be taken with replacement, each sample having the same number of subjects per treatment group as the original dataset. The probability of being observed at each visit, $\hat{\pi}_{ij}$, should then be calculated using PROC LOGISTIC and the overall probabilities for each subject i of being observed at visit j should be calculated as $\pi_{ij} = \prod_{a=1}^{j} \hat{\pi}_{ia}$. The inverse of the unconditional probabilities, π_{ij}, are the weights that should be used in the first GLM. The SAS code to perform this analysis for the insomnia data is provided in Appendix 8.C. It is similar to that for the mania example in Section 8.5 and so will not be repeated here.

```
*The response of interest is the change from baseline;

DATA tst_boot_vert;
    SET tst_boot_vert;
    tstc= tst - tst_0;
RUN;

*Step 2: Run a weighted GLM (to get the IPW predictions) this model
should be based on all variables if dataset has (fully observed)
baseline and post-baseline variables;

ODS LISTING CLOSE;
PROC MIXED DATA= tst_boot_vert ORDER=data;
    CLASS trt visit;
    MODEL tstc=base_mss trt visit trt*visit/SOLUTION
    OUTP=first_glm_out;
    BY replicate;
    WEIGHT prob;
RUN;
QUIT;
ODS LISTING;
```

SAS Code Fragment 8.10   Imputation model for each bootstrap sample.

Because the response for the insomnia data is continuous we can control for random differences between the two treatment groups at baseline by including the baseline TST score in our models. As often in clinical trials, we will use as the efficacy parameter the change from baseline in the response variable. SAS Code Fragment 8.10 shows how the change in TST from baseline (called *tstc* below) and the imputation model is calculated for the insomnia data.

Both the imputation and final analysis models can be calculated using, for example, PROC MIXED (although the model is a linear regression and not a mixed model). As in the mania example, the predicted change in *tst* from baseline should be used as the new response variable for the final analysis model (see SAS Code Fragment 8.11).

The DR estimates of the mean and standard error of the treatment effects and difference in the change of these effects from baseline can be calculated at the final visit using PROC MEANS as shown in Section 8.5. The results of this analysis for the insomnia data at the final visit can be seen in Table 8.3.

Comparing these results with those of the MI Method 3 performed in Chapter 6 (see Table 6.2), we can see that overall both mean estimates are quite close with the DR method estimating a mean difference of 21.3 and MI a difference of 19.3. Both analyses also conclude that there is evidence to suggest a significant difference in treatment levels at the final visit (p-value = 0.0039 and 0.0025 for DR and MI, respectively).

```
*set new response to be the predicted response from the previous GLM;

DATA tst_boot_vert;
    MERGE tst_boot_vert first_glm_out(KEEP=pred replicate subjid
    visit);
    BY replicate visit subjid;
    tstc=pred;
    DROP pred;
RUN;


PROC SORT DATA=tst_boot_vert;
    BY replicate DESCENDING trt DESCENDING visit;
RUN;
*Run final analysis model using only the relevant covariates;

ODS LISTING CLOSE;
PROC MIXED DATA=tst_boot_vert  order=data;
    CLASS trt visit;
    MODEL tstc= base_mss trt visit trt*visit /SOLUTION
    OUTP=final_analysis_out;
    BY replicate;
    LSMEANS trt*visit /CL DIFF=CONTROL("1" "5");
    ODS OUTPUT DIFFS=diffs LSMEANS=lsms;
RUN;
QUIT;
ODS LISTING;
```

SAS Code Fragment 8.11   Final analysis model to calculate the treatment change from baseline.

Table 8.3   Results for Vansteelandt *et al.* method for insomnia dataset: least-squares means (LSMEANS) estimate of treatment effects (change from baseline in TST) and the difference between treatments at Visit 5.

TRT level	LSMEANS TRT estimate	Std. error TRT	TRT difference, LSMEANS estimate	Std. error	p-value
1	62.4	4.7			
2	83.6	5.3	21.3	7.4	0.0039

Appendix 8.A How to implement Vansteelandt *et al.* method for mania dataset (binary response)

Mania dataset: Vansteelandt *et al.* method "by hand"

```
*The following code will run the Vansteelandt et al. method for the
Mania Dataset with binary response;
```

```
*Create 100 bootstrap samples with replacement. Each bootstrap sample
is the same size as the original data;

ODS LISTING CLOSE;
PROC SURVEYSELECT DATA=maniah  METHOD = urs SAMPSIZE= 1100
   REP=100 SEED=883960001 OUT=ymrs_boot_samples OUTHITS;
RUN;
ODS LISTING;

DATA ymrs_boot_samples;
  SET ymrs_boot_samples;
  DROP numberhits;
RUN;

*Create missingness indicators for each visit rij which take the
value 1 if the response is observed and 0 if not;

%MACRO create_missing_indicators();
   DATA ymrs_boot_samples;
   SET ymrs_boot_samples;
   %DO i=1 %TO 5;
     IF resp_&i NE . THEN r_&i = 1;ELSE r_&i = 0;
   %END;
   OUTPUT;
RUN;
%mend create_missing_indicators;
%create_missing_indicators();

*Run logistic regression for each visit;

ODS LISTING CLOSE;
PROC LOGISTIC DATA=ymrs_boot_samples DESCENDING;
   CLASS trt resp_0 country;
   MODEL r_2=base_ymrs resp_0 trt country;
   BY replicate;
   OUTPUT OUT=p_2 P=prob_2;
   ODS OUTPUT CONVERGENCESTATUS =convstat;
RUN;
QUIT;
ODS LISTING;

*if subject was missing at previous visit then delete that
observation, probability at Visit 2 is conditional on being observed
at Visit 1;

DATA ymrs_boot_temp;
   SET ymrs_boot_samples;
   IF r_2 EQ 0 THEN DELETE;
RUN;
```

```
*Estimate the probability of being observed at Visit 3;
ODS LISTING CLOSE;

PROC LOGISTIC DATA= ymrs_boot_temp DESCENDING;
   CLASS trt resp_0 resp_1 country;
   MODEL r_3= base_ymrs resp_0 resp_2 trt country;
   BY replicate;
   OUTPUT OUT=p_3 P=prob_3;
   ODS OUTPUT CONVERGENCESTATUS =convstat;
RUN;
QUIT;
ODS LISTING;

DATA ymrs_boot_temp;
   SET ymrs_boot_temp;
   IF r_3 EQ 0 THEN DELETE;
RUN;

*Estimate the probability of being observed at Visit 4;
ODS LISTING CLOSE;
PROC LOGISTIC DATA= ymrs_boot_temp DESCENDING;
   CLASS resp_0 resp_2 resp_3 trt country;
   MODEL r_4= base_ymrs resp_0 resp_2 resp_3 trt country;
   BY replicate;
   OUTPUT OUT=p_4 P=prob_4;
   ODS OUTPUT CONVERGENCESTATUS =convstat;
RUN;
QUIT;
ODS LISTING;

*The default model for the final visit doesn't converge so instead we
use baseline values and trt only;

ODS LISTING CLOSE;
PROC LOGISTIC DATA= ymrs_boot_temp DESCENDING;
   CLASS resp_0;
   MODEL r_5= base_ymrs resp_0;
   BY replicate;
   OUTPUT OUT=p_5 P=prob_5;
   ODS OUTPUT CONVERGENCESTATUS =convstat;
RUN;
QUIT;
ODS LISTING;

*Before merging probabilities for each visit first need to sort them;

%MACRO sortdata();
%DO i = 2 %TO 5;
```

```
PROC SORT DATA = p_&i;
   BY replicate subjid trt;
RUN;

DATA p_&i;
   SET p_&i;
   KEEP replicate subjid trt prob_&i;
RUN;
%END;
%MEND sortdata;
%sortdata();
```

*Calculate the product of the probabilities of being observed from Visits 1 to j-1;

*PROC LOGISTIC for Visit 1 didn't converge so pooled probability is sqrt(prob_2). Perform this calculation;

```
DATA p_2;
   SET p_2;
   prob_2=SQRT(prob_2);
RUN;
```

*Start with the probability of being observed at the first visit. The overall probability of being observed at Visit 2 is the probability of being observed at Visit 1*Visit 2 as the data are monotone missing;

```
DATA overall_probability;
   SET p_2;
   prob_1=prob_2;
   prob_2 = prob_1*prob_2;
RUN;
```

*Likewise for Visit 3 the overall probability of being observed at Visit 3 is the probability of being observed at Visit 1*Visit 2*Visit3 as the data are monotone missing;

```
DATA overall_probability;
   MERGE overall_probability p_3;
   BY replicate subjid trt;
   *prob 2 is now prob_1*prob2;
   prob_3 = prob_2*prob_3;
RUN;
```

*The same applies for visit 4;
```
DATA overall_probability;
   MERGE overall_probability p_4;
```

```
   BY replicate subjid trt;
   *prob 3 is now prob_1*prob2*prob_3;
   prob_4 = prob_3*prob_4;
RUN;


*And also for visit 5;
DATA overall_probability;
   MERGE overall_probability p_5;
   BY replicate subjid trt;
   *prob 4 is now prob_1*prob2*prob_3*prob_4;
   prob_5 = prob_4*prob_5;
RUN;


*Calculate the inverse probability of being observed at each visit;
%MACRO get_inverse_prob();
DATA overall_probability;
SET overall_probability;
   %DO i = 1 %TO 5;
     prob_&i = 1/prob_&i;
   %END;
RUN;
%MEND get_inverse_prob;
%get_inverse_prob();


*Append inverse probabilities to the original dataset;
PROC SORT DATA=YMRS_BOOT_SAMPLES;
   BY replicate subjid trt;
RUN;
PROC SORT DATA=overall_probability;
   BY replicate subjid trt;
RUN;


DATA ymrs_boot_samples;
   MERGE ymrs_boot_samples overall_probability;
   BY replicate subjid trt;
RUN;


*Convert the data back to vertical format;
DATA ymrs_boot_vert;
  SET ymrs_boot_samples;
  %MACRO makevert();
  %DO i=1 %TO 5;
    resp=resp_&i;
      r=r_&i;
      prob=prob_&i;
    visit=&i;
    OUTPUT;
      DROP resp_&i R_&i prob_&i;
```

```
   %END;
  %MEND makevert;
  %makevert();
RUN;


*Make sure data are sorted appropriately;
PROC SORT DATA=ymrs_boot_vert;
   BY replicate descending trt descending visit;
RUN;


*Run a weighted GLM (to get the IPW predictions) this model should be
based on all variables if dataset has (fully observed) baseline and
post-baseline variables;

ODS LISTING CLOSE;
PROC GLIMMIX DATA=ymrs_boot_vert;
   CLASS trt visit country;
   MODEL resp=base_ymrs country trt trt*visit/DIST=binomial LINK=logit;
   BY replicate;
   WEIGHT prob;
   OUTPUT OUT=first_glm_out PRED(ILINK)=pred ;
RUN;
ODS LISTING;


*Now take the predicted response from dataset "first_glm_out" and use
it as the new response;

PROC SORT DATA=first_glm_out;
   BY replicate visit subjid;
RUN;


PROC SORT DATA= ymrs_boot_vert;
   BY replicate visit subjid;
RUN;


*set new response to be the predicted response from the previous GLM;

DATA ymrs_boot_vert;
   MERGE ymrs_boot_vert first_glm_out(keep=pred replicate subjid
visit);
   BY replicate visit subjid;
   resp=pred;
   DROP pred;
RUN;


PROC SORT DATA=ymrs_boot_vert;
   BY replicate DESCENDING trt DESCENDING visit;
RUN;
```

*Run the second logistic regression using the predicted probability of being observed obtained from the first logistic regression. To do this, need to use the binomial notation where the probability is the number of successes and 1 is the number of trials;

```
DATA ymrs_boot_vert;
   SET ymrs_boot_vert;
   denom=1;
RUN;
```

*Run final analysis model using only the covariates for which coefficient are required (in this case treatment effects are each visit);

```
ODS LISTING CLOSE;
PROC GLIMMIX DATA=ymrs_boot_vert;
   CLASS trt visit;
   MODEL resp/denom=trt visit trt*visit/DIST=binomial LINK=logit;
   BY replicate;
   LSMEANS trt*visit /odds ODDSRATIO CL DIFF=control("1" "5");
   OUTPUT OUT=YMRS_Final_Analysis_out PRED(ILINK)=pred;
   ODS OUTPUT DIFFS=diffs LSMEANS=lsms;
RUN;
QUIT;
ODS LISTING;
```

*Calculate overall estimates of mean and standard error of treatment effect at final visit;
*Dataset "lsms" contains the estimates of the treatment effect for each visit over the 100 bootstrap samples. We are interested in the final visit;

```
DATA lsms;
   SET lsms;
   IF visit NE 5 THEN DELETE;
RUN;
```

```
PROC SORT DATA=lsms;
   BY trt;
RUN;
```

*Get the mean and standard error of estimates over the bootstrap samples to get the overall bootstrapped estimate;

```
PROC MEANS DATA=lsms;
   VAR estimate;
   BY trt;
```

```
     *stddev gives the bootstrap standard error of the overall estimate
     (this is the same as working out the formula given in section 8.4)
     See appendix 8.B for proof.;
     OUTPUT OUT=lsm_estimates MEAN=lsm STDDEV=se;
RUN;


*Show estimates of the difference in the treatment groups;
DATA diffs;
   SET diffs;
   IF visit NE 5 THEN DELETE;
RUN;


PROC MEANS DATA=diffs;
   VAR estimate;
   OUTPUT OUT=trt_diff_estimates MEAN=trt_diff STDDEV=diff_SE;
RUN;


*calculate the p-value of treatment difference at last visit;
DATA trt_diff_estimates;
   SET trt_diff_estimates;
   t_Value= trt_diff/diff_SE;
   p_value=(1-probt(abs(t_value),5490))*2;
RUN;


*odds ratio of estimates;
DATA lsm_estimates;
   SET lsm_estimates;
   or=exp(lsm);
RUN;


DATA trt_diff_estimates;
   SET trt_diff_estimates;
   or =exp(trt_diff);
RUN;
```

Identical implementation via a SAS macro by the authors, available from DIA pages at missingdata.org.uk

```
%INCLUDE "vansteelandt_method.sas";
%INCLUDE "VansteelandtSubMacros.sas";
%vansteelandt_method(datain=maniav, trtname=trt, subjname=subjid,
   visname=visit, basecont=%str(base_YMRS), baseclass=%str(country),
   postclass=%str(),seed=883960001,nboot=100,visit_basecont_5=%str
   (base_YMRS,visit_baseclass_5=%str(RESP_0),primaryname=resp,
   analcovarcont=%str(), analcovarclass=%str(),trtref=1,
   dataout=test_vans_predicted, resout=test_vans_results
                     );
```

Appendix 8.B SAS code to calculate estimates from the bootstrapped datasets

Bootstrap SE as per equation in Section 8.4.2.1 are equivalent to PROC MEANS using the option "STDDEV" for mania example

```
/*ASIDE: The following code will show the estimate of the standard
error using the formula in section 8.4 is the same as that from using
the stddev option in PROC MEANS for the LS means of treatment at the
final visit*/

    DATA bootse;
      MERGE lsm_estimates (KEEP=trt lsm) lsms;
      BY trt;
    RUN;

    DATA bootse;
      SET bootse;
      diff=estimate-lsm;
      *to calculate the numerator[θ\hat(b)- θ\hat(.)]^2;
      diff2=diff*diff;
      KEEP trt lsm estimate diff diff2;
    RUN;

    PROC MEANS DATA=bootse;
      VAR diff2;
      BY trt;
      *Calculate  Σ_(b=1)^B[θ\hat(b)- θ\hat(.)]^2;
      OUTPUT OUT=lsm_sum SUM=sumls;
    RUN;

    DATA lsm_sum;
      SET lsm_sum;
      *Calculate  Σ_(b=1)^B[θ\hat(b)- θ\hat(.)]^2/B-1
      B is 10;
      sumls=sumls/9;
    RUN;

    DATA lsm_sum;
      SET lsm_sum;
*Calculate the standard error of the estimates  [Σ_(b=1)^B[θ\hat(b)-
θ\hat(.)]^2/B-1]^1/2;
      sumls=sqrt(sumls);
      *sumls gives the same estimate of the standard error as above in
      proc means (See dataset "lsm_estimates");
    RUN;
```

Appendix 8.C How to implement Vansteelandt *et al.* method for insomnia dataset

Insomnia dataset: Vansteelandt *et al.* method "by hand" (continuous response)

```
*The following code will run the Vansteelandt et al. method for the
Mania dataset;

*Create 100 bootstrap samples with replacement. Each bootstrap sample
is the same size as the original data (640 observations);

ODS LISTING CLOSE;
PROC SURVEYSELECT DATA=sleeph  METHOD = urs SAMPSIZE= 640
   REP=100 SEED=883960001 OUT=tst_boot_samples OUTHITS;
RUN;
ODS LISTING;

DATA tst_boot_samples;
  SET tst_boot_samples;
  DROP numberhits;
RUN;

*Create missingness indicators for each visit Rij which take the
value 1 if the response is observed and 0 if not;
%MACRO create_missing_indicators();
DATA tst_boot_samples;
   SET tst_boot_samples;
   %DO i=1 %TO 5;
       IF tst_&i NE . THEN r_&i = 1;ELSE r_&i = 0;
   %END;
   OUTPUT;
RUN;
%MEND create_missing_indicators;

%create_missing_indicators();

*First visit was fully observed and so proc logistic cannot be run,
so the probability of being observed at visit 1 is 1 the first logistic
regression is for visit 2;

*Run logistic regression for each visit;
ODS LISTING CLOSE;
PROC LOGISTIC DATA=tst_boot_samples DESCENDING;
   CLASS trt;
   MODEL r_2=tst_0 base_mss trt;
   BY replicate;
   OUTPUT OUT=p_2 P=prob_2;
```

```
      ODS OUTPUT CONVERGENCESTATUS =convstat;
RUN;
QUIT;
ODS LISTING;


*if subject was missing at previous visit then delete that observation,
probability at visit 3 is conditional on being observed at visit 1
and visit 2;

DATA tst_boot_temp;
   SET tst_boot_samples;
   IF r_2 EQ 0 THEN DELETE;
RUN;


ODS LISTING CLOSE;
PROC LOGISTIC DATA=tst_boot_temp DESCENDING;
   CLASS trt;
   MODEL r_3= tst_0 tst_2 base_mss trt;
   BY replicate;
   OUTPUT OUT=p_3 P=prob_3;
   ODS OUTPUT CONVERGENCESTATUS =convstat;
RUN;
QUIT;
ODS LISTING;


DATA tst_boot_temp;
   SET tst_boot_temp;
   IF r_3 EQ 0 THEN DELETE;
RUN;


ODS LISTING CLOSE;
PROC LOGISTIC DATA=tst_boot_temp DESCENDING;
   CLASS trt;
   MODEL r_4= tst_0 tst_2 tst_3 base_mss trt;
   BY replicate;
   OUTPUT OUT=p_4 P=prob_4;
   ODS OUTPUT CONVERGENCESTATUS =convstat;
RUN;
QUIT;
ODS LISTING;


DATA tst_boot_temp;
   SET tst_boot_temp;
   IF r_4 EQ 0 THEN DELETE;
RUN;


ODS LISTING CLOSE;
PROC LOGISTIC DATA=tst_boot_temp DESCENDING;
```

```
   CLASS trt;
   MODEL r_5= tst_0 tst_2 tst_3 tst_4 base_mss trt;
   BY replicate;
   OUTPUT OUT=p_5 P=prob_5;
   ODS OUTPUT CONVERGENCESTATUS =convstat;
RUN;
QUIT;
ODS LISTING;
```

```
*Before merging probabilities for each visit first need to sort them;
```

```
%MACRO sortdata();
%DO i = 2 %TO 5;
PROC SORT DATA = p_&i;
   BY replicate subjid trt;
RUN;
```

```
DATA p_&i;
   SET p_&i;
   KEEP replicate subjid trt prob_&i;
RUN;
%END;
%MEND sortdata;
%sortdata();
```

```
*Calculate the product of the probabilities of being observed from
visits 1 to j-1;
```

```
*As the first visit was fully observed, give each subject a probability
of 1 make a dataset with probabilities 1 for each subject;
```

```
DATA p_1;
   SET p_2 (KEEP=replicate subjid trt);
   prob_1=1;
RUN;
```

```
DATA overall_probability;
   MERGE p_1 p_2;
   BY replicate subjid trt;
   *the overall probability of being observed at visit 2 is the
   probability of being observed at visit 1*visit 2, as the data
   are monotone missing;
   prob_2 = prob_1*prob_2;
RUN;
```

```
*Likewise for visit 3 the overall probability of being observed at
visit 3 is the probability of being observed at visit 1*visit 2*visit3
as the data are monotone missing;
```

```
DATA overall_probability;
   MERGE overall_probability p_3;
   BY replicate subjid trt;
   *prob 2 is now prob_1*prob2;
   prob_3 = prob_2*prob_3;
RUN;

*The same applies for visit 4;
DATA overall_probability;
   MERGE overall_probability p_4;
   BY replicate subjid trt;
   *prob 3 is now prob_1*prob2*prob_3;
   prob_4 = prob_3*prob_4;
RUN;

*And also for visit 5;
DATA overall_probability;
   MERGE overall_probability p_5;
   BY replicate subjid trt;
   *prob 4 is now prob_1*prob2*prob_3*prob_4;
   prob_5 = prob_4*prob_5;
RUN;

*Calculate the inverse probability of being observed at each visit;

%MACRO get_inverse_prob();
DATA overall_probability;
SET overall_probability;
   %DO i = 1 %TO 5;
       prob_&i = 1/prob_&i;
   %END;
RUN;
%MEND get_inverse_prob;
%get_inverse_prob();

*Append inverse probabilities to the original dataset;

PROC SORT DATA=tst_boot_samples;
   BY replicate subjid trt;
RUN;
PROC SORT DATA=overall_probability;
   BY replicate subjid trt;
RUN;
DATA tst_boot_samples;
   MERGE tst_boot_samples overall_probability;
   BY replicate subjid trt;
RUN;
```

```
*Convert the data back to vertical format;

DATA tst_boot_vert;
  SET tst_boot_samples;
  %MACRO makevert();
    %DO i=1 %TO 5;
      tst=tst_&i;
        r=r_&i;
        prob=prob_&i;
      visit=&i;
      OUTPUT;
       DROP tst_&i r_&i prob_&i;
    %END;
  %MEND makevert;
  %makevert();
RUN;

*Make sure data are sorted appropriately;

PROC SORT DATA=tst_boot_vert;
   BY replicate descending trt descending visit;
RUN;

*The response of interest is the change from baseline;
DATA tst_boot_vert;
   SET tst_boot_vert;
   tstc= tst - tst_0;
RUN;

*Run a weighted GLM (to get the IPW predictions) this model should be
based on all variables if dataset has (fully observed) baseline and
post-baseline variables;

ODS LISTING CLOSE;
PROC MIXED DATA= tst_boot_vert ORDER=data;
   CLASS trt visit;
   MODEL tstc=base_mss trt visit trt*visit/SOLUTION OUTP=first_glm_out;
   BY replicate;
   WEIGHT prob;
RUN;
QUIT;
ODS LISTING;

*Now take the predicted response from dataset "first_glm_out" and use
it as the new response;

PROC SORT DATA=first_glm_out;
   BY replicate visit subjid;
RUN;
```

```
PROC SORT DATA=tst_boot_vert;
   BY replicate visit subjid;
RUN;


*set new response to be the predicted response from the previous GLM;

DATA tst_boot_vert;
   MERGE tst_boot_vert first_glm_out(keep=pred replicate subjid visit);
   BY replicate visit subjid;
   tstc=pred;
   DROP pred;
RUN;


PROC SORT DATA=tst_boot_vert;
   BY replicate DESCENDING trt DESCENDING visit;
RUN;


*Run final analysis model using only the covariates for which coefficient
are required (in this case treatment effects are each visit);

ODS LISTING CLOSE;
PROC MIXED DATA=tst_boot_vert  order=data;
   CLASS trt visit;
   MODEL tstc= base_mss trt visit trt*visit /SOLUTION
   OUTP=final_analysis_out;
   BY replicate;
   LSMEANS trt*visit /CL DIFF=control("1" "5");
   ODS OUTPUT DIFFS=diffs LSMEANS=lsms;
RUN;
QUIT;
ODS LISTING;


*Get overall estimates of mean and variance of treatment effect at
final visit;

*Dataset "lsms" contains the estimates of the treatment effect for
each visit over the 100 bootstrap samples. We are interested in the
final visit;

DATA lsms;
   SET lsms;
   IF visit NE 5 THEN DELETE;
RUN;


PROC SORT DATA=lsms;
   BY trt;
RUN;
```

```
*Get the mean and standard error of estimates over the bootstrap
samples to get the overall bootstrapped estimate;

PROC MEANS DATA=lsms;
   VAR estimate;
   BY trt;
   *stddev gives the bootstrap standard error of the overall estimate
   (this is the exact same as working out the formula given in
   section 8.4) See appendix 8.B for proof.;
   OUTPUT OUT=lsm_estimates MEAN=lsm STDDEV=se;
RUN;


*Show estimates of the difference in the treatment groups;

DATA diffs;
   SET diffs;
   IF visit NE 5 THEN DELETE;
RUN;

PROC MEANS DATA=diffs;
   VAR estimate;
   OUTPUT OUT=trt_diff_estimates MEAN=trt_diff STDDEV=diff_SE;
RUN;


*calculate the p-value of treatment difference at last visit;

DATA trt_diff_estimates;
   SET trt_diff_estimates;
   t_Value= trt_diff/diff_SE;
   p_value=(1-probt(abs(t_value),5490))*2;
RUN;


PROC CONTENTS DATA = trt_diff_estimates; RUN;
```

Identical implementation via a SAS macro by the authors, available from DIA pages at missingdata.org.uk

```
%INCLUDE "vansteelandt_method.sas";
%INCLUDE "VansteelandtSubMacros.sas";
%vansteelandt_method(
   datain=sleepv, trtname=trt, subjname=subjid, visname=visit,
   basecont=%str(base_mss),    seed=883960001, nboot=100,debug=0,
   primaryname=tst, analcovarcont=%str(base_mss), trtref=1,
   dataout=Sleep_vans_predicted, resout=Sleep_vans_results
   );
```

References

Carpenter JR, Kenward MG (2006) A comparison of multiple imputation and doubly robust estimation for analyses with missing data. *Journal of the Royal Statistical Society Series A* **169**: 571–584.

Daniel R, Kenward MG (2012) A method for increasing the robustness of multiple imputation. *Computational Statistics and Data Analysis* **56**: 1624–1643.

Efron B, Tibshirani RJ (1993) *An Introduction to the Bootstrap*. Chapman and Hall/CRC, Boca Raton, FL.

Freund RJ, Wilson WJ, Sa P (2006) *Regression Analysis: Statistical Modelling of a Response Variable*. Academic Press, San Diego, CA.

Kang JDY, Schafer JL (2007) Demystifying double robustness: a comparison of alternative strategies for estimating a population mean from incomplete data. *Statistical Science* **22**(4): 523–539.

Molenberghs G, Kenward MG (2007) *Missing Data in Clinical Studies*. John Wiley & Sons Ltd., West Sussex.

Robins J, Rotnitzky A, Zhao L (1994) Estimation of regression coefficients when some regressors are not always observed. *Journal of the American Statistical Association* **89**(427): 846–866.

Tchetgen E (2009) A simple implementation of doubly robust estimation in logistic regression with covariates missing at random. *Journal of Epidemiology* **20**: 391–394.

Teshome B, Molenberghs G, Sotto C, Kenward MG (2011) Doubly robust and multiple-imputation-based generalized estimating equations. *Journal of Biopharmaceutical Statistics* **21**: 202–225.

Vansteelandt S, Carpenter J, Kenward MG (2010) Analysis of incomplete data using inverse probability weighting and doubly robust estimators. *Methodology: European Journal of Research Methods for the Behavioral and Social Sciences* **6**(1): 37–48.

Table of SAS Code Fragments

8.1   Take a bootstrap sample.

8.2   Simple macro to create missingness indicators.

8.3   Code to calculate the probability of being observed at the first visit.

8.4   Code to calculate the probability of being observed at the first or the second visit.

8.5   Code to calculate the unconditional probability of being observed at each visit.

8.6   Calculate the inverse probability of being observed.

8.7   Convert the dataset to vertical format and run the weighted imputation model.

8.8   Set the predicted outcome from the imputation model as the new response and run the final analysis model.

8.9   Use LSMEANS to get the treatment effect at the final visit for each bootstrap sample and PROC MEANS to get the overall estimate of treatment effect.

8.10 Imputation model for each bootstrap sample.

8.11 Final analysis model to calculate the treatment change from baseline.

Bibliography

Agresti A (2002) *Categorical Data Analysis*, 2nd edn. John Wiley & Sons, New York.

Allison PD (2000) Multiple imputation for missing data: a cautionary tale. *Sociological Methods and Research* **28**: 301–309.

Allison PD (2002) *Missing Data*. Sage, Newbury Park, CA.

Allison PD (2005) *Imputation of Categorical Variables with PROC MI*. Proceedings of the Thirtieth Annual SAS® Users Group International Conference, available at http://www2.sas.com/proceedings/sugi30/113-30.pdf, accessed 7 July 2013.

Altshuler L, Suppes T, Black D, Nolen W, Keck P, Frye M, McElroy S, Kupka R, Grunze H, Walden J, Leverich G, Denicoff K, Luckenbaugh D, Post R (2003) Impact of anti-depressant discontinuation after acute bipolar depression remission on rates of depressive relapse at 1-year follow-up. *American Journal of Psychiatry* **160**: 1252–1262.

Barnard J, Rubin DB (1999) Small-sample degrees of freedom with multiple imputation. *Biometrika* **86**: 948–955.

Bernaards CA, Belin TR, Schafer JL (2007) Robustness of multivariate normal approximation for imputation of incomplete binary data. *Statistics in Medicine* **26**: 1368–1382.

Bhatt NB, Gudo ES, Semá C, Bila D, Di Mattei P, Augusto O, Garsia R, Jani IV (2009) Loss of correlation between HIV viral load and CD4+ T-cell counts in HIV/HTLV-1 co-infection in treatment naïve Mozambican patients. *International Journal of STD and AIDS* **20**(12): 863–868.

Blumer J, Findling R, Welchung J, Soubrane C, Reed M (2009) Controlled clinical trial of zolpidem for the treatment of insomnia associated with attention-deficit/hyperactivity disorder in children 6 to 17 years ot age. *Pediatrics* **123**(5): e770–e776, available at http://pediatrics.aappublications.org/content/123/5/e770.long, accessed 18 June 2013.

Bodner TE (2008) What improves with increased missing data imputations? *Structural Equation Modeling* **15**(4): 651–675.

Bollen KA, Stine RA (1992) Bootstrapping goodness-of-fit measures in structural equation models. *Sociological Methods and Research* **21**: 205–229.

Boulware LE, Liu Y, Fink NE, Coresh J, Ford DE, Klag MJ, Powe NR (2006) Temporal relation among depression symptoms, cardiovascular disease events, and mortality in end-stage renal disease: contribution of reverse causality. *Clinical Journal of American Society of Nephrology* **1**(3): 496–504.

Clinical Trials with Missing Data: A Guide for Practitioners, First Edition. Michael O'Kelly and Bohdana Ratitch.
© 2014 John Wiley & Sons, Ltd. Published 2014 by John Wiley & Sons, Ltd.

Bowden C, Mosolov S, Hranov L, Chen E, Habil H, Kongsakon R, Manfredi R, Lin H-N (2010) Efficacy of valproate versus lithium in mania or mixed mania: a randomized, open 12-week trial. *International Clinical Psychopharmacology* **25**: 60–67.

Brand JPL (1999) Development, implementation and evaluation of multiple imputation strategies for the statistical analysis of incomplete data sets. Ph.D. dissertation, Erasmus University, Rotterdam.

Bunouf P, Grouin J-M, Molenberghs G (2012) Analysis of an incomplete binary outcome derived from frequently recorded longitudinal continuous data: application to daily pain evaluation. *Statistics in Medicine* **31**: 1554–1571.

Burnham KP, Anderson DR (2002) *Model Selection and Multimodel Inference*, 2nd edn. Springer-Verlag, New York.

Burzykowski T, Carpenter J, Coens C, Evans D, France L, Kenward M, Lane P, Matcham J, Morgan D, Phillips A, Roger J, Sullivan B, White I, Yu L-M; of the Statisticians in the Pharmaceutical Industry (PSI) Missing Data Expert Group (2009) Missing data: discussion points from PSI missing data expert group. *Pharmaceutical Statistics* **9**: 288–297.

Cardiovascular and Renal Drugs Advisory Committee AdComm Bulletin (2012) *Supplemental New Drug Application (sNDA) 202439/S–002, XARELTO (rivaroxaban), by Janssen Pharmaceuticals, Inc, for use in combination with aspirin or with aspirin + clopidogrel or ticlopidine, to reduce risk of thrombotic cardiovascular events in patients with acute coronary syndrome (ST Elevation Myocardial Infarction [STEMI], Non-ST Elevation Myocardial Infarction [NSTEMI], or Unstable Angina [UA])*, IDRAC Thomson Reuters No. 143271. http://www.idrac.com/viewing.asp?ref=US00143271, accessed 22 March 2013

Carosi G, Lazzarin A, Stellbrink H, Moyle G, Rugina S, Staszewski S, Givens N, Ross L, Granier C, Ait-Khaled M, Leather D, Nichols WG (2009) Study of once-daily versus twice-daily fosamprenavir plus ritonavir administered with abacavir/lamivudine one daily in antiretroviral-naïve HIV-1-infected adult subjects. *HIV Clinical Trials* **10**(6): 356–367.

Carpenter JR, Kenward MG (2006) A comparison of multiple imputation and doubly robust estimation for analyses with missing data. *Journal of the Royal Statistical Society, Series A* **169**: 571–584.

Carpenter JR, Kenward MG (2007) Missing data in randomised controlled trials – a practical guide. National Health Service Co-ordinating Center for Research Methodology, Birmingham, available at www.hta.nhs.uk/nihrmethodology/reports/1589.pdf, accessed 18 June 2013.

Carpenter JR, Kenward MG (2013) *Multiple Imputation and its Application*. John Wiley & Sons Ltd., West Sussex.

Carpenter JR, Roger JH, Kenward MG (2013) Analysis of longitudinal trials with protocol deviation: a framework for relevant, accessible assumptions and inference via multiple imputation. *Journal of Biopharmaceutical Statistics*, **23**(6):1352–1371. DOI: 10.1080/10543406.2013.834911

Casella G, George EI (1992) Explaining the Gibbs sampler. *The American Statistician* **46**: 167–174.

Cassidy EL, Baird E, Sheikh JI (2001) Recruitment and retention of elderly patients in clinical trials. *American Journal of Geriatric Psychiatry* **9**: 136–140.

Cavanagh J, Smyth R, Goodwin G (2004) Relapse into mania or depression following lithium discontinuation: a 7 year follow-up. *Acta Psychiatrica Scandinavica* **109**: 91–95.

Chen F (2011) Missing no more: using the PROC MCMC procedure to model missing data. SAS Global Forum 2013, available at http://support.sas.com/resources/papers/proceedings13/436-2013.pdf, accessed 29 November 2013.

Cohen J (1988) *Statistical Power Analysis for the Behavioral Sciences*, 2nd edn. Lawrence Erlbaum Associates.

Collins LM, Schafer JL, Kam C-M (2001) A comparison of inclusive and restrictive strategies in modern missing data procedures. *Psychological Methods* **6**: 330–351.

Committee for Proprietary Medicinal Products (2001) Points to consider on missing data, available at http://www.ema.europa.eu/docs/en_GB/document_library/Scientific_guideline/2009/09/WC500003641.pdf, accessed 18 June 2013.

Cook R, Weisberg S (1982) *Applied Regression Including Computing and Graphics*. John Wiley & Sons Ltd., New York.

Cowles MK, Carlin BP (1996) Markov chain Monte Carlo convergence diagnostics: a comparative review. *Journal of the American Statistical Association* **91**: 883–904.

Daniel R, Kenward MG (2012) A method for increasing the robustness of multiple imputation. *Computational Statistics and Data Analysis* **56**: 1624–1643.

Daniels M, Hogan J (2008) *Missing Data in Longitudinal Studies*. Chapman & Hall, Boca Raton, FL.

Davis SM, Stroup TS, Koch GG, Davis CE, Rosenheck RA, Lieberman JA (2011) Time to all-cause treatment discontinuation as the primary outcome in the Clinical Antipsychotic Trials of Intervention Effectiveness (CATIE) schizophrenia study. *Statistics in Biopharmaceutical Research* **3**(2): 253–265.

Demirtas H, Freels SA, Yucel RM (2008) Plausibility of multivariate normality assumption when multiply imputing non-Gaussian continuous outcomes: a simulation assessment. *Journal of Statistical Computation and Simulation* **78**: 69–84.

Dempster AP, Laird NM, Rubin DB (1977) Maximum likelihood from incomplete data via EM algorithm. *Journal of the Royal Statistical Society, Series B* **39**: 1–38.

Draper N, Smith H (1981) *Applied Regression Analysis*. John Wiley & Sons Ltd., New York.

Efron B, Tibshirani RJ (1993) *An Introduction to the Bootstrap*. Chapman & Hall/CRC, Boca Raton, FL.

Eli Lilly and Company (2008) An efficacy study of compound LY2624803 in the treatment of patients with chronic insomnia (SLUMBER), available at http://clinicaltrials.gov/ct2/results?term=NCT00784875&Search=Search, accessed 18 June 2013.

Emre M, Aarsland D, Albanese A, Byrne J, Deuschl G, De Deyn P, Durif F, Kulisevsky J, van Laar T, Lees A, Poewe W, Robillard A, Rosa M, Wolters E, Quarg P, Tekin P, Lane R (2004) Rivastagmine for dementia associated with Parkinson's disease. *New England Journal of Medicine* **351**: 2509–2518.

Enders CK (2002) Applying the Bollen-Stine bootstrap for goodness-of-fit measures to structural equation models with missing data. *Multivariate Behavioral Research* **37**: 359–377.

Enders CK (2010) *Applied Missing Data Analysis*. The Guilford Press, New York.

Eron J, Yeni P, Gathe Jr J, Estrada V, DeJesus E, Staszewski S, Khuong-Josses MA, Yau L, Vavro C, Lim ML (2006) The KLEAN study of fosamprenavir-ritonavir versus lopinavir-ritonavir, each in combination with abacavir-lamivudine, for initial treatment of HIV infection over 48 weeks: a randomised non-inferiority trial. *Lancet* **368**: 476–482.

European Medicines Agency (2008a) Guideline on the clinical development of medicinal products for the treatment of HIV infection. EMEA/CPMP/EWP/633/02 Rev.2, available at http://www.ema.europa.eu/docs/en_GB/document_library/Scientific_guideline/2009/09/WC500003460.pdf, accessed 22 March 2013.

European Medicines Agency (2008b) Appendix to the guideline on the evaluation of anticancer medicinal products in man (CHMP/EWP/205/95 REV. 3): methodological considerations for using progression-free survival (PFS) as primary endpoint in confirmatory trials for registration, EMEA/CHMP/EWP/27994/2008, available at http://www.ema.europa.eu/docs/en_GB/document_library/Other/2009/12/WC500017749.pdf, accessed 23 June 2013.

European Medicines Agency (2010) Guideline on missing data in confirmatory clinical trials. EMA/CPMP/EWP/1776/99 Rev.1, available at http://www.ema.europa.eu/docs/en_GB/document_library/Scientific_guideline/2010/09/WC500096793.pdf, accessed 23 June 2013.

Fahn S, Elton RL; UPDRS Development Committee (1987) Unified Parkinson's disease rating scale. In: S Fahn, CD Marsden, DB Calne, M Goldstein (eds), *Recent Developments in Parkinson's Disease*. Macmillan, Florham Park, NJ, pp. 153–163.

Freedman DA (2006) On the so-called "Huber sandwich estimator" and "robust standard errors." *The American Statistician* **60**: 299–302.

Freund RJ, Wilson WJ, Sa P (2006) *Regression Analysis: Statistical Modelling of a Response Variable*. Academic Press, San Diego, CA.

Gardiner JC, Luo ZH, Roman LA (2009) Fixed effects, random effects and GEE: what are the differences? *Statistics in Medicine* **28**: 221–239.

Gelman A, Raghunathan TE (2001) Discussion of Arnold *et al.* "Conditionally Specified Distributions". *Statistical Science* **16**: 249–274.

Gelman A, Rubin DB (1992) Inference from iterative simulation using multiple sequences. *Statistical Science* **7**: 457–472.

Glynn R, Laird N, Rubin DB (1986) Selection modeling versus mixture modeling with nonignorable nonresponse. In: H Wainer (ed.), *Drawing Inferences from Self-selected Samples*. Springer-Verlag, New York.

Glynn R, Laird N, Rubin DB (1993) Multiple imputation in mixture models for nonignorable nonresponse with follow-ups. *Journal of the American Statistical Association* **88**: 984–993.

Goria MN (1992) On the fourth root transformation of chi-square. *Australian Journal of Statistics* **34**(1): 55–64.

Gottschall AC, West SG, Enders CK (2012) A comparison of item-level and scale-level multiple imputation for questionnaire batteries. *Multivariate Behavioral Research* **47**(1): 1–25.

Graham JW, Olchowski AE, Gilreath TD (2007) How many imputations are really needed? Some practical clarifications of multiple imputation theory. *Prevention Science* **8**: 206–213.

Graham JW, Schafer JL (1999) On the performance of multiple imputation for multivariate data with small sample size. In: R Hoyle (ed.), *Statistical Strategies for Small Sample Research*. Sage, Thousand Oaks, CA.

Guico-Pabia C, Fayyad R, Soares C (2012) Assessing the relationship between functional impairment/recovery and depression severity. *International Clinical Psychopharmacology* **27**: 1–7.

Hartley HO, Hocking RR (1971) The analysis of incomplete data. *Biometrics* **27**: 783–808.

Hauser R, Auinger P; Parkinson Study Group (2011) Determination of minimal clinically important change in early and advanced Parkinson's disease. *Movement Disorders* **26**: 813–818.

Hedeker D (2012) Missing data in longitudinal studies, available at http://www.uic.edu/classes/bstt/bstt513/missbLS.pdf, accessed 20 June 2013.

Hedeker D, Gibbons R (2006) *Longitudinal Data Analysis*. John Wiley & Sons Ltd., New York.

Heitjan F, Little RJA (1991) Multiple imputation for the fatal accident reporting system. *Applied Statistics* **40**: 13–29.

Holm K, Goa K (2000) Zolpidem: an update of its pharmacology, therapeutic efficacy and tolerability in the treatment of insomnia. *Drugs* **59**: 865–889.

Horton NJ, Lipsitz SR (2001) Multiple imputation in practice: comparison of software packages for regression models with missing variables. *The American Statistician* **55**: 244–254.

Horton NJ, Lipsitz SR, Parzen M (2003) A potential for bias when rounding in multiple imputation. *The American Statistician* **57**: 229–232.

Huber P (1967) The behaviour of maximum likelihood estimates under nonstandard conditions. In *Proceedings of the 5th Berkeley Symposium on Mathematical Statistics and Probability* **1**: 221–233.

Hughes S, Harris J, Flack N, Cuffe RL (2012) The statistician's role in the prevention of missing data. *Pharmaceutical Statistics* **11**: 410–416.

Hurvich CM, Tsai CL (1989) Regression and time series model selection in small samples. *Biometrika* **76**: 297–307.

International Committee of Medical Journal Editors (2010) Uniform requirements for manuscripts submitted to biomedical journals, available at http://www.icmje.org/urm _full.pdf, accessed 22 March 2013.

International Conference on Harmonisation of Technical Requirements for Registration of Pharmaceuticals for Human Use (1998) Statistical principles for clinical trials: E9, available at http://www.emea.europa.eu/docs/en_GB/document_library/Scientific _guideline/2009/09/WC500002928.pdf, accessed 23 June 2013.

Jungquist C, Tra Y, Smith M, Pigeon W, Matteson-Rusby S, Xia Y, Perlis M (2012) The durability of cognitive behavioral therapy for insomnia in patients with chronic pain. *Sleep Disorders*, available at http://www.hindawi.com/journals/sd/2012/679648/, accessed 20 June 2013.

Kang JDY, Schafer JL (2007) Demystifying double robustness: a comparison of alternative strategies for estimating a population mean from incomplete data. *Statistical Science* **22**(4): 523–539.

Keene O (2010) Intent-to-treat analysis in the presence of off-treatment or missing data. *Pharmaceutical Statistics* **10**: 191–195.

Kelleher T, Thiry A, Wilber R, Cross A (2001) Missing data methods in HIV clinical trials: regulatory guidance and alternative approaches. *Drug Information Journal* **35**: 1363–1371.

Kenward MG (2011) Handling dropout and withdrawal in longitudinal clinical trials, presented at Biostatistics Network Symposium: "Contemporary statistical methods in medical research", 15th September 2011, available at http://www.ucl.ac.uk/statistics/biostatistics -network/talks/TalkKenward.pdf, accessed 17 July 2013.

Kenward MG, Carpenter JR (2009) Multiple imputation. In: M Davidian, G Fitzmaurice, G Molenberghs, G Verbeke (eds), *Longitudinal Data Analysis: A Handbook of Modern Statistical Methods*. Chapman & Hall, London, pp. 477–500.

Kenward MG, Roger JH (1997) Small sample inference for fixed effects from restricted maximum likelihood. *Biometrics* **53**: 983–997.

Kenward MG, White IR, Carpenter JR (2010) Should baseline be a covariate or dependent variable in analyses of change from baseline in clinical trials? by Liu GF, Lu K, Mogg R, Mallick M, Mehrotra DV in Statistics in Medicine 2009; 28: 2509–2530. *Statistics in Medicine* **29**: 1455–1456.

Koch GG, Amara IA, Forster J, McSorley D, Peace KE (1993) Statistical issues in the design and analysis of ulcer healing and recurrence studies. *Drug Information Journal* **27**: 805–824.

Koch GG, Davis SM, Anderson RL (1998) Methodological advances and plans for improving regulatory success for confirmatory studies. *Statistics in Medicine* **17**(15–16): 1675–1690.

Krystal A, Erman M, Zammit G, Soubrane C, Roth T; ZOLONG Study Group (2008) Long-term efficacy and safety of zolpidem extended-release 12.5 mg, administered 3 to 7 nights per week for 24 weeks, in patients with chronic primary insomnia: a 6-month, randomized, double-blind, placebo-controlled, parallel-group, multicenter study. *Sleep* **31**: 79–90.

Landis RJ, Heyman ER, Koch GG (1978) Average partial association in three-way contingency tables: a review and discussion of alternative tests. *International Statistical Review* **46**: 237–254.

Lavori PW, Dawson R, Shera D (1995) A multiple imputation strategy for clinical trials with truncation of patient data. *Statistics in Medicine* **14**: 1913–1925.

Lee KJ, Carlin JB (2010) Multiple imputation for missing data: fully conditional specification versus multivariate normal imputation. *American Journal of Epidemiology* **171**(5): 624–632.

Leite WL, Beretvas N (2010) The performance of multiple imputation for Likert-type items with missing data. *Journal of Modern Applied Statistical Methods* **9**(1): 64–74.

Liang K-Y, Zeger S (1986) Longitudinal data analysis using generalized linear models. *Biometrika* **73**(1): 13–22.

Liang K-Y, Zeger S (2000) Longitudinal data analysis of continuous and discrete responses for pre-post-designs. *Sankhya Indian Journal of Statistics* **62B**: 134–148.

Lieberman JA, Stroup TS, McEvoy JP, Swartz MS, Rosenheck RA, Perkins DO, Keefe RSE, Davis SM, Davis CE, Lebowitz BD, Severe J, Hsiao JK (2005) Effectiveness of antipsychotic drugs in patients with chronic schizophrenia. *The New England Journal of Medicine* **353**(12): 1209–1223.

Lin Q, Xu L for the Eli Lilly and Company Advanced Analytic Missing Data Hub (2012) shared_parameter1.sas, available at http://missingdata.lshtm.ac.uk/dia/Selection%20Model_20120726.zip, accessed 20 June 2013.

Lipkovich I, Houston J, Ahl J (2008) Identifying patterns in treatment response profiles in acute bipolar mania: a cluster analysis approach. *BMC Psychiatry* **8**: 65, available at http://www.ncbi.nlm.nih.gov/pmc/articles/PMC2515837, accessed 18 June 2013.

Little RJA (1993) Pattern-mixture models for multivariate incomplete data. *Journal of the American Statistical Association* **88**: 125–134.

Little TD, Howard WJ, McConnell EK, Stump KN (2011) Missing data in large data projects: two methods of missing data imputation when working with large data projects, available at http://crmda.dept.ku.edu/resources/kuantguides/11_ImputationWithLargeDataSets.pdf, accessed 7 July 2013.

Little RJA, Rubin DB (2002) *Statistical Analysis with Missing Data*, 2nd edn. John Wiley & Sons Ltd., New York.

Little RJA, Yau L (1996) Intent-to-treat analysis in longitudinal studies with dropouts. *Biometrics* **52**: 1324–1333.

Liu GF, Lu K, Mogg R, Mallick M, Mehrotra DV (2009) Should baseline be a covariate or dependent variable in analyses of change from baseline in clinical trials? *Statistics in Medicine* **28**: 2509–2530.

Liu GF, Zhan X (2011) Comparisons of methods for analysis of repeated binary responses with missing data. *Journal of Biopharmaceutical Statistics* **21**: 371–392.

MacKinnon JG, White H (1985) Some heteroskedasticity-consistent covariance matrix estimators with improved finite sample properties. *Journal of Econometrics* **29**: 305–325.

Magruder KM, Ouyang B, Miller S, Tilley BC (2009) Retention of under-represented minorities in drug abuse treatment studies. *Clinical Trials* **6**: 252–260.

Mallinckrodt CH (2013) *Preventing and Treating Missing Data in Longitudinal Clinical Trials*. Cambridge University Press, Cambridge.

Mallinckrodt CH, Clark WS, David SR (2001a) Accounting for dropout bias using mixed-effects models. *Journal of Biopharmaceutical Statistics* **11**(1–2): 9–21.

Mallinckrodt CH, Clark WS, David SR (2001b) Type I error rates from mixed effects model repeated measures versus fixed effects ANOVA with missing values imputed via last observation carried forward. *Drug Information Journal* **35**: 1215–1225.

Mallinckrodt CH, Kaiser CJ, Watkin JG, Molenberghs G, Carroll RJ (2004) The effect of correlation structure on treatment contrasts estimated from incomplete clinical trial data with likelihood-based repeated measures compared with last observation carried forward ANOVA. *Clinical Trials* **1**: 477–489.

Mallinckrodt CH, Lane PW, Schnell D, Peng Y, Mancuso J (2008) Recommendation for the primary analysis of continuous endpoints in longitudinal clinical trials. *Drug Information Journal* **42**: 303–319.

Mallinckrodt CH, Sanger TM, Dubé S, DeBrota DJ, Molenberghs G, Carroll RJ, Potter WZ, Tollefson GD (2003) Assessing and interpreting treatment effects in longitudinal clinical trials with missing data. *Biological Psychiatry* **53**: 754–760.

Mantel N, Haenszel W (1959) Statistical aspects of the analysis of data from retrospective studies of disease. *Journal of the National Cancer Institute* **22**: 719–748.

Mayer G, Wang-Weigand S, Roth-Schechter B, Lehmann R, Staner C, Partinen M (2009) Efficacy and safety of 6-month nightly ramelteon administration in adults with chronic primary insomnia. *Sleep* **32**: 351–360.

Medpage Today Bulletin (2012) Acute coronary syndrome: FDA panel narrowly rejects Xarelto for ACS, available at http://www.medpagetoday.com/Cardiology/AcuteCoronarySyndrome/32888, accessed 16 July 2013.

Meng X-L (1994) Multiple imputation inferences with uncongenial sources of input. *Statistical Science* **9**: 538–558.

Mergl R, Henkel V, Allgaier A, Kramer D, Hautzinger M, Kohnen R, Coyne J, Hegerl U (2011) Are treatment preferences relevant in response to serotonergic antidepressants and cognitive-behavioral therapy in depressed primary care patients? Results from a randomized controlled trial including a patients' choice arm. *Psychotherapy and Psychosomatics* **80**: 39–47.

Molenberghs G, Kenward MG (2007) *Missing Data in Clinical Studies*. John Wiley & Sons Ltd., West Sussex.

Moreno-Black G, Shor-Posner G, Miguez MJ, Burbano X, O'Mellan S, Yovanoff P (2004) "I will miss the study, God bless you all": participation in a nutritional chemoprevention trial. *Ethnicity and Disease* **14**: 469–475.

Myers W (2000) Handling missing data in clinical trials: an overview. *Drug Information Journal* **34**: 525–533.

National Research Council, Panel on Handling Missing Data in Clinical Trials, Committee on National Statistics, Division of Behavioral and Social Sciences and Education (2010) *The Prevention and Treatment of Missing Data in Clinical Trials*. The National Academies Press, Washington, DC, available at http://www.nap.edu/catalog.php?record_id=12955, accessed 16 July 2013.

Office of Human Research Protections (2008) Guidance on important considerations for when participation of human subjects in research is discontinued. Washington, DC, available at http://www.hhs.gov/ohrp/documents/200811guidance.pdf, accessed 23 June 2013.

O'Neill RT (2011) The Prevention and Treatment of Missing Data in Clinical Trials, Some FDA Background, presentation at the *Prevention and Treatment of Missing Data in Clinical Trials* course sponsored by Johns Hopkins School of Public Health; Iselin, New Jersey.

Oudshoorn CGM, van Buuren S, Rijckevorsel JLA (1999) Flexible Multiple Imputation by Chained Equations of the AVO-95 Survey. *TNO Prevention and Health*, TNO Report G/VGZ/99.045.

Parkinson Study Group (2004a) A controlled, randomized delayed-start study of rasagiline in early Parkinson disease. *Archives of Neurology* **61**: 561–566.

Parkinson Study Group (2004b) Levodopa and the progression of Parkinson's disease. *New England Journal of Medicine* **351**: 2498–2508.

Peduzzi P, Concato J, Kemper E, Holford TR, Feinstein AR (1996) A simulation study of the number of events per variable in logistic regression analysis. *Journal of Clinical Epidemiology* **49**(12): 1373–1379.

Permutt T (2011) Regulatory Considerations, presentation at the *Prevention and Treatment of Missing Data in Clinical Trials course* sponsored by Johns Hopkins School of Public Health; Iselin, New Jersey.

Post R, Altshuler L, Frye M, Suppes T, McElroy S, Keck P, Leverich G, Kupka R, Nolen W, Luckenbaugh D, Walden J, Grunze H (2005) Preliminary observations on the effectiveness of levetiracetam in the open adjunctive treatment of refractory bipolar disorder. *Journal of Clinical Psychiatry* **66**: 370–374.

Post F, Moyle G, Stellbrink H, Domingo P, Podzamczer D, Fisher M, Norden AG, Cavassini M, Rieger A, Khuong-Josses MA, Branco T, Pearce HC, Givens N, Vavro C, Lim ML (2010) Randomized comparison of renal effects, efficacy, and safety with once-daily abacavir/lamivudine versus tenofovir/emtricitabine, administered with efavirenz, in antiretroviral-naïve, HIV-1-infected adults: 48-week results from the ASSERT study. *Journal of Acquired Immune Deficiency Syndrome* **55**(1): 49–57.

Pulido F, Baril JG, Staszewski S, Khuong-Josses MA, Yau L, Vavro C, Lim ML (2007) Long-term efficacy and safety of fosamprenavir + ritonavir (FPV/r) versus lopinavir/ritonavir (LPV/r) over 96 weeks. *47th Annual Interscience Conference on Antimicrobial Agents and Chemotherapy,* Chicago, IL. Abstract H-361.

Purdue Pharma LP (2007) A study of zolpidem tartrate sublingual tablet in adult patients with insomnia, available at http://clinicaltrials.gov/ct2/results?term=NCT00466193 &Search=Search, accessed 18 June 2013.

Raghunathan TE, Lepkowski JM, Van Hoewyk J, Solenberger P (2001) A multivariate technique for multiply imputing missing values using a sequence of regression models. *Survey Methodology* 27(1): 85–95.

Ratitch B (2012a) Fitting control-based imputation (using monotone sequential regression) macro documentation, available at http://missingdata.lshtm.ac.uk/dia/PMM%20Delta %20Tipping%20Point%20and%20CBI_20120726.zip, accessed 20 June 2013.

Ratitch B (2012b) Tipping point analysis with delta-adjusting imputation (using monotone sequential regression) macro documentation, available at http://missingdata.lshtm.ac.uk/dia/ PMM%20Delta%20Tipping%20Point%20and%20CBI_20120726.zip, accessed 20 June 2013.

Ratitch B, O'Kelly M (2011) Implementation of pattern-mixture models using standard SAS/STAT procedures. In *Proceedings of Pharmaceutical Industry SAS User Group*, Nashville, available at http://pharmasug.org/proceedings/2011/SP/PharmaSUG-2011-SP04 .pdf, accessed 23 June 2013.

Ratitch B, O'Kelly M, Tosiello R (2013) Missing data in clinical trials: from clinical assumptions to statistical analysis using pattern mixture models. *Pharmaceutical Statistics* 12: 337–347, available at http://onlinelibrary.wiley.com/doi/10.1002/pst.1549/pdf, accessed 20 June 2013.

Robins J, Gill, R (1997) Non-response models for the analysis of non-monotone ignorable missing data. *Statistics in Medicine* 16: 39–56.

Robins J, Rotnitzky A, Zhao L (1994) Estimation of regression coefficients when some regressors are not always observed. *Journal of the American Statistical Association* 89(427): 846–866.

Robinson KA, Dennison CR, Wayman DM, Pronovost PJ, Needham DM (2007) Systematic review identifies number of strategies important for retaining study participants. *Journal of Clinical Epidemiology* 60: 757–765.

Roger JH (2010) Discussion of Incomplete and Enriched Data Analysis and Sensitivity Analysis, presented by Geert Molenberghs. *Drug Information Association (DIA) Meeting, Special Interest Area Communities (SIAC) - Statistics.*

Roger JH (2012) Fitting pattern-mixture models to longitudinal repeated-measures data, available at http://missingdata.lshtm.ac.uk/dia/Five_Macros20120827.zip, accessed 20 June 2013.

Roger JH, Ritchie S, Donovan C, Carpenter JR (2008) Sensitivity Analysis for Longitudinal Studies with Withdrawal. *PSI Conference*, available at http://www.psiweb.org/docs/ 2008finalprogramme.pdf, accessed 20 June 2013.

Rosenbaum PR, Rubin DB (1983) The central role of the propensity score in observational studies for causal effects. *Biometrika* 70: 41–55.

Roth T, Walsh J, Krystal A, Wessel T, Roehrs T (2005) An evaluation of the efficacy and safety of eszopiclone over 12 months in patients with chronic primary insomnia. *Sleep Medicine* 6: 487–495.

Rubin DB (1976) Inference and missing data. *Biometrika* **63**: 581–592.

Rubin DB (1978) Multiple imputation in sample surveys – a phenomenological Bayesian approach to nonresponse. *Proceedings of the Survey Research Methods Section of the American Statistical Association* **1**: 20–34.

Rubin DB (1987) *Multiple Imputation for Nonresponse in Surveys.* John Wiley & Sons Ltd., New York.

Rubin DB (1996) Multiple imputations after 18+ years. *Journal of the American Statistical Association* **91**(434): 473–489.

Rubin DB, Schenker N (1986) Multiple imputation for interval estimation from simple random samples with ignorable response. *Journal of the American Statistical Association* **81**: 366–374.

SAS Institute Inc. (2011a) *SAS/STAT® 9.3 User's Guide: The GLIMMIX Procedure (Chapter).* SAS Institute Inc., Cary, NC.

SAS Institute Inc. (2011b) *SAS/STAT® 9.3 User's Guide: The MIXED Procedure (Chapter).* SAS Institute Inc., Cary, NC.

SAS Institute Inc. (2011c) *SAS/STAT® 9.3 User's Guide: The GENMOD Procedure (Chapter).* SAS Institute Inc., Cary, NC.

SAS Institute Inc. (2011d) *SAS/STAT® 9.3 User's Guide.* SAS Institute Inc., Cary, NC.

Schafer JL (1997) *Analysis of Incomplete Multivariate Data.* Chapman & Hall, New York.

Schafer JL (1999) Multiple imputation: a primer. *Statistical Methods in Medical Research* **8**: 3–15.

Schafer JL (2003) Multiple imputation in multivariate problems when the imputation and analysis models differ. *Statistica Neerlandica* **57**: 19–35.

Schafer JL, Graham JW (2002) Missing data: our view of the state of the art. *Psychological Methods* **7**: 147–177.

Schafer JL, Olsen MK (1998) Multiple imputation for multivariate missing-data problems: a data analyst's perspective. *Multivariate Behavioral Research* **33**: 545–571.

Scharfstein D, Robins J (2002) Estimation of the failure time distribution in the presence of informative censoring. *Biometrika* **89**: 617–634, available at http://www.jstor.org/stable/4140606, accessed 23 June 2013.

Schenker N, Taylor JMG (1996) Partially parametric techniques for multiple imputation. *Computational Statistics and Data Analysis* **22**: 425–446.

Schenkman M, Ellis T, Christiansen C, Barón A, Tickle-Degnen L, Hall A, Wagenaar R (2011) Profile of functional limitations and task performance among people with early- and middle-stage Parkinson disease. *Physical therapy* **91**: 1338–1354.

Seed M, Juarez M, Alnatour R (2009) Improving recruitment and retention rates in preventive longitudinal research with adolescent mothers. *Journal of Child and Adolescent Psychiatric Nursing* **22**: 150–153.

Senturia YD, McNiff MK, Baker D, Gergen P, Mitchell H, Joseph C, Wedner HJ (1998) Successful techniques for retention of study participants in an inner-city population. *Controlled Clinical Trials* **19**: 544–554.

Shulman LM, Gruber-Baldini AL, Anderson KE, Fishman PS, Reich SG, Weiner WJ (2010) The clinically important difference on the unified Parkinson's disease rating scale. *Archives of Neurology* **67**(1): 64–70.

Siddiqui O, Hung HMJ, O'Neil R (2009) MMRM vs. LOCF: a comprehensive comparison based on simulation study and 25 NDA datasets. *Journal of Biopharmaceutical Statistics* **19**: 227–246.

Smith K, Patel P, Fine D, Bellos N, Sloan L, Lackey P, Kumar PN, Sutherland-Phillips DH, Vavro C, Yau L, Wannamaker P, Shaefer MS; HEAT Study Team (2009) Randomized, double-blind, placebo-matched, multicentre trial of abacavir/lamivudine or tenofovir/emtricitabine with lopinavir/ritonavir for initial HIV treatment. *AIDS* **23**(12): 1547–1556.

Squires K, Young B, DeJesus E, Bellos N, Murphy D, Sutherland-Phillips DH, Zhao HH, Patel LG, Ross LL, Wannamaker PG, Shaefer MS; ARIES Study Team (2010) Safety and efficacy of a 36-week induction regimen of abacavir/lamivudine and ritonavir-boosted atazanavir in HIV-infected patients. *HIV Clinical Trials* **11**(2): 69–79.

Stine R (1989) An introduction to bootstrap methods: Examples and ideas. *Sociological Methods and Research* **18**: 243–291.

Tangen CT, Koch GG (1999) Complementary nonparametric analysis of covariance for logistic regression in a randomized clinical trial setting. *Journal of Biopharmaceutical Statistics* **9**(1): 45–66.

Tanner MA, Wong WH (1987) The calculation of posterior distributions by data augmentation (with discussion). *Journal of the American Statistical Association* **82**: 528–550.

Tchetgen E (2009) A simple implementation of doubly robust estimation in logistic regression with covariates missing at random. *Journal of Epidemiology* **20**: 391–394.

Teshome B, Molenberghs G, Sotto C, Kenward MG (2011) Doubly robust and multiple-imputation-based generalized estimating equations. *Journal of Biopharmaceutical Statistics* **21**: 202–225.

Thijs H, Molenberghs G, Michiels B, Verbeke G, Curran D (2002) Strategies to fit pattern-mixture models. *Biostatistics* **3**: 245–265.

Tohen M, Greil W, Calabrese J, Sachs G, Yatham L, Oerlinghauser B, Koukopoulos A, Cassano G, Grunze H, Licht R, Dell'Osso L, Evans A, Risser R, Baker R, Crane H, Dossenbach M, Bowden C (2005) Olanzapine versus lithium in the maintenance treatment of bipolar disorder: a 12-month, randomized, double-blind, controlled clinical trial. *American Journal of Psychiatry* **162**: 1281–1290.

U.S. Food and Drug Administration, Center for Drug Evaluation and Research (2004) *Approval Package for Application Number 21-446,* available at http://www.accessdata.fda.gov/drugsatfda_docs/nda/2004/021446_Lyrica%20Capsules_medr.PDF, accessed 16 July 2013.

U.S. Food and Drug Administration (2008) *Guidance for sponsors, clinical investigators, and IRBs: data retention when subjects withdraw from FDA-regulated clinical trials,* Rockville, available at www.fda.gov/downloads/RegulatoryInformation/Guidances/UCM126489.pdf, accessed 23 June 2013.

U.S. Food and Drug Administration (2010) *FDA executive summary prepared for the March 19, 2010 meeting of the Circulatory System Devices Panel: P090013, REVO MRI SureScan Pacing System, Medtronic, Inc.,* available at http://www.fda.gov/downloads/advisorycommittees/committeesmeetinmaterials/medicaldevices/medicaldevicesadvisorcommittee/circulatorysystemdevicespanel/ucm204715.pdf, accessed 18 June 2013.

U.S. Food and Drug Administration (2013) *Briefing document, Pulmonary Allergy Drugs Advisory Committee Meeting: NDA 204-275: fluticasone furoate and vilanterol inhalation powder for the long-term, maintenance treatment of airflow obstruction and for reducing exacerbations in patients with chronic obstructive pulmonary disease (COPD)*, available at http://www.fda.gov/downloads/AdvisoryCommittees/CommitteesMeetingMaterials/Drugs/Pulmonary-AllergyDrugsAdvisoryCommittee/UCM347929.pdf, accessed 23 June 2013.

van Buuren S (2007) Multiple imputation of discrete and continuous data by fully conditional specification. *Statistical Methods in Medical Research* **16**: 219–242.

van Buuren S (2012) *Flexible Imputation of Missing Data*. Chapman & Hall/CRC Press, Boca Raton, FL.

van Buuren S, Brand JPL, Groothuis-Oudshoorn CGM, Rubin DB (2006) Fully conditional specification in multiple imputation. *Journal of Statistical Computation and Simulation* **76**: 1049–1064.

van Buuren S, Oudshoorn CGM (1999) *Flexible multivariate imputation by MICE*. TNO-rapport PG 99.054. TNO Prevention and Health, Leiden, available at http://www.stefvanbuuren.nl/publications/Flexible%20multivariate%20-%20TNO99054%201999.pdf, accessed 7 July 2013.

van Ginkel JR, Van der Ark LA, Sijtsma K (2007a) Multiple imputation for item scores when test data are factorially complex. *British Journal of Mathematical and Statistical Psychology* **60**: 315–337.

van Ginkel JR, Van der Ark LA, Sijtsma K (2007b) Multiple imputation of test and questionnaire data and influence on psychometric results. *Multivariate Behavioral Research* **42**: 387–414.

Vansteelandt S, Carpenter J, Kenward MG (2010) Analysis of incomplete data using inverse probability weighting and doubly robust estimators. *Methodology: European Journal of Research Methods for the Behavioral and Social Sciences* **6**(1): 37–48.

Verbeke G, Molenberghs G (1997) *Linear Mixed Models in Practice: A SAS-oriented Approach. Lecture Notes in Statistics 126*. Springer-Verlag, New York.

Verbeke G, Molenberghs G (2000) *Linear Mixed Models for Longitudinal Data*. Springer-Verlag, New York.

Villacorta V, Kegeles S, Galea J, Konda KA, Cuba JP, Palacios CF, Coates TJ; NIMH Collaborative HIV/STD Prevention Trial Group (2007) Innovative approaches to cohort retention in a community-based HIV/STI prevention trial for socially marginalized Peruvian young adults. *Clinical Trials* **4**: 32–41.

Von Hippel PT (2009) How to impute interactions, squares, and other transformed variables. *Sociological Methodology* **39**(1): 265–291.

Walter M, Hart S (2001) Methods employed to retain an urban population: experience of the Inner-City Asthma Study (ICAS). *Controlled Clinical Trials* **22**: 35S.

White H (1982) Maximum likelihood estimation of misspecified models. *Econometrica* **50**: 1–26.

White IR, Royston P, Wood AM (2011) Multiple imputation using chained equations: issues and guidance for practice. *Statistics in Medicine* **30**: 377–399.

Wilson EB, Hilferty MM (1931) The distribution of chi-square. *Proceedings of the National Academy of Sciences of the United States of America* **17**: 684–688.

Wolfinger R, O'Connell M (1993) Generalized linear mixed models: a pseudo-likelihood approach. *Journal of Statistical Computation and Simulation* **48**: 233–243.

Xu L, Lin Q (2012) Shared parameter model for informative missing data, available at http://missingdata.lshtm.ac.uk/dia/Selection%20Model_20120726.zip, accessed 20 June 2013.

Yan X, Lee S, Li N (2009) Missing data handling methods in medical device clinical trials. *Journal of Biopharmaceutical Statistics* **19**: 1085–1098, available at http://www.tandfonline.com/doi/pdf/10.1080/10543400903243009, accessed 23 June 2013.

Yan X, Li H, Gao Y, Gray G (2008) Case study: sensitivity analysis in clinical trials. *AdvaMed/FDA conference*, available at http://www.amstat.org/sections/sigmedd/Advamed/advamed08/presentation/Yan_sherry.pdf, accessed 20 June 2013.

Yucel RM, He Y, Zaslavsky AM (2008) Using calibration to improve rounding in imputation. *The American Statistician* **62**: 1–5.

Zheng W, Lin Q; Eli Lilly and Company Advanced Analytic Missing Data Hub (2012) *Sensitivity Analysis on Incomplete Longitudinal Data with Selection Model*, available at http://missingdata.lshtm.ac.uk/dia/Selection%20Model_20120726.zip, accessed 20 June 2013.

Zook PM, Jordan C, Adams B, Visness CM, Walter M, Pollenz K, Logan J, Tesson E, Smartt E, Chen A, D'Agostino J, Gern JE (2010) Retention strategies and predictors of attrition in an urban pediatric asthma study. *Clinical Trials* **7**: 400–410.

Index

Bold page numbers refer to SAS code fragments, figures, or tables.

Clinical Trials with Missing Data: A Guide for Practitioners, First Edition. Michael O'Kelly and Bohdana Ratitch.
© 2014 John Wiley & Sons, Ltd. Published 2014 by John Wiley & Sons, Ltd.

selection models, 15, 61. *See also*
  Selection models
shared parameter models, 15, 61.
  See also Shared parameter
  models
plausibility of, 87–88
primary analysis under assumption
  of, 17, 86
reasons to avoid, 87
Missing values. *See also* Multiple
  imputation, modeling uncertainty
  about imputed values
definition, 4, 34
explicit imputation of, 185
plot summarizing, **286**, **291**, **296**,
  302, **305**, **313**, **316**, **319**
uncertainty of imputation of, 186
Missingness. *See also* Missing
  completely at random, Missing at
  random, Missing not at random
definition, 4
descriptive presentation of, 113–114,
  141–145, **146**
  sample protocol text describing,
    124–125
ignorable, 5. *See also* Missing
  completely at random; Missing
  at random
intermediate, *see* Missingness,
  non-monotone
intermittent, *see* Missingness,
  non-monotone
mechanism, 4, 191
model of, 4, 370, 374, 380–381
  logistic regression, 114, 380
  unconditional probability of being
    observed in, 380–381, **386**
monotone, 3, 61, 192–193, 195, 197,
  198–199, 244, 249, 285, 382
non-monotone, 3, 61, 63, 64,
  192–193, 195, 198–199, 244,
  249, 284, 382. *See also*
  Imputation model, multivariate
  normal distribution use for
assumptions for, 268, 269
handling of, 268

partial imputation for, 198–199,
  200, 210–212, **210**, 245, 285,
  285
patterns by
  reasons for discontinuation, 81,
    141, 143, **143**, **146**
  visit of discontinuation, 142, 144,
    144, **146**
patterns of, 3–4, 141–144, 192–195,
  193, 195, 196, 244
probability of, 248
types of, 4–5
Mixed linear model, 131
Mixed model for repeated measures,
  13, 75, 131, 187, **149**. *See also*
  Parkinson's disease example
baseline adjustment, 147
bias compared to last observation
  carried forward, 131–132,
  140
caution regarding correctness of
  assumptions, 59
convergence, 147–148
covariance structures, 135–139
  AR(1), 138
  compound symmetry, 135, 161
    heterogeneous, 135
  heterogeneous, 286
  spatial, 137–139
  spatial power, 138, **158**, 158–160
    plus random subject effect,
      138–139
  Toeplitz, 136–137
    heterogeneous, 137, 156–158
  unstructured, 135–236, 150–156
effect size calculation, 164–166
interaction in
  baseline by visit, 147, 148
  treatment by site by visit, 163–164
  treatment by subgroup by visit,
    162, **162**
  treatment by visit, 133, 146–147,
    171
mathematical specification, 132–135
missing-at-random assumption
  implemented via, 13, 86, 140

Statistics in Practice

Human and Biological Sciences

Earth and Environmental Sciences

Buck, Cavanagh and Litton – Bayesian Approach to Interpreting Archaeological Data
Chandler and Scott – Statistical Methods for Trend Detection and Analysis in the
    Environmental Statistics
Glasbey and Horgan – Image Analysis in the Biological Sciences
Haas – Improving Natural Resource Management: Ecological and Political Models
Haas – Introduction to Probability and Statistics for Ecosystem Managers
Helsel – Nondetects and Data Analysis: Statistics for Censored Environmental Data
Illian, Penttinen, Stoyan and Stoyan – Statistical Analysis and Modelling of Spatial Point
    Patterns
Mateu and Muller (Eds) – Spatio-Temporal Design: Advances in Efficient Data Acquisition
McBride – Using Statistical Methods for Water Quality Management
Webster and Oliver – Geostatistics for Environmental Scientists, Second Edition
Wymer (Ed.) – Statistical Framework for RecreationalWater Quality Criteria and Monitoring

Industry, Commerce and Finance

Aitken – Statistics and the Evaluation of Evidence for Forensic Scientists, Second Edition
Balding – Weight-of-evidence for Forensic DNA Profiles
Brandimarte – Numerical Methods in Finance and Economics: AMATLAB-Based
    Introduction, Second Edition
Brandimarte and Zotteri – Introduction to Distribution Logistics
Chan – Simulation Techniques in Financial Risk Management
Coleman, Greenfield, Stewardson and Montgomery (Eds) – Statistical Practice in Business
    and Industry
Frisen (Ed.) – Financial Surveillance
Fung and Hu – Statistical DNA Forensics
Gusti Ngurah Agung – Time Series Data Analysis Using EViews
Jank and Shmueli (Ed.) – Statistical Methods in e-Commerce Research
Kenett (Ed.) – Operational Risk Management: A Practical Approach to Intelligent Data
    Analysis
Kenett (Ed.) – Modern Analysis of Customer Surveys: With Applications using R
Kenett and Zacks – Modern Industrial Statistics: With Applications in R, MINITAB and JMP,
    Second Edition
Kruger and Xie – Statistical Monitoring of Complex Multivariate Processes: With
    Applications in Industrial ProcessControl
Lehtonen and Pahkinen – Practical Methods for Design and Analysis of Complex Surveys,
    Second Edition
Ohser and Mücklich – Statistical Analysis of Microstructures in Materials Science
Pasiouras (Ed.) – Efficiency and Productivity Growth: Modelling in the Financial Services
    Industry
Pourret, Naim and Marcot (Eds) – Bayesian Networks: A Practical Guide to Applications
Ruggeri, Kenett and Faltin – Encyclopedia of Statistics and Reliability
Taroni, Aitken, Garbolino and Biedermann – Bayesian Networks and Probabilistic Inference
    in Forensic Science
Taroni, Bozza, Biedermann, Garbolino and Aitken – Data Analysis in Forensic Science

Printed and bound by CPI Group (UK) Ltd, Croydon, CR0 4YY

27/10/2024

14580208-0002

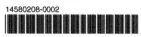